Nancy L. Roth, PhD
Linda K. Fuller, PhD
Editors

Women and AIDS
Negotiating Safer Practices, Care, and Representation

Pre-publication
REVIEWS,
COMMENTARIES,
EVALUATIONS . . .

D0148995

"**W**omen and AIDS: Negotiating Safer Practices, Care, and Representation* addresses the unique problems of women, and particularly women of color. The book's mission is nothing less than to prevent the spread of AIDS among women. It does so by identifying and characterizing the obstacles that prevent women from employing safer sex practices, realizing more effective health care, and discussing women's experiences with AIDS. To overcome these problems, specific and extremely useful negotiation strategies are described. Composed of twelve chapters by outstanding feminist scholars, the best thinking in this area is represented in this volume, and the editors have done an outstanding job of unifying these chapters into one coherent book. Must reading—a tour de force!"

James W. Chesebro, PhD
Professor, Department
of Communication,
Indiana State University,
Terre Haute, IN

"**H**oorah for an intelligent book focusing on women—who are the current wave of the HIV epidemic. We all need to better understand the co-factors of risk (from desire to power) in order to develop and support both effective HIV prevention and care strategies, and women in their roles and in their choices for safety and healing.

Roth and Fuller remind us that HIV issues of prevention and management are complex and difficult—attention must be paid to these complexities in order for our strategies to succeed. This book is a must-read for AIDS educators, administrators, policy makers and HIV Prevention Community Planning Group members nationwide.

As we better understand the context and subtext of women's motivations and decisions, we may better be able to assist women to increase their sense of personal agency in these crucial negotiations and in finding effectiveness in their own voices."

Fern Goodhart, MS, CHES
Director of Health Education,
Rutgers University Student
Health Services,
Princeton, NJ

"**T**he book is most relevant, addressing many of the key issues concerning HIV/AIDS prevention, transmission, treatment, and support facing women today. The chapters provide broad coverage of important social issues concerning women and AIDS, clearly describing the powerful role of human communication in responding to these complex issues. I particularly appreciate the sensitivity in the book's chapters to different cultural perspectives on AIDS and the focus on empowering women to confront health risks. This book is of great value to students, social scientists, health care providers, people living with HIV/AIDS, and women who are at risk for contracting HIV/AIDS. I commend the book's editors and chapter authors for their excellent, pertinent, and timely scholarship."

Gary L. Kreps, PhD
Dean of the School
of Communication,
Hofstra University,
Hempstead, NY

The Harrington Park Press
An Imprint of The Haworth Press, Inc.

Women and AIDS
Negotiating Safer Practices, Care, and Representation

HAWORTH Innovations in Feminist Studies
Esther Rothblum, PhD and Ellen Cole, PhD
Senior Co-Editors

New, Recent, and Forthcoming Titles:

Women and AIDS
Negotiating Safer Practices, Care, and Representation

Nancy L. Roth, PhD
Linda K. Fuller, PhD
Editors

The Harrington Park Press
An Imprint of The Haworth Press, Inc.
New York • London

Published by

The Harrington Park Press, an imprint of The Haworth Press, Inc., 10 Alice Street, Binghamton, NY 13904-1580

Cover design by Marylouise E. Doyle.

The Library of Congress has catalogued the hardcover version of this book as:

Women and AIDS : negotiating safer practices, care, and representation / Nancy L. Roth, Linda K. Fuller, editors.
     p. cm.
    Includes bibliographical references and index.
    ISBN 0-7890-6014-0 (alk. paper)
    1. AIDS (Disease)—Prevention. 2. Women—Diseases—Prevention. 3. Women—Health and hygiene. 4. Negotiation. 5. Safe sex in AIDS prevention. I. Roth, Nancy, 1936- . II. Fuller, Linda K.
RA644.A25W646 1997
616.97'9205'082—dc21

                                                      97-16980
                                                        CIP

To the Nashville, Tennessee HIV/AIDS community—Many thanks for sharing your wisdom with us.

Nancy L. Roth

For my part, this book is dedicated to the following women who are out there in the trenches *doing* something about AIDS: Jeanne Blake, Charline Boudreau, Jean Carlomusto, Rita DeSouza, Barbara Hammer, Vivian Kleiman, Anne Lewis, Patricia Livingstone, Jennifer Lytton, Juanita Mohammed, Paula Mozen, Beverly Peterson, Mimi Plevin-Foust, Ann Poritzky, Gini Reditker, Cynthia Roberts, Meg Saegebarth, and Deborah Wasser.

Linda K. Fuller

CONTENTS

ABOUT THE EDITORS

Nancy L. Roth, PhD, is a Communication Specialist at Hoffmann-La Roche in Nutley, New Jersey. Previously, she was Assistant Professor in the Department of Communication at Rutgers University. While her primary research areas are issues of gender, identity, and policy in health communication, she has also written extensively about HIV/AIDS. Her work has been published in journals such as the *Journal of Psychology and Human Sexuality, Organization Science,* the *Howard Journal of Communications,* and *Employee Rights and Responsibilities Journal.* She has also written chapters for several edited books, including *The Psychology of Sexual Orientation* (L. Diamant, Ed.), *Communicating about Communicable Diseases* (L. K. Fuller and L. McPherson-Shilling, Eds.), and *Health Workers and AIDS* (L. Bennett, D. Miller, and M. Ross, Eds.).

Linda K. Fuller, PhD, is Associate Professor in the Communications Department at Worcester State College. She is the author/editor of 18 books, including *The Cosby Show: Audiences, Impact, Implications* (1992), *Community TV in the U.S.* (1994), *Communicating about Communicable Diseases* (1994), *Media-Mediated Relationships* (1996), and the five-volume series *Beyond the Stars: Studies in American Popular Film* (1990-1996). Dr. Fuller has also written more than 200 professional publications and conference reports, and in 1996, she served as a Fulbright Senior Fellow at Nanyang Technological University in Singapore.

CONTRIBUTORS

Mary Alderson, PhD, was the first coordinator of Project SHARE.

Deborah L. Brimlow is in the AIDS Education and Training Center for Texas and Oklahoma, School of Public Health, University of Texas, PO Box 20186, Houston, TX 77225.

Deborah J. Cohen is a PhD candidate at Rutgers University. She is interested in support group and therapy communication and is currently looking at the communication that arises in women's infertility support groups.

Carol Collins is a PhD candidate in the School of Communication, Information, and Library Studies at Rutgers University. Her research interests include African-American biography, African-American young adult literature, and African-American young adult biography.

Pamela Emmons, RN, is the current coordinator of Project Share and the nurse recruiter for the Meharry/Vanderbilt AIDS Clinical Trials Unit.

John Nguyet Erni is the author of *Unstable Frontiers: Technomedicine and the Cultural Politics of "Curing" AIDS* (University of Minnesota Press, 1994). He teaches courses in media and cultural studies and on AIDS in the Department of Communication, University of New Hampshire. He is the recipient of the 1996-1997 Gustafson Fellowship from the Center for the Humanities at UNH for his work on a book about AIDS in Thailand, sexual politics, and the global vectors of orientalism.

Frank Hatcher, PhD, is Associate Professor of Microbiology at Meharry Medical College. He was the principle investigator on the grant that funded Project SHARE.

Katie Hogan was the recipient of the 1996 Pergamon-National Women's Studies Association Award for Graduate Scholarship in Women's Studies. She is a doctoral candidate in English at Rutgers University, where she teaches women's studies and basic composition. Her dissertation, "The Angel in the House: Gender, AIDS, and the Politics of Sentimental Representation," contributes to long-standing feminist debates on literary sentimentality by analyzing the consequences of sentimental representations of women in AIDS literature and popular culture. In addition to her dissertation, her recent publications on gender and HIV argue for an explicit feminist standpoint in the cultural and literary criticism on AIDS.

T. Todd Imahori, PhD, is Associate Professor of Speech and Communication Studies at San Francisco State University. His area of specialization is Intercultural Communication, particularly in the areas of intercultural communication competence, cross-cultural communication between Japan and the United States, Asian-American/Pacific Islander communication, and communication and ethnic diversity. His work has appeared in *International and Intercultural Communication Annual Vol. 18, International Journal of Intercultural Relations,* and *Western Journal of Communication,* among others.

Lorraine D. Jackson, PhD, is Assistant Professor of Speech Communication at the California Polytechnic State University in San Luis Obispo where she teaches courses in health communication, gender and communication, and communication theory. Her recent experimental research, published in *Health Communication,* assesses the effects of a communication intervention designed to promote patient adherence with treatment. Dr. Jackson's other research interests and publications include promoting safer-sex behavior, health message design, ethical communication in medicine, and women's health issues. Currently, she is co-editing (with B. K. Duffy) *Health Communication Research: A Guide to Developments and Directions,* to be published by Greenwood Press in 1997.

Diane M. Kimoto, PhD, is Assistant Professor of Speech Communication in the College of Communication at the University of Alabama. Her research has focused around several key themes: (1) How we can understand persons and how they affect one another in social interaction, particularly in reference to HIV/AIDS and deception, and (2) How we can understand and explore the rich, personal, and interpersonal dynamics of cultural interactions and cross-generational relationships.

Linda C. Lederman, PhD, is a professor in the Department of Communication at Rutgers University.

Gina Ann Margillo, MA, is Public Health Community Coordinator for the California Department of Health Services. In this capacity, she develops and implements culture-specific health programs with at-risk communities across the state of California. She presented an earlier version of this study at the annual meeting of the National Council for International Health in Alexandria, VA in July 1995.

Barbara Nabrit-Stephens, MD, is the pediatrician for all the babies in the research project associated with Project SHARE. She is in private practice in Nashville, Tennessee.

Myra Shoub Nelson is a PhD candidate in the School of Communication, Information, and Library Studies at Rutgers University. Her research focuses on communication about chronic illness. She and Dr. Roth have collaborated on a number of projects concerning HIV/AIDS and communication.

Marcela Raffaelli, PhD, is Assistant Professor of Psychology and Ethnic Studies at University of Nebraska-Lincoln. After receiving her PhD from the University of Chicago in 1990, she was involved in developing and evaluating AIDS-prevention programs for at-risk populations, including Brazilian street youth and residents of U.S. inner cities. Her current research interests include examining cultural influences on the sexual behavior of Latina women; she also studies parent-child communication about sexual topics and developmental processes among children and adolescents living and working on the streets of Latin American cities.

Michael W. Ross is in the Center for Health Promotion Research and Development, School of Public Health, University of Texas.

Michael J. Selby received his PhD in Clinical Psychology from The University of Memphis in 1988, and completed a postdoctoral fellowship in Neuropsychology at the UCLA Neuropsychiatric Institute and Hospital in 1989. He is currently Associate Professor in the Department of Psychology, California State University, San Luis Obispo, and a member of the medical staff with the California Department of Corrections. Dr. Selby maintains an active research program, and is the author of a number of articles and presentations on a variety of topics, including the effects of AIDS, drug abuse, and multiple sclerosis on brain functioning; the relationship between hostility and depression; drug abuse and eating disorders; and the prediction of violence.

David F. Shaw is a doctoral candidate in Media Studies at the University of Colorado at Boulder. His research interests include visual communication and mass-mediated and popular imagery. He is currently writing a dissertation on the AIDS Memorial Quilt.

Mary Ann South, MD, is Kellogg Professor of Pediatrics at Meharry Medical College and the principle investigator for the Meharry/Vanderbilt ACTG.

Mariana Suarez-Al-Adam received her Master's Degree from Rutgers University in 1995. Her thesis explored how psychological and physical abuse influences Latino women's ability to protect themselves from HIV infection. She is also interested in examining folk medicine use by HIV-infected Hispanics.

Gust A. Yep, PhD, teaches in the Department of Speech and Communication Studies at San Francisco State University (SFSU). Before joining SFSU, he was Associate Professor of Communication Studies and Interim Director of the Institute for Asian-American and Pacific Asian Studies at the California State University in Los Angeles (CSLA). His work has appeared as chapters in *Communicating About Communicable Diseases* (edited by L. K. Fuller and L. McPherson-Shilling), *Media-Mediated Relationships* (edited by L. K. Fuller), *Cross-Cultural Perspectives on HIV/AIDS Education* (edited by D. C. Umeh), *Combating Heterosexism and Homophobia* (edited by J. T. Sears and W. L. Williams), and *Hispanic Psychology: Critical Issues in Theory and Research* (edited by A. M. Padilla), as well as articles in a number of scholarly publications including *AIDS Education and Prevention, Hispanic Journal of Behavioral Sciences, International Quarterly of Community Health Education, Journal of American College Health,* and *Journal of Social Behavior and Personality,* among others. He is also a member of the Editorial Board for the *Journal of Social Behavior and Personality.* Dr. Yep was nominated three times for the Outstanding Professor Award at CSLA and joined the list of outstanding American educators in *Who's Who Among America's Teachers* (1994).

Introduction

The Women's National AIDS Resource estimates that by the year 2000, the number of HIV-positive women will equal the number of HIV-positive men. Further, the Centers for Disease Control and Prevention (CDC) reports that in the United States, while women currently represent 14 percent of AIDS statistics, the HIV-infection rate of women is increasing at four times the rate of men. Currently, AIDS is the top killer of young African-American women, and is fast becoming a leading cause of death for women aged 18 to 45. However, as of 1990, more than 65 percent of the women who had died from HIV-related causes had never received an official AIDS diagnosis, and until 1993, the Social Security Administration had denied benefits to women whose HIV-related illnesses were outside of the CDC's male models of AIDS.

Although we as women constitute the highest at-risk population, and although we are predicted to leave more than 80,000 orphans by the turn of the century, women and our concerns have only recently been addressed in the AIDS literature. Increasingly, our voices are being heard as AIDS activists (ACT UP, 1992; Doyal, Naidoo, and Wilson, 1994; Lester, 1989; Patton, 1994; Pearlburg, 1991; Watstein and Laurich, 1991), as givers and receivers of medical advice (U.S. Public Health Service, 1987; American College Health Association, 1988; Berer, 1993; Corea, 1994; Cox, 1995; Norwood, 1987; Santee, 1988), and as counselors (Patton and Kelly, 1987; Kaplan, 1988; Richardson, 1989; Bury, Morrison, and McLachlan, 1992; Squire, 1993). We address concerns about children (Cohen and Durham, 1993), women of color (Crawford et al., 1992; Sabatier, 1988), sex workers (Alexander, 1988), and families (Macklin, 1994). We also tell personal stories about our AIDS-related experiences (Peavey, 1990; Rieder and Ruppelt, 1988; Rudd and Taylor, 1992).

This volume is the first to address women and AIDS from a communication perspective, although others have explored

HIV/AIDS and communication in general (Edgar, Fitzpatrick, and Freimuth, 1992; Fuller, 1996; Fuller and Shilling, 1995; Lupton, 1994; Murphy and Poirier, 1993). In the absence of a cure or vaccine, communication is central to efforts to stem the spread of the HIV virus and to care for those who are already infected. The ways that HIV and those infected and affected by the virus are constructed, communicatively affects transmission/prevention, caregiver-patient relationships, and medical outcomes. Media representations play a large role in popular perceptions of the disease and those infected and affected by it.

The essays in this collection explore women's "negotiation" of safer sex and intravenous drug use practices; women's "negotiation" of the health care system as patients, medical research subjects, and caregivers; and women's "negotiation" of HIV-related media representations as producers, consumers, and objects of representation.

In the first section, we address issues related to women's negotiation of safer sexual and IV drug use practices with partners and potential partners. We use the term "negotiation" in its most common sense: "to deal or bargain with others." The essays call into question the concept of negotiation in relationships where negotiating partners have unequal physical, economic, and social power. Cultural constructions of sex and drug-sharing relationships are explored in a variety of communities.

In the second section, we extend the meaning of negotiation to include the sense of "moving through or around," in reference to the U.S. health care system. These chapters investigate HIV-positive incarcerated women's encounters with prison health care, women's experiences as HIV medical study staff and patients, and women's processes as carers for HIV-positive patients. These chapters challenge traditional assumptions about relationships between carers and patients and the meaning of patient compliance.

In the third section, we extend our understanding of negotiation yet again to include the connotation "to manage, transact, or conduct," in reference to the media. In this section, we explore how women use the media for HIV-related social action, to promote women's views of HIV and sexuality, and to commemorate the loss of loved ones. We also interpret how women, particularly women of color, are represented by the media in the context of HIV/AIDS.

In a time when women are increasingly affected and infected by the HIV virus, against which our most powerful tools are discursive, this book indicates some barriers to negotiating safer practices, some obstructions in negotiating the health care system, and some hazards in negotiating the media. This book raises important and painful questions about gender, race, and class issues that are exacerbated by the epidemic. Yet, these essays also provide guidance for communicating through and around these obstacles and for discursively reducing them. It is our hope that our work will help more women to successfully negotiate safer practices, appropriated care, and media representation.

REFERENCES

ACT UP/New York. (1992). *Women, AIDS, and Activism.* Boston: South End Press.

Alexander, P. (1988). *Prostitutes Prevent AIDS: A Manual for Health Educators.* San Francisco: California Prostitutes Education Project.

American College Health Association, (1988). *Women & AIDS.* Rockville, MD: ACHA.

Berer, M. (1993). *Women and HIV/AIDS: An International Resource Book.* New York: Pandora.

Bury, J., Morrison, V., and McLachlan, S. (Eds.). (1992). *Working with Women with AIDS: Medical, Social, and Counselling Issues.* New York: Tavistock/Routledge.

Cohen, F.L. and Durham, J.D. (Eds.). (1993). *Women, Children, and HIV/AIDS.* New York: Springer Publishing Co.

Corea, G. (1994). *The Invisible Epidemic: The Story of Women and AIDS.* New York: Perennial.

Cox, L. (1995). "Microbicide—A woman's weapon for fighting AIDS." *The New York News,* (November/December): 3.

Crawford, A. et al. (Eds.). (1992). *Our Lives in Balance: U.S. Women of Color and the AIDS Epidemic.* Latham, NY: Kitchen Table Women of Color Press.

Doyal, L., Naidoo, J., and Wilson, T. (Eds.). (1994). *AIDS: Setting a Feminist Agenda.* Bristol, PA: Taylor & Francis.

Edgar, T., Fitzpatrick, M.A., and Freimuth, V. (Eds.). (1992). *AIDS: A Communication Perspective.* Hillsdale, NJ: Lawrence Erlbaum.

Fuller, L.K. (Ed.). (1996). *Media-Mediated AIDS.* Amherst, MA: HRD Press.

Fuller, L.K. and McPherson-Shilling, L. (Eds.). (1995). *Communicating About Communicable Diseases.* Amherst, MA: HRD Press.

Kaplan, H.S. (1988). *The Real Truth About Women and AIDS.* New York: Simon and Schuster.

Lester, B. (1989). *Women and AIDS: A Practical Guide for Those Who Help Others.* New York: Continuum.

Lupton, D. (1994). *Moral Threats and Dangerous Desires: AIDS in the News Media.* London: Taylor & Francis.

Macklin, E. (Ed.). (1994). *AIDS and Families.* Binghamton, NY: The Haworth Press.

Murphy, T.F. and Poirier, S. (Eds.). (1993). *Writing AIDS: Gay Literature, Language, and Analysis.* New York: Columbia University Press.

Norwood, C. (1987). *Advice for Life: A Woman's Guide to AIDS Risks and Prevention.* New York: Pantheon.

Patton, C. (1994). *Last Served? Gendering the HIV Pandemic.* London: Taylor & Francis.

Patton, C. and Kelly, J. (1987). *Making It: A Woman's Guide to Sex in the Age of AIDS.* Ithaca, NY: Firebrand Books.

Pearlburg, G. (1991). *Women, AIDS, & Communities: A Guide for Action.* Metuchen, NJ: Women's Action Alliance and the Scarecrow Press, Inc.

Peavey, F. (1990). *A Shallow Pool of Time: An HIV+ Woman Grapples with the AIDS Epidemic.* Philadelphia: New Society.

Richardson, D. (1989). *Women and the AIDS Crisis.* London: Pandora.

Rieder, I. and Ruppelt, P. (Eds.). (1988). *AIDS: The Women.* San Francisco: Cleis Press.

Rudd, A. and Taylor, D. (1992). *Positive Women: Voices of Women Living with AIDS.* Seattle: Seal Press.

Sabatier, R. (Ed.). (1988). *Blaming Others: Prejudice, Race, and Worldwide AIDS.* Philadelphia: New Society Publishers.

Santee, B. (1988). *Women and AIDS: The Silent Epidemic.* New York: Women and AIDS Resource Network.

Squire, C. (Ed.). (1993). *Women and AIDS: Psychological Perspectives.* Newbury Park, CA: Sage.

U.S. Public Health Service. (1987). *Women and AIDS: Initiatives of the Public Health Service.* Washington DC: GPO.

Watstein, S. and Laurich, R.A. (1991). *AIDS and Women: A Sourcebook.* Phoenix: Oryz Press.

PART I:
NEGOTIATING SAFER PRACTICES

Chapter 1

Reconsidering the HIV/AIDS Prevention Needs of Latino Women in the United States

Marcela Raffaelli
Mariana Suarez-Al-Adam

INTRODUCTION

The change in contraceptive technology in the 1960s helped to shift the focus of responsibility for contraceptive decision making to women. The same focus on females is being pursued with AIDS prevention, although women cannot control condom use. (Worth, 1989, p. 306)

Wherever women are culturally and economically subordinate to men, they cannot control or even readily negotiate safer sex, including condom use and lifelong mutual fidelity. (Merson, 1993, p. 1267)

[P]erhaps the most critical feature of many behavior changes that might prevent the sexual transmission of HIV is that they require the cooperation of another person, namely, the woman's sex partner. (O'Leary and Jemmott, 1995, p. 3)

He told me that I was being disrespectful of him. He said, "After twenty-six years . . . I'm not garbage and I'm not with

Correspondence should be addressed to Marcela Raffaelli, Department of Psychology, University of Nebraska, Lincoln, NE 68588-0308.

other women. Maybe it's you who's infected. I'm not at risk."
He left the house and when he came home he was drunk.
(Puerto Rican woman describing her partner's reaction to her
bringing up condom use; Suarez, 1995, p. 58)

The HIV/AIDS epidemic represents an ever-increasing threat to
Latino[1] populations in the United States, with women being most
affected by this deadly disease. In this chapter, we explore the
challenges Latino women face as they attempt to reduce their risk of
sexual transmission of HIV, the virus that causes AIDS. Our main
interest lies in examining how the economic, cultural, and social
realities of women's lives contribute to their risk of HIV infection
and constrain their ability to reduce that risk. Because there is
neither a cure for AIDS nor a vaccination to block HIV transmission, prevention of infection is the main objective of the global
AIDS strategy (WHO, 1992). Discussions of HIV prevention
among women typically emphasize the need to develop an unobtrusive female-controlled method that kills HIV and other pathogens
while permitting conception (e.g., Stein, 1990; Worth, 1989). However, development of such a method has remained elusive, and
current prevention efforts focus largely on promoting consistent
condom use, which has been identified as the most effective HIV
prevention strategy other than abstinence or a lifelong mutually
monogamous relationship with an uninfected partner (Kaemingk and
Bootzin, 1990; WHO, 1992). Secondary strategies such as reducing
the number of partners appear to be less effective (Reiss and Leik,
1989), particularly when the risk status of partners is difficult to
ascertain.

The quotations at the start of this chapter highlight the challenges
women face as they attempt to reduce their risk of HIV infection by
negotiating safer sex with their partners. In common with women
all over the world, Latino women may be unable to assert themselves in their sexual relationships and may have great difficulty
making the behavior changes needed to reduce the risk of HIV
transmission. The magnitude of the challenges faced by Latino
women is evident in the fact that, unlike most other population
groups, Latino women have not increased their use of condoms
(e.g., Remez, 1993; Stewart, 1993). One large-scale longitudinal

survey of non-Hispanic white, black, and Hispanic heterosexuals living in San Francisco revealed that Hispanic women were the only ethnic/gender group to show no increase in condom use over time (Catania et al., 1993). Assessments at two time points one year apart revealed that the proportion of Hispanic women reporting occasional condom use did not change (20 percent versus 21 percent), whereas the proportion of black women who sometimes used condoms increased from 21 percent to 26 percent. In fact, consistent condom use among Hispanic women actually *decreased* from 8 percent at Wave I to 3 percent at Wave II, compared to an increase from 5 percent to 14 percent among black women.

The lack of behavioral change among the general population of Latino women is reflected in epidemiological surveillance data. In 1993, the AIDS case rate for Hispanic women was 6.4 times higher than the rate for non-Hispanic white women, and the rate for Hispanic men was 2.6 times higher than for non-Hispanic white men (CDC, 1994). Although Hispanic women represent just under 10 percent of the U.S. female population (U.S. Bureau of the Census, 1995), they account for 20 percent of cumulative female AIDS cases (CDC, 1995); Hispanic men represent 10.6 percent of the U.S. male population and 16.8 percent of cumulative male AIDS cases. To date, heterosexual transmission accounts for a larger proportion of diagnosed AIDS cases among Hispanic women (44 percent) than either white (37 percent) or black (33 percent) women (CDC, 1995), and the proportion of AIDS cases attributable to heterosexual transmission has increased from 27 percent in 1984 to 34 percent in 1987 (Holmes, Karon, and Kreiss, 1990) and 47 percent in the period of 1994 through 1995 (CDC, 1995). Among certain Latino subgroups, sexual intercourse has long been the main transmission route, as can be seen when female AIDS cases reported since the start of the epidemic are examined by birthplace. Although injection drug use (IDU) is the predominant exposure category among Latino women born in the United States (56 percent) and Puerto Rico (46 percent), it accounts for under a quarter of cases among women born in other Latin American countries where heterosexual intercourse is the main exposure category (Diaz et al., 1993).

Latinos constitute the fastest growing ethnic group in the United States (Marin, 1993), and the proportion of Latino women affected by heterosexual transmission of HIV can be expected to increase. These statistics reinforce the need for information in which to ground preventive interventions for Latino populations, especially women. This chapter focuses on factors that put Latino women at continued risk of HIV infection and attempts to identify alternatives to risk reduction strategies which focus on the individual. It is divided into four main sections. In the first section, we identify factors that contribute to Latino women's risk of HIV infection and assess how realistic it is to advocate that women "negotiate" safer sex with their partners. In the middle sections, we summarize the results of HIV prevention efforts and discuss the limited applicability of traditional approaches to HIV prevention to disenfranchised women. In the final section, we discuss directions for future intervention efforts and attempt to identify approaches that hold promise in reducing Latino women's risk of HIV infection. Because women who are at risk from injection drug use face different issues than women whose main source of risk is heterosexual intercourse, we focus primarily on issues related to the sexual transmission of HIV.

FACTORS THAT AFFECT LATINO WOMEN'S ABILITY TO IMPLEMENT RISK REDUCTION MEASURES

A number of factors contribute to Latino women's risk of HIV infection and limit the extent to which they can reduce that risk (for a discussion of issues confronting women in general, see Amaro, 1995; Heise and Elias, 1995; O'Leary et al., 1993; Weiss and Gupta, 1993; Worth, 1989; Wyatt, 1994). In addition to risk factors that are common to women from all ethnic groups (such as poverty and violence), Latino women living in the United States confront additional challenges, including cultural factors that delineate appropriate sexual behavior and constrain women's power in their sexual relationships, and the pressures of immigration and acculturation. Although these factors are discussed separately below, it is important to recognize that in real life, they are intertwined and may interact in complex ways.

Poverty

Socioeconomic status can contribute both directly and indirectly to an increased risk of HIV infection among women (Mays and Cochran, 1988; O'Leary et al., 1993). Many poor women have inadequate access to health care and information about prevention of HIV and other sexually transmitted diseases, which puts them at direct risk of infection (Quinn and Cates, 1992). Poor women may also feel so overwhelmed by the stress of daily life that protecting themselves from HIV/AIDS is low on their list of priorities (Kalichman, Hunter, and Kelly, 1992; Nyamathi and Vasquez, 1989). In addition, it has been proposed that stress may lead to a direct risk of HIV infection because some women cope with stress by engaging in sexual activity (Kalichman et al., 1995) or injecting drugs (Nyamathi, Stein, and Brecht, 1995). Finally, impoverished women may lack the resources to leave a relationship with a high-risk partner, and others may depend on sex as a survival activity (Mays and Cochran, 1988). Thus, poverty limits women's options and may diminish their motivation to change high risk behavior or their ability to insist that partners comply with requests for condom use.

Latino populations are disproportionately represented among disenfranchised populations in the United States, and are thus at a higher risk of HIV infection. With the exception of Cuban-Americans, Hispanics are more likely than non-Hispanic whites to be poor, attend inadequate schools, to not complete high school, to be unemployed, and suffer from increased morbidity and mortality rates (Torres, 1991). These various factors contribute to an increased risk of HIV infection among some Latino women, and may limit their ability to implement risk reduction efforts.

Cultural Factors

Another set of factors that may make it difficult for Latino women to reduce their risk of HIV infection are cultural norms that define appropriate behavior and regulate gender roles. In any discussion of cultural norms, it is important to recognize that norms define ideals rather than actual behavior, that individuals will vary in their adherence to norms, and that it is important not to overstate the role cultural factors play in explaining individual behavior

(De La Cancela, 1989). It is also important to recognize that the meaning of a behavior differs for those raised in the culture and those observing it from outside (LeVine, 1984). Finally, the extent to which different Hispanic subgroups will subscribe to these norms will differ (Fernandez, 1995).

Recognizing these caveats, there is a good degree of consensus on characteristics of traditional Hispanic culture that may contribute to the risk of HIV infection, especially culturally defined gender roles that define and limit the behavior of men and women. As discussed below, these culturally defined gender roles can be expected to influence women's ability to negotiate safer sex in a number of ways; in particular, Latino women who attempt to introduce condom use into a relationship may experience difficulties (Forrest et al., 1993; Kenen and Armstrong, 1992; Nyamathi et al., 1995; Stewart, 1993).

One aspect of Hispanic culture that may limit the degree to which women can implement safer sex strategies involves the degree to which they and their partners subscribe to traditional gender roles of *machismo* and *marianismo*. These idealized gender roles are complementary and opposite, with men being considered strong, rational, virile, and independent while women are thought of as submissive, sentimental, chaste, and dependent (e.g., Comas-Diaz, 1987; Gilmore and Uhl, 1987; Goldwert, 1985; Magana and Magana, 1992; Marin, 1988; Panitz et al., 1983; Thompson, 1991; Wiest, 1983). The concept of *machismo* is an important and often misunderstood aspect of Hispanic gender role expectations, with traditional *machismo* incorporating responsibilities as well as rights. Male responsibilities include providing economically for the family, defending its welfare, and procreating children to carry on the family name. A man's rights include controlling the behavior of family members and having authority over them. Males are socialized to be sexually active and virile, and extramarital activity is considered a male prerogative.

The complement to *machismo* is *marianismo*. Whereas boys are taught to be active and in control of those around them, girls are taught to be self-sacrificing and dutiful, and to bow to the will of the men in their lives (first their fathers, and later their husbands). In contrast to boys, who are expected to be sexually active, girls are taught the importance of female virginity before marriage and faithfulness afterward. This sexual double standard results in dichotomization of women into "good" and "bad," with "good" women (mothers and wives) being disinterested in sex and ignorant about sexual matters and "bad" women being sexually available and knowledgeable. Women who attempt to introduce condom use into a relationship may be going against traditional gender roles in several ways, including defying the male prerogative of controlling family members' behavior and exhibiting knowledge about, and interest in, sexual behavior.

Although in recent years, a number of authors have challenged traditional depictions of Hispanic gender roles as stereotypical and invalid (e.g., Amaro, 1988b; De La Cancela, 1989; Singer et al., 1990), there is evidence that features of these idealized roles are reflected in the attitudes and behavior of at least some Latino subgroups. First, research on male and female roles within the family supports the notion that although many Latino families are more egalitarian than traditional depictions would imply, there is also evidence of male domination and control. For example, Powell (1995) reported that in a group of 29 Mexican men living in the United States, 58 percent agreed that "a wife should do whatever her husband wants" and 69 percent agreed that "husbands should make all the important decisions in a marriage."

A second body of evidence supporting the reality of culturally defined gender roles exists in the finding that as a group, Latino women are dissatisfied with their sex lives. In a study of 137 Mexican-American women, Amaro (1988b) found that some aspects of stereotypical gender beliefs held true; for example, the majority of women (66 percent) agreed that sex is more of a duty than a pleasure for women, and few (6 percent) said they enjoyed or felt happy in their sexual relationship. Similarly, Worth (1989) reported that impoverished Puerto Rican women who participated in a group program in New York were dissatisfied with their sex lives and complained about their partners' sexual behavior.

A third example points to research on communication styles which reveals that Mexican women's preferred strategies to deal with unwelcome requests from their intimate partners tended to reflect conventional gender role expectations (Belk et al., 1988).

Finally, research on sexual behavior suggests that many Latino men and women adhere to culturally defined gender role expectations. For example, Latino women engage in lower levels of sexual activity than either non-Hispanic white or black women (Grimstead et al., 1993), and Latino men engage in higher levels. These separate strands of research converge to support the notion that traditional gender roles play a part in regulating the sexual behavior of Latino men and women.

Another aspect of many Latino women's lives, consistent with traditional gender role expectations, is that their partners may engage in sexual activity with other partners. Compared to other ethnic groups, Hispanic men are more likely to have multiple sexual partners (Billy et al., 1993); further, if married, Hispanic men are more likely to engage in extramarital activity (Choi, Catania, and Dolcini, 1993; Marin, Gomez, and Hearst, 1993). It has also been suggested that cultural definitions of *machismo* permit a man to retain his male identity even if he engages in same-sex activity, as long as he takes the "active" (insertive) role (Carrier, 1976; Carrier, 1985; Magana and Carrier, 1991; Parker and Carballo, 1990). Although same-sex activity may not be as common as ethnographic research suggests, U.S. surveys reveal that Latino men are more likely than men from other ethnic groups to report homosexual contact and Latino women are more likely to report having a main partner who has sex with men. In a nationally representative survey of men aged 20 to 39, 4.8 percent of Hispanic men, compared to 2 percent of non-Hispanic men, reported same-gender sexual contact in the past ten years; 2.8 percent of Hispanic men (versus 1 percent of non-Hispanics) reported only same-gender contact, meaning that 2 percent had engaged in sexual activity with both same and opposite sex partners (Billy et al., 1993).

A study of 620 nonpregnant women living in southern Florida revealed that Hispanic women were more likely than non-Hispanic women to report unprotected sex with a bisexual main partner (23 percent versus 13 to 14 percent of white, American-born black, and Haitian women) (Harrison et al., 1990). These U.S. findings are reinforced by research with Mexican populations. One study of Mexican men in a town on the U.S.-Mexican border revealed that 27 percent of men who engaged in same-sex activity had also engaged in vaginal intercourse during the past month (Ramirez et al., 1994). Another group of researchers also found that 27 percent of men recruited at "gay" locations (e.g., gay discos, bars, parks frequented by gay men) in six Mexican cities had engaged in sex with both male and female partners in the previous year (Izazola-Licea et al., 1991). This research suggests that Latino women have a higher probability than non-Latino women of having a nonmonogamous sex partner, making condom use in primary relationships a necessary safeguard for many women. Yet, other features of traditional Hispanic culture make the introduction of condoms problematic.

One factor limiting women's ability to negotiate safer sex with their partners is that several aspects of Latino culture make it difficult for men and women to discuss sexual topics (e.g., Forrest et al., 1993). This reflects expectations that males be knowledgeable and assume the dominant role in sexual encounters, and females be ignorant and assume the subordinate role. It also reflects a broader cultural reticence regarding sexual topics (O'Donnell, San Doval, Vornfett, and De Jong, 1994; Singer et al., 1990). This cultural taboo is evident in a study examining to whom HIV-positive men disclosed their diagnosis; 69 percent of Spanish-speaking Hispanics, compared to 88 percent of English-speaking Hispanics and 96 percent of whites, had disclosed their serostatus to their intimate partner (Mason et al., 1995). Another study revealed that fewer Latino men and women had discussed AIDS-preventive behaviors with their sex partner during the past year (35 percent of Latinos versus 49 percent of African Americans and 65 percent of whites) (Singer et al., 1990). In addition, sexual communication, which has emerged as a predictor of condom use in most populations (e.g., Catania et al., 1989; for a review, see Fisher and Fisher, 1992), does not appear to play a similar role among Latinos. In fact, one study revealed that higher levels of condom use among Latino men were associated with "*not discussing* [italics added] condom use with wives or girlfriends" and believing that "talking about condoms destroys romance" (Mikawa et al., 1992, p. 430). The nature and function of sexual communication among Latino couples is little understood, and research on this topic is urgently needed; however, it is clear that talking about sex is often unacceptable, so efforts to communicate directly about sexuality and HIV/AIDS prevention are likely to be problematic.

Related to this reticence regarding sexual topics is a resistance to condom use and a preference for "unobtrusive" methods of birth control in most Latino groups. Surveys of family planning methods used by married couples in Latin America (conducted during the 1980s) reveal that the only country where more than 3 percent of married couples used condoms was Costa Rica, where 13 percent of couples reported condom use (Robey et al., 1992, Table 2). It should be noted, however, that nonuse of condoms among Latin populations does not appear to be linked to religious prohibitions as has been suggested (e.g., Ickovics and Rodin, 1992). These same surveys reveal that contraceptive prevalence was over 50 percent in most Latin countries (including Mexico), but female sterilization and oral contraceptives were the most common method. It appears that in the United States, Latinos have maintained negative attitudes toward condoms (e.g., Singer et al., 1990) as well as a preference for unobtrusive methods of birth control (e.g., Amaro, 1988b). Latinos in the United States are less likely to report condom use than members of other ethnic groups (Catania et al., 1992; Lauver et al., 1995; O'Donnell, San Doval, Vornfett, and O'Donnell, 1994). A nationally representative survey of never-married American women revealed that only 24.5 percent of Hispanic women among those surveyed had ever used condoms, compared to 48.6 percent of white women and 28.2 percent of black women (Remez, 1993). A study of 15-to-24-year-old men and women in Detroit revealed that Hispanics were less likely than African Americans to report ever using condoms with main, secondary, and casual partners (Ford, Rubenstein, and Norris, 1994). Not surprisingly, Latinos have more negative attitudes toward condoms than other ethnic groups. For example, in another study, 38 percent of Hispanic men and 27 percent of Hispanic women (compared to 19 percent of African-American men and 14 percent of African-American women) agreed that "[c]ondoms are too much trouble to use," and Hispanic men were twice as likely as African-American men (24.5 percent versus 12.6 percent) to agree that "[m]ost women use some other kind of birth control, so condoms aren't necessary" (O'Donnell, San Doval,

Vornfett, and O'Donnell, 1994, p. 144). Unfamiliarity with condoms and resistance to their use is a major barrier for women to overcome.

Perhaps a greater challenge to women's attempts to implement condom use is the fact that Latino men have more negative condom attitudes than women (Marin et al., 1993; San Doval et al., 1995), and qualitative research reveals that Latino men hold negative perceptions of women who carry condoms or request condom use (Forrest et al., 1993). This is thought to reflect the fact that condoms have traditionally been associated with "illicit" sexual relationships, and are more acceptable in nonprimary relationships (e.g., Marin, Gomez, and Hearst, 1993). For example, Hispanic men recruited at a sexually transmitted disease clinic were less likely to report intending to use condoms the next time they had sex with a primary (54 percent) as compared to a nonprimary (90 percent) partner (San Doval et al., 1995). An additional barrier to condom use is that a woman's request that a main sexual partner use a condom may be perceived as proof of distrust, infidelity, or disrespect (Amaro, 1988b). In the clinic sample recruited by San Doval and colleagues (San Doval et al., 1995), most men (93 percent) said they would use a condom if their primary partner "insisted"; however, responses to other questions administered in this same study suggest that their partners would have substantial barriers to overcome. Over one-tenth of the men (13 percent) said they would be angry if their primary partner "[t]ried to talk me into using condoms," and only about one-third (35 percent) agreed that it "[i]s okay for *my* sex partner to carry condoms" (San Doval et al., 1995, p. 392). Considering that this study population was actively seeking care at a sexually transmitted disease clinic, we can predict that attitudes in the general population will be even less supportive of condom use in primary relationships.

In sum, various factors related to traditional Hispanic culture—including gender role expectations, the sexual double standard, norms regarding sexual communication, and preferred contraceptive practices—may contribute in different ways to Latino women's risk of HIV infection, and differ in how these factors influence women's ability to negotiate safer sex with their partners. Traditional barriers to HIV/AIDS risk reduction may diminish as individuals become more acculturated; however, adapting to a new culture

may lead to different challenges and sources of risk. We turn next to an examination of how these factors may influence Latino women's ability to implement risk reduction measures.

Immigration and Acculturation Stress

Acculturation is the process by which migrants learn about and adapt to the host culture (e.g., Marin and Marin, 1991). Although there is a good deal of debate over how to operationalize and measure acculturation (e.g., Fernandez, 1995; Negy and Woods, 1992), most theorists agree that it is an important factor in describing the life experience of Latinos. Acculturation is significant in discussions of HIV/AIDS prevention because the acculturation process is linked to risk status in a number of ways. At the most basic level, immigrants to the United States may be unable to speak English and have difficulty communicating with social service agencies or health care providers, making it difficult to obtain health services and information. Studies consistently show that less acculturated Hispanics have lower levels of AIDS-related knowledge than more acculturated Hispanics (Epstein et al., 1994; Marin and Marin, 1990; Nyamathi et al., 1993; Rapkin and Erickson, 1990). Second, immigrants must often deal with prejudice, discrimination in housing, and limited employment options, all of which limit their economic opportunities and lead to increased life stress. Finally, the acculturation process has been identified as a significant source of stress for both individuals and families (Padilla, 1980; Vega and Miranda, 1985). Perhaps most important, immigrants are exposed to new models of behavior and situations that may challenge traditional beliefs and norms which cause friction between family members.

Traditional Hispanic culture has been described as both a protector and risk factor for Latino women. Less acculturated women tend to be at lower risk of HIV infection from their own behavior; for example, they have fewer sex partners (Marin et al., 1993; Nyamathi et al., 1993; Rapkin and Erickson, 1990; Sabogal et al., 1995). On the other hand, less acculturated women may be at risk from their partners' behavior and from traditional attitudes toward condom use. In one study of women, 72 percent of less acculturated Hispanics, compared to 54 percent of more acculturated Hispanics, and 37 percent of African-Americans, reported that their partner did

not like to use condoms (Nyamathi et al., 1995). If they adhere to traditional gender role expectations, Latino women may be reluctant or unable to initiate discussions of condom use or HIV prevention. Acculturation to the mainstream Anglo culture may be linked to an increase in women's power in their personal relationships. One study that included a sample of young, highly acculturated Hispanic women who were either injection drug users or partners of IDUs revealed that women reported a high degree of power in their personal relationships and many reported being successful in persuading their partners to use condoms (Kline, Kline, and Oken, 1992). However, among non-IDU populations, highly acculturated Latino women are often at increased risk of HIV infection from their own sexual behavior. Higher levels of acculturation have consistently been linked to an increase in the number of sex partners among Hispanic women (Marin et al., 1993; Nyamathi et al., 1993; Rapkin and Erickson, 1990; Sabogal et al., 1995). At the same time, condom use has remained low even among more acculturated Latinos; Marin and colleagues (Marin et al., 1993) reported that 71 percent of English-speaking Hispanic women never used condoms, compared to 53 percent of non-Hispanic white women (79 percent of Spanish-speaking women reported never using condoms). Thus, it appears that in the process of acculturation, Latino women may be shedding some of the behavioral restraints imposed by traditional gender roles, but may not be able to give up more deep-seated rules governing sexual behavior and partner relationships.

The process of acculturation and of adjusting to a new way of life may also be a source of stress for the larger family unit, especially if migration results in economic disruption and unemployment (DeAngelis, 1995). Upon migration to the United States, many Latino men can no longer be the sole economic providers for the family (Wurzman, 1982). In traditional Hispanic society, when a man cannot provide for his family, he is no longer viewed as a real man by himself or others, and as a consequence, he will suffer loss of dignity and self-respect (Panitz et al., 1983). It has been suggested that under conditions of extreme stress, some Hispanic males may compensate for the loss of family authority by exhibiting "a rigid and maladaptive tyrannical and hypermasculine facade" (De La Cancela, 1986, p. 295; see also DeAngelis, 1995). This reaction to

stress will probably have repercussions for women's ability to protect themselves from HIV infection, and in extreme cases, may be
linked to domestic abuse.

Domestic Violence

It is important to note at the outset that rates of domestic violence
are comparable in Hispanic and non-Hispanic families when factors
such as urbanization, low income, and age are controlled (Straus
and Smith, 1990). In addition, research on domestic abuse in various Latin American countries reveals that levels of abuse are no
higher than in other countries around the world (Heise, Pitanguy,
and Germain, 1994). However, as is true in most segments of society, a significant number of Latino women are in abusive relationships that limit their ability to control their own behavior. One U.S.
study revealed that one out of eight Hispanic husbands physically
abused their wives during the previous year (Straus and Smith,
1990). Impoverished Latino women appear to be at higher risk of
domestic violence, as suggested by a study of 48 women receiving
general (not abuse-related) services at two community-based organizations serving impoverished Latino populations (Suarez, Raffaelli, and O'Leary, 1995). Two-thirds of the women had experienced at least one act of physical violence from their current sex
partner at some point in the relationship: 61 percent of the women
had been pushed or shoved; 33 percent slapped; 29 percent kicked,
bitten, or hit; and 11 percent threatened with a knife or gun. When
asked why their partner had physically abused them, some women
attributed the violence to their partner's desire to control them. For
example, one women said her partner slapped her because "he
wants to have full control of me" and another said her partner's
behavior had "taught me to control myself better. I don't instigate
him anymore." Other women explicitly linked the abuse to their
own failure to behave in a culturally appropriate way; for example,
one women said her partner abused her because she did not "treat
him the way that a good Puerto Rican girl raised in Puerto Rico
would treat her husband."

Because *machismo* condones the control of women, it has been
proposed as a factor in spousal abuse (Loizos, 1978; Straus, 1983).
Although this issue has not been systematically investigated, a

study of barriers to condom use found that one-third of less acculturated Hispanic women said they were afraid of getting hurt if they asked their partner to use condoms (compared to 12 percent of acculturated Hispanics and 20.5 percent of African Americans (Nyamathi et al., 1995). The small-scale abuse study described above also asked women to rate their partner on a hypermasculinity scale and found significant correlations between hypermasculinity and both psychological and physical abuse (Suarez, 1995). Without investigating this issue more directly, it is impossible to draw conclusions about linkages between *machismo* and abuse; however, it is clear that a significant proportion of Latino women experience abuse in their intimate relationships.

Women who experience or fear abuse are at risk of HIV infection for several reasons. These women will probably be less able to assert themselves, since abused women are reluctant to risk angering their partner by suggesting that condoms be used (Amaro, 1995; Worth, 1989). In addition, abuse may take the form of rape or other coerced sexual activity which precludes HIV-prevention measures (Heise, Pitangay, and Germain, 1994). Finally, physical and psychological abuse have been linked in the general population to negative outcomes including depression and low self-esteem (Campbell, 1989; Ferraro, 1979; Mitchell and Hodson, 1983), and passivity and lack of assertion (Launius and Lindquist, 1988), all of which may interfere with a woman's motivation and ability to protect herself from HIV. Thus, women who are in abusive relationships or who fear negative partner reactions will be less able to engage in risk reduction behavior.

The social, economic, and cultural realities of Latino women's lives present serious challenges to risk reduction efforts. Many Latino women live in poverty and lack adequate access to health care and information, necessary precursors to behavior change. In addition, Latino women may experience culturally sanctioned inequality in their personal relationships and lack support for risk reduction efforts. Even if a woman knows or suspects that her partner engages in sexual activity outside the relationship, her subordinate status will likely leave her unable to insist on preventive measures. For the subset of women who experience or fear abuse, attempts to negotiate condom use or discuss HIV prevention may lead to physical harm. These challenges are considerable, and raise the question of whether HIV/AIDS prevention programs can be successful in helping Latino women implement and maintain behavior change in their sexual relationships. We turn now to an examination of the available research on this topic.

TRADITIONAL APPROACHES TO HIV PREVENTION

Risk reduction interventions promoting consistent condom use and other safer sex strategies have resulted in dramatic behavior change in specific U.S. populations, most notably among self-identified gay men living in urban settings (e.g., Catania et al., 1991; Ekstrand and Coates, 1990; Kelly et al., 1989; Silvestre et al., 1993; Stall, Coates, and Hoff, 1988; Winkelstein et al., 1987). Unfortunately, the success of similar interventions in promoting behavioral change among women is less impressive.

It is only recently that HIV prevention efforts have focused on women; initial efforts targeted current or past injection drug users (IDU), who make up the majority of women diagnosed with AIDS to date. Changes in sexual behavior have been reported in studies targeting women involved with drugs, although the number of studies including Latino women has been small. One study testing the efficacy of a skills-building approach in reducing sexual risk behavior among 91 female methadone patients (64 percent Hispanic) found positive but modest gains two weeks after the intervention ended (Schilling et al, 1991). Most notably, women in the intervention group were more likely to obtain, carry, and use condoms and to report feeling comfortable talking to their partners about safe sex. In addition, 64 percent of the intervention group, compared to 36 percent of the control group, reported sexual behavior change at the two-week follow-up; a 15-month follow-up of 62 women revealed that some gains were maintained, including condom use, comfort discussing sexual issues, and positive attitudes toward HIV/AIDS prevention (El-Bassel and Schilling, 1992). Unfortunately, this study did not report results by ethnicity, so it is impossible to tell whether Latino women were as likely to report behavior change as non-Latino women.

Heterosexual women who are not injection drug users have only recently become the target of intervention efforts, and few of these interventions have been published (Moore, Harrison, and Doll, 1994). A small number of intervention programs involving primarily African-American women have demonstrated significant (but modest) sexual behavior change including redemption of condom coupons (considered a measure of behavioral intentions) (Solomon and DeJong, 1989) and changes in condom use (Hobfall et al., 1994). The most impressive outcomes were reported by Kelly and his colleagues (1994), who found that women who participated in a skills training intervention showed significant gains from baseline to a three-month follow-up. For example, women in the intervention group reported an increase in the proportion of intercourse acts during which a condom was used (from 26 percent at baseline to 56 percent at follow-up, compared to an increase from 26 percent to 32 percent among control group participants). The proportion of women reporting any condom use increased from 43 percent to 66 percent among the intervention group, but did not change among control group participants. This research suggests that well-designed interventions have the potential to bring about behavior change among at least some women; what is still unknown is whether Latino women will also benefit from comparable behavior change programs.

Few sexual risk reduction studies have included enough Latino women to examine ethnicity effects. Those studies that report on Latino women separately reveal only very minor changes, although few intensive interventions comparable to that conducted by Kelly and colleagues (1994) have been implemented. A brief (12-minute) educational intervention implemented at WIC clinics increased Latino women's levels of AIDS information and AIDS-related attitudes from pretest to an immediate posttest; however, at a retest two to three months after participation, gains in AIDS-related attitudes had disappeared and no significant differences in the behavior of experimental and control group members were observed (Flaskerud and Nyamathi, 1990). A more lengthy intervention developed by these same researchers targeted Latino women recruited at homeless shelters and drug-treatment programs (Nyamathi et al., 1994). Women received either a "specialized" intervention consisting of a

two-hour gender and culturally sensitive program of AIDS education and skills building conducted by Latino staff or a "traditional"
intervention consisting of a one-hour education program. Two-
week follow-up assessments revealed that women in the specialized
group were less likely to report IDU but were no less likely to report
having sex with multiple partners (8.5 percent compared to 6.1
percent of women in the traditional group). Unfortunately, this
study did not assess condom use, so it is impossible to know
whether women increased their condom use as a result of participating in the intervention.

Other interventions targeting Latino women are in the implementation or data analysis phase and their results have not yet been
published (e.g., O'Donnell, San Doval, Vornfett, and O'Donnell,
1994; Weeks et al., 1995). Given the fairly modest results obtained
in interventions targeting African-American and non-Hispanic
white American women, it will be surprising if dramatic results are
obtained. As is being increasingly recognized, even the best
designed prevention programs are of limited success in promoting
behavior change among women who are at greatest risk (Amaro,
1995; Heise and Elias, 1995; O'Leary and Jemmott, 1995). We turn
next to an examination of the limitations of traditional HIV-prevention approaches.

Limitations of Traditional Approaches to HIV Prevention

Amaro (1995) identified three main features of models of sexual
behavior on which HIV prevention programs have been based that
limit their applicability to women. First, models tend to be individualistic, neglecting the broader social and cultural contexts in which
sexual behavior is embedded. Second, models tend to assume that
sexual activity is under an individual's control, ignoring the fact
that sexual encounters are often initiated impulsively or may be
coercive. Finally, models tend to ignore the extent to which sexual
behavior is constrained by culturally determined factors, including
gender roles, sexual values, and norms that typically result in
inflexible sexual repertoires and create a power differential between
men and women.

These factors all limit the usefulness of models in explaining
women's sexual choices and predicting risk-taking behavior. In

fact, there is mounting evidence that psychosocial variables found to predict the sexual behavior of men have limited predictive value for women (Amaro, 1995; Catania et al., 1992; for a review, see Moore, Harrison, and Doll, 1994). For example, one study examined a wide range of social and psychological predictors of HIV risk behavior among 671 primarily African-American women living in low-income housing projects in five U.S. cities (Sikkema et al., 1996). Predictor variables included HIV knowledge, age, personal risk perception, number of recent conversations with sex partners about condoms and AIDS concerns, alcohol and substance use, peer norms, risk reduction behavioral intentions, and condom barrier beliefs—variables that have been predictive in studies of male sexual behavior. In this analysis, most women (81 percent) at low risk were correctly classified by the study variables but only about half (52 percent) of women at high risk were correctly classified, suggesting that additional factors not included in current models of sexual behavior influence women's high-risk sexual behavior.

Another issue that is often ignored in prevention programs is that many women's only risk is engaging in unprotected sexual activity with one sexual partner, and the dynamics of steady relationships differ from casual or new relationships. Another analysis of the housing project data (Wagstaff et al., 1995) revealed that women who had a single partner they perceived as risky (i.e., the women were "sure" or "pretty sure" their sex partner had other partners or injected drugs) were less likely to report condom use at last intercourse than women who had multiple partners (28 percent versus 53 percent) and less likely to report talking to partners about condom use than women who had multiple partners (55 percent versus 73 percent). The two groups of women expressed similar levels of intentions to use condoms, and had equal perceptions of risk; however, these intentions and perceptions did not translate into behavior among women who were monogamous even if they knew or suspected their partners were at risk. Finally, an often ignored issue is that condom use relies not only on the cooperation of a male partner (which may be difficult to obtain) but also prevents conception, making condom use doubly problematic for many women (see Carovano, 1991; Worth, 1989).

The limitations of traditional approaches to HIV prevention are magnified among Latino women. Of particular relevance to current risk reduction recommendations is the fact that, even if they feel vulnerable and want to change their behavior, many Latino women will be unable to "negotiate" safer sex with their partners. As described earlier, condoms are not widely used as a birth control method among Latino populations and have traditionally been associated with illicit relationships. In addition, because it is not a cultural norm for couples to discuss sexual matters, women may be reluctant to introduce the topic of condoms or attempt to negotiate safer sex with sexual partners. A woman's attempts to discuss HIV prevention in general, and condom use in particular, may be seen as inappropriate or disrespectful of the male prerogative to control the couple's sexual activity, and be taken as evidence for lack of trust. These barriers to condom use are considerable, as can be seen in the finding that 45 percent of 83 Latino women surveyed in Florida said they would not use a condom even if they knew their partner was infected with HIV, compared to 15 percent of white and 20 percent of black women (Harrison et al., 1990).

Most theorists agree that the complex interplay of economic, cultural, and social forces that define the realities of Latino women's lives present special challenges that risk reduction efforts have not been able to meet. The crux of the matter is summed up by Magana and Magana (1992): "[G]iven the subservient status of the Latino woman, it is difficult to come up with realistic strategies to help her protect herself" (p. 40). Despite this bleak reality, there are promising developments in the theoretical and applied literature on HIV/AIDS prevention that deserve further attention when considering the prevention needs of Latino women.

DIRECTIONS FOR FUTURE INTERVENTION EFFORTS

In recent years, there have been a number of conceptual and practical developments that hold promise for increasing the success of future HIV prevention efforts with Latino women. One area where advances are being made is the conceptual front, as theorists and researchers recognize the limited utility of existing models in explaining the sexual behavior of heterosexual women. By incorporating explicit discussions of how gender and power dynamics influence sexual behavior, and exploring how risk behavior is influenced by these factors, the applicability of models to women's behavior will increase (Amaro, 1995). Research on what individual, partner, socioeconomic, and cultural variables predict risk and preventive behavior among subgroups of Latino women are needed. It is also imperative that the topic of sexual decision making in Latino couples be addressed directly, rather than inferring how couples negotiate sexual decisions from studies of other aspects of family decision making or distribution of power (Hurtado, 1995). In addition, qualitative research is needed to understand quantitative research findings.

The importance of conducting qualitative research was demonstrated in a study of Mexican-American men which showed that acculturation operates selectively on sexual behavior (Carrier and Magana, 1991; Magana and Carrier, 1991). In-depth field research revealed that the homosexual behavior of Mexican-American men followed either the Mexican pattern (i.e., strong role separation with emphasis on anal intercourse) or the Anglo-American pattern (i.e., less role separation with more flexible sexual repertoire). What determined the pattern men followed was the ethnicity of their early sexual partners rather than time spent in the United States or language preference (typical measures of acculturation). This finding suggests the need to get beyond simple "demographic" variables and look for ways of examining the life experience of individuals.

Another conceptual development is the growing recognition of the importance of working on the community as well as the individual level (e.g., Kelly et al., 1993). Community-level interventions incorporating mass media, outreach, and diffusion strategies as well as clinic-based programs were highly successful in bringing about changes in the gay community (Coates, 1990). Although the United States has been resistant to utilize the mass media as a channel for disseminating HIV-prevention information, promoting norms supporting prevention, and bringing about other desired group changes, there is evidence from around the world that social marketing approaches can play a significant role in HIV/AIDS prevention (Ling et al., 1992).[2] Person-to-person outreach is also an effective way of promoting risk reduction; one intervention program for gay men successfully utilized popular community members as behavioral change agents (Kelly et al., 1992). Perhaps most important, by directing efforts at community members, prevention programs can involve current and future sex partners of intervention participants as well as the participants themselves. This is especially important for women, who may feel alienated and unduly burdened when they (rather than their sex partners) are the target of condom promotion efforts (Worth, 1989).

Prevention programs that focus exclusively on women and place the responsibility for behavior change on them ignore half of the (hetero) sexual equation (Ehrhardt, 1992; Flaskerud and Uman, 1993). Many Latino women are at risk because they lack power in their personal relationships; thus, it is imperative to target intervention efforts at men as well as women. In addition, because research suggests that Latino men control the decision to use condoms (e.g., Mikawa et al., 1992), it is counterproductive to focus condom promotion efforts exclusively on women. Given the fact that condom use is often not accepted in primary relationships, several scholars have suggested the compromise strategy of promoting consistent condom use with secondary partners (e.g., Marin, Gomez, and Hearst, 1993; San Doval et al., 1995). This would circumvent many of the barriers to introducing condoms into an ongoing relationship where conception might be desired, draw on culturally valued notions of responsibility to the family, and take advantage of the fact that condom use with secondary partners is acceptable to most Latino men.

Ultimately, however, if women are at risk as the result of their inferior social status or culturally determined expectations that are not amenable to short-term change, interventions must take this fact into account. On the pragmatic level, prevention programs for Latino women should acknowledge that condom use is a desired but not always attainable goal and give women other options that they can use. In a thought-provoking review of women-centered prevention methods, Erica Gollub (1995) attributes the continued emphasis on male condoms to "the misguided search for the *perfect* method" (p. 65). She points out that condoms may be the most effective way to prevent HIV transmission, but "for a woman with a partner who says no, they are 0 percent effective" (Gollub, 1995, p. 74). Because of this, Gollub urges that prevention programs give women information on the full range of available prevention methods (in a hierarchy reflecting degree of risk) so that they may choose what works best for them.

Other scholars and advocates have argued that interventions should be aimed at changing the reality of women's lives by improving their status in society. Empowerment approaches typically being women together to work toward common goals (e.g., Amaro, 1995). The potential impact of an empowerment approach is described by Heise and Elias (1995), who report on how two groups of Indian women reacted to a film on women and HIV. One group was withdrawn, embarrassed, and expressed fears of bringing up the topic of condoms with their husbands. The second group reacted differently; the women "felt capable and entitled to discuss condom use with their husbands and recommended holding a community meeting to discuss the dangers of the new disease" (Heise and Elias, 1995, p. 940). This dramatic difference was due to the fact that the second group had been participating in a community organization project for six years and was used to acting collectively to address common problems. Empowerment approaches aimed at helping women gain more control over their sexual lives have been successful among inner-city women in the United States (e.g., Levine et al., 1993). Although empowerment approaches have not been applied to HIV prevention in Latino communities, some aspects of community empowerment approaches will probably be applicable to Latino populations (for a discussion, see De La Cancela, 1989), although care must be taken to ensure that interventions are appropriate to the specific Latino community for which they are developed.

A final promising development in the prevention literature is the growth of a more sophisticated awareness of how cultural forces influence individual behavior. Although program planners have long stressed that prevention programs must be culturally sensitive, many programs for Latinos "translate" or at most, "adapt" interventions originally developed for non-Latino populations (Marin, 1993). Culture goes beyond language; however, it represents a powerful internalized force that is "experienced by the person as needs or obligations . . . " (D'Andrade, 1984, p. 97). Through the process of socialization, individuals learn the rules of their culture and come to experience an internal pressure to obey those rules; failure to follow cultural directives is experienced as anxiety provoking (D'Andrade, 1984). Another characteristic of culture that is often ignored is that it incorporates both rational and nonrational (emotional) elements (D'Andrade, 1984; LeVine, 1984). Prevention programs cannot treat culturally derived values, beliefs, and norms as little more than opinions or facts that can be changed to conform to a more "correct" or acceptable version. Cultural meaning systems have a deeply felt and complex psychological reality that must be taken into account when developing interventions.

Gerardo Marin (1993) identified three characteristics of culturally appropriate interventions: interventions are based on values of the target group; strategies reflect the group's subjective culture; and strategies fit the preferred behavioral repertoire of the target group. Theorists have identified a number of cultural values that should be taken into account when considering the HIV/AIDS prevention needs of Latino populations (Marin, 1988; Marin, 1989). These include *familismo,* an emphasis on the family as the primary source of social support and identity; *simpatia,* an emphasis on smooth interpersonal relationships; *personalismo,* a preference for personal relationships and individual contact; and *respeto,* the need to maintain respectful hierarchical relationships. Two examples from Latin America demonstrate that by identifying themes that resonate with the target population, prevention programs can have widespread effects. In Mexico, formative research revealed that female commercial sex workers were concerned about the impact of HIV on their children rather than themselves. Mothers worried about who would care for their children if they became infected with HIV; thus, the intervention materials appealed to sex workers as mothers and urged them to stay healthy for their children's sake. Evaluations indicated significant increases in condom use, from 39 percent of women in the month before the project to 66 percent six months after its end (Liskin et al., 1989). In Colombia, after a radio campaign featured the slogan "To love with responsibility is also a man's concern," the proportion of listeners reporting that condoms were embarrassing, disrespectful to the home, vulgar, or not satisfying declined by up to 40 percentage points (Liskin et al., 1990).

These examples illustrate the effectiveness of messages incorporating culturally appropriate themes.

A second characteristic of culturally appropriate interventions is that strategies fit the target group's subjective culture. For example, many Latino men who have same-sex partners do not self-identify as "gay" or "bisexual," so they will not be reached by prevention messages aimed at these populations and may underestimate their risk of HIV infection (Magana and Magana, 1992; Marin, 1988; Marin, 1989). Special interventions will be needed to reach Latino men who have sex with both men and women, and these interventions must be couched in terms that are meaningful to the population. The third characteristic of culturally appropriate interventions identified by Marin, that interventions adhere to the preferred behavioral repertoire of the target population, is demonstrated in a project conducted by O'Donnell and colleagues (O'Donnell, San Doval, Vornfett, and DeJong, 1994). During the formative research phase of an intervention project with Hispanics, these researchers learned that participants did not want to change traditional patterns of reticence on sexual topics; rather, they wanted to learn how to protect themselves *without* explicit discussions. Thus, rather than focusing on changing communication patterns and trying to teach participants to talk to their partners about sex, the intervention modeled nonverbal (and minimally verbal) strategies to achieve condom use.

These simple examples all share a common theme: prevention programs reflect the values and needs of the target population. By involving members of the intended audience in the planning stages of intervention development and being open to their values and needs rather than coming in with a predetermined agenda, program planners can increase the effectiveness of their intervention. It is especially important to avoid "importing" strategies that have been successful in other population groups. For example, safer-sex eroticization (successful in promoting condom use among Anglo-American gay men) may not be as effective in a population where sex is regarded as a woman's duty rather than a source of pleasure. Instead, it might be more acceptable to emphasize the contraceptive (Amaro, 1988b) or health (Fernandez, 1995) benefits of condom use. By using cultural norms, attitudes, and values as "enablers" rather than barriers, prevention planners can increase the effectiveness of their intervention programs.

Latino women in the United States, like women all around the world, are at risk of HIV infection in large part from their inferior status both in society and in their own culture. This chapter has identified some of the main factors that limit Latino women's ability to implement risk reduction measures and attempted to identify potential intervention approaches. In the short run, there is an urgent need to develop interventions that reflect the social, cultural, and economic realities of Latino women's lives and give them realistic options that they can implement without jeopardizing their relationships or their personal safety. In the long run, fundamental changes in how men and women are viewed and expected to behave will be necessary to stem the AIDS epidemic among Latino populations.

NOTES

1. The term "Latino" is used to refer to populations of Latin American origin of descent (Hayes-Bautista and Chapa, 1986); the term "Hispanic" (a census term which excludes Latinos of non-spanish origin) is used to report data utilizing this label, or more narrowly, to refer to aspects of Latino culture that can be traced back to Spanish origins. It is important to note that both these umbrella terms encompass a number of subgroups with distinct historical, political, economic, and racial differences (Amaro, 1988a); however, most scholars agree that Latino subgroups share historical and cultural features that result in significant commonalities, particularly with regard to HIV-prevention needs (e.g., Magana and Magana, 1992; Marin, 1988).

2. For a discussion of reasons for resistance to public education efforts in the United States, see Ehrhardt (1992).

REFERENCES

Amaro, H. (1988a). Considerations for prevention of HIV infection among Hispanic women. *Psychology of Women Quarterly, 12*, 429-443.

Amaro, H. (1988b). Women in the Mexican-American community: Religion, culture, and reproductive attitudes and experiences. *Journal of Community Psychology, 16*, 6-20.

Amaro, H. (1995). Love, sex, and power: Considering women's realities in HIV prevention. *American Psychologist, 50*(6), 437-447.

Belk, S. S., Garcia-Falconi, R., Hernandez-Sanchea, J. E., and Snell, W. E. (1988). Avoidance strategy use in the intimate relationships of women and men from Mexico and the United States. *Psychology of Women Quarterly, 12*, 165-174.

Billy, J. O. G., Tanfer, K., Grady, W. R., and Klepinger, D. H. (1993). The sexual behavior of men in the United States. *Family Planning Perspectives, 25*(2), 52-60.

Campbell, J. (1989). A test of two explanatory models of women's responses to battering. *Nursing Research, 38*(1), 18-25.

Carovano, K. (1991). More than mothers and whores: Redefining the AIDS prevention needs of women. *International Journal of Health Services, 21*(1), 131-142.

Carrier, J. M. (1976). Cultural factors affecting urban Mexican male homosexual behavior. *Archives of Sexual Behavior, 5*, 103-124.

Carrier, J. M. (1985). Mexican male bisexuality. *Journal of Homosexuality, 11*, 75-85.

Carrier, J. M., and Magana, J. R. (1991). Use of ethnosexual data on men of Mexican origin for HIV/AIDS prevention programs. *Journal of Sex Research, 28*(2), 189-202.

Catania, J. A., Coates, T. J., Kegeles, S., Fullilove, M. T., Peterson, J., Marin, B., Siegel, D., and Hulley, S. (1992). Condom use in multi-ethnic neighborhoods of San Francisco: The population-based AMEN (AIDS in Multi-Ethnic Neighborhoods) Study. *American Journal of Public Health, 82*(2), 284-287.

Catania, J. A., Coates, T. J., Peterson, J., Dolcini, M. M., Kegeles, S., Siegel, D., Golden, E., and Fullilove, M. T. (1993). Changes in condom use among black, Hispanic, and white heterosexuals in San Francisco: The AMEN cohort survey. *The Journal of Sex Research, 30*(2), 121-128.

Catania, J. A., Coates, T. J., Stall, R., Bye, L., Kegeles, S. M., Capell, F., Henne, J., McKusick, L., Morin, S., Turner, H., and Pollack, L. (1991). Changes in condom use among homosexual men in San Francisco. *Health Psychology, 10*, 190-199.

Catania, J. A., Dolcini, M.M., Coates, T. J., Kegeles, S. M., Greenblatt, R.M., Puckett, S., Corman, M., and Miller, J. (1989). Predictors of condom use and multiple partnered sex among sexually active adolescent women: Implications for AIDS-related health interventions. *The Journal of Sex Research, 26*(4), 514-524.

CDC. (1994). AIDS among racial/ethnic minorities—United States, 1993. *MMWR, 43*, 644-647, 652-655.

CDC. (1995). *HIV/AIDS surveillance report, 7*(1). Atlanta: Centers for Disease Control and Prevention.

Choi, K., Catania, J. A., and Dolcini, M. M. (1993). Extramarital sex and HIV risk behavior among U.S. adults: Results from the National AIDS Behavioral Survey. *American Journal of Public Health, 84*(12), 2003-2007.

Coates, T. J. (1990). Strategies for modifying sexual behavior for primary and secondary prevention of HIV disease. *Journal of Consulting and Clinical Psychology, 58*(1), 57-69.

Comas-Diaz, L. (1987). Feminist therapy with Hispanic/Latin women: Myth or reality? *Women and Therapy*, 6(4), 39-61.

D'Andrade, R. G. (1984). Cultural meaning systems. In R. A. Shweder and R. A. LeVine (Eds.), *Culture theory: Essays on mind, self, and emotion*, 88-119. New York: Cambridge University Press.

DeAngelis, T. (1995). Adapting to new cultures, challenges. *APA Monitor*, July, 48-49.

De La Cancela, V. (1986). A critical analysis of Puerto Rican machismo: Implications for clinical practice. *Psychotherapy*, 23(2), 291-296.

De La Cancela, V. (1989). Minority AIDS prevention: Moving beyond cultural perspectives towards sociopolitical empowerment. *AIDS Education and Prevention*, 1(2), 141-153.

Diaz, T., Buehler, J. W., Castro, K. G., and Ward, J. W. (1993). AIDS trends among Hispanics in the United States. *American Journal of Public Health*, 83(4), 504-509.

Ehrhardt, A. A. (1992). Trends in sexual behavior and the HIV pandemic (Editorial). *American Journal of Public Health*, 82(11), 1459-1461.

Ekstrand, M. L. and Coates, T. J. (1990). Maintenance of safer sexual behaviors and predictors of risky sex: The San Francisco Men's Health Study. *American Journal of Public Health*, 80, 973-977.

El-Bassel, N. and Schilling, R. F. (1992). 15-month follow-up of women methadone patients taught skills to reduce heterosexual HIV transmission. *Public Health Reports*, 107(5), 500-504.

Epstein, J. A., Dusenbury, L., Botvin, G. J., and Diaz, T. (1994). Acculturation, beliefs about AIDS, and AIDS education among New York City Hispanic parents. *Hispanic Journal of Behavioral Sciences*, 16(3), 342-354.

Fernandez, M. I. (1995). Latins and AIDS: Challenges to HIV prevention efforts. In A. O'Leary and L. S. Jemmott (Eds.), *Women at risk: Issues in the primary prevention of AIDS*, 159-174. New York: Plenum Press.

Ferraro, K. J. (1979). Physical and emotional battering: Aspects of managing hurt. *California Sociologist*, 2, 134-149.

Fisher, J.D. and Fisher, W.A. (1992). Changing AIDS-risk behavior. *Psychological Bulletin*, 111(3), 455-474.

Flaskerud, J. H. and Nyamathi, A. M. (1990). Effects of an AIDS education program on the knowledge, attitudes and practices of low income black and Latina women. *Journal of Community Health*, 15(6), 343-355.

Flaskerud, J. H. and Uman, G. (1993). Directions for AIDS education for Hispanic women based on analyses of survey findings. *Public Health Reports*, 108(3), 298-304.

Ford, K., Rubenstein, S., and Norris, A. (1994). Sexual behavior and condom use among urban, low-income, African-American and Hispanic youth. *AIDS Education and Prevention*, 6(3), 219-229.

Forrest, K. A., Austin, D. M., Valdes, M. I., Fuentes, E. G., and Wilson, S. R. (1993). Exploring norms and beliefs related to AIDS prevention among California Hispanic men. *Family Planning Perspectives*, 25(3), 111-117.

Gilmore, D. and Uhl, S. C. (1987). Further notes on Andalusian machismo. *Journal of Psychoanalytical Anthropology, 10*(4), 341-360.

Goldwert, M. (1985). Mexican machismo: The flight from femininity. *Psychoanalytic Review, 72*(1), 161-169.

Gollub, E. L. (1995). Women-centered prevention techniques and technologies. In A. O'Leary and L. S. Jemmott (Eds.), *Women at Risk: Issues in the Primary Prevention of AIDS*, 43-82. New York: Plenum Press.

Grimstead, O. A., Faigeles, B., Binson, D., and Eversley, R. (1993). Sexual risk for human immunodeficiency virus infection among women in high-risk cities. *Family Planning Perspectives, 25*(6), 252-256, 277.

Harrison, D. F., Wambach, K. G., Byers, J. B., Imershein, A. W., Levine, P., Maddox, K., Quadagno, D. M., Fordyce, M. L., and Jones, M. A. (1990). AIDS knowledge and risk behaviors among culturally diverse women. *AIDS Education and Prevention, 3*(2), 79-89.

Hayes-Bautista, D. E., and Chapa, J. (1986). Latino terminology: Conceptual bases for standardized terminology. *American Journal of Public Health, 77*(1), 61-68.

Heise, L. L. and Elias, C. (1995). Transforming AIDS prevention to meet women's needs: A focus on developing countries. *Social Science and Medicine, 40*(7), 931-943.

Heise, L. L., Pitanguy, J., and Germain, A. (1994). *Violence against women: The hidden health burden.* Washington: The World Bank.

Hobfall, S. E., Jackson, A. P., Lavin, J., Britton, P. J., and Shepherd, J. B. (1994). Reducing inner-city women's AIDS risk activities: A study of single, pregnant women. *Health Psychology, 13*(5), 397-403.

Holmes, K. K., Karon, J. M., and Kreiss, J. (1990). The increasing frequency of heterosexually acquired AIDS in the United States, 1983-1988. *American Journal of Public Health, 80*(7), 858-862.

Hurtado, A. (1995). Variations, combinations, and evolutions: Latino families in the United States. In R. E. Zambrana (Ed.), *Understanding Latino Families: Scholarship, Policy, and Practice,* 40-61. Thousand Oaks, CA: Sage.

Ickovics, J. R. and Rodin, J. (1992). Women and AIDS in the United States: Epidemiology, natural history, and mediating mechanisms. *Health Psychology, 11*(1), 2-16.

Izazola-Licea, J. A., Valdespino-Gomez, J. L., Gortmaker, S. L., Townsend, J., Becker, J., Palacios-Martinez, M., Mueller, N. E., and Sepulveda-Amor, J. (1991). HIV-1 seropositivity and behavioral and sociological risks among homosexual and bisexual men in six Mexican cities. *Journal of Acquired Immune Deficiency Syndromes, 4*, 614-622.

Kaemingk, K. L. and Bootzin, R. R. (1990). Behavior change strategies for increasing condom use. *Evaluation and Program Planning, 13*, 47-54.

Kalichman, S. C., Adair, V., Somlai, A. M., and Weir, S. S. (1995). The perceived social context of AIDS: Study of inner-city sexually transmitted disease clinic patients. *AIDS Education and Prevention, 7*(4), 298-307.

Kalichman, S. C., Hunter, T. L., and Kelly, J. A. (1992). Perceptions of AIDS susceptibility among minority and nonminority women at risk for HIV infection. *Journal of Consulting and Clinic Psychology, 60*(5), 725-732.

Kelly, J. A., Murphy, D. A., Sikkema, K. J., and Kalichman, S. C. (1993). Psychological interventions to prevent HIV infection are urgently needed: New priorities for behavioral research in the second decade of AIDS. *American Psychologist, 48*(10), 1023-1034.

Kelly, J. A., Murphy, D. A., Washington, C. D., Wilson, T. S., Koob, J. J., Davis, D. R., Ledezma, G., and Devantes, B. (1994). The effects of HIV/AIDS intervention groups for high-risk women in urban clinics. *American Journal of Public Health, 84*(12), 1918-1922.

Kelly, J. A., St. Lawrence, J. S., Hood, H. V., and Brasfield, T. L. (1989). Behavioral intervention to reduce AIDS risk activities. *Journal of Consulting and Clinic Psychology, 57*(1), 60-67.

Kelly, J. A., St. Lawrence, J. S., Stevenson, L. Y., Hauth, A. C., Kalichman, S. C., Diaz, Y. E., Brasfield, T. L., Koob, J. J., and Morgan, M. G. (1992). Community HIV/AIDS risk reduction: The effects of endorsement by popular people in three cities. *American Journal of Public Health, 82*(11), 1483-1489.

Kenen, R. H. and Armstrong, K. (1992). The why, when, and whether of condom use among female and male drug users. *Journal of Community Health, 17*(5), 303-317.

Kline, A., Kline, E., and Oken, E. (1992). Minority women and sexual choice in the age of AIDS. *Social Science and Medicine, 34*(4), 447-457.

Launius, M. H. and Lindquist, C. U. (1988). Learned helplessness, external locus of control and passivity in battered women. *Journal of Interpersonal Violence, 3*(3), 307-318.

Lauver, D., Armstrong, K., Marks, S., and Schwarz, S. (1995). HIV risk status and preventive behaviors among 17,619 women. *Journal of Obstetric, Gynecologic, and Neonatal Nursing, 24*(1), 33-39.

Levine, O. H., Britton, P. J., James, T. C., Jackson, A. P., Hobfoll, S. E., and Lavin, J. P. (1993). The empowerment of women: A key to HIV prevention. *Journal of Community Psychology, 21*, 320-334.

LeVine, R. A. (1984). Properties of culture: An ethnographic view. In R. A. Shweder and R. A. LeVine (Eds.), *Culture theory: Essays on Mind, Self, and Emotion,* 67-87. New York: Cambridge University Press.

Ling, J. C., Franklin, B. A. K., Lindsteadt, J. F., and Gearon, S. A. N. (1992). Social marketing: Its place in public health. *Annual Review of Public Health, 13*, 341-362.

Liskin, L., Church, C. A., Piotrow, P. T., and Harris, J. A. (1989). AIDS Education—A beginning, *Population Reports, Series L, No. 8.* Baltimore: Johns Hopkins University, Population Information Program.

Liskin, L., Wharton, C., Blackburn, R., and Kestelman, P. (1990). Condoms—now more than ever, *Population Reports, Series H, No. 8.* Baltimore: Johns Hopkins University, Population Information Program.

Loizos, P. (1978). Violence and the family: Some Mediterranean examples. In M. P. Martin (Ed.), *Violence and the Family*, 183-195. Chichester, England: Wiley.

Magana, J. R. and Carrier, J. M. (1991). Mexican and Mexican-American male sexual behavior and spread of AIDS in California. *Journal of Sex Research*, *28*(3), 425-441.

Magana, J. R. and Magana, H. A. (1992). Mexican-Latino children. In M. L. Stuber (Ed.), *Children and AIDS*, 33-43. Washington: American Psychiatric Press.

Marin, B. (1988). *AIDS Prevention in non-Puerto Rican Hispanics*. Rockville, MD: NIDA.

Marin, B. V., Gomez, C. A., and Hearst, N. (1993). Multiple heterosexual partners and condom use among Hispanics and non-Hispanic whites. *Family Planning Perspectives*, *25*(4), 170-174.

Marin, B. V. and Marin, G. (1990). Effects of acculturation on knowledge of AIDS and HIV among Hispanics. *Hispanic Journal of Behavioral Sciences*, *12*(2), 110-121.

Marin, B. V., Tschann, J. M., Gomez, C. A., and Kegeles, S. M. (1993). Acculturation and gender differences in sexual attitudes and behaviors: Hispanic vs. non-Hispanic white unmarried adults. *American Journal of Public Health*, *83*(12), 1759-1761.

Marin, G. (1989). AIDS prevention among Hispanics: Needs, risk behaviors, and cultural values. *Public Health Reports*, *104*(5), 411-415.

Marin, G. (1993). Defining culturally appropriate community interventions: Hispanics as a case study. *Journal of Community Psychology*, *21*, 149-161.

Marin, G. and Marin, B. V. (1991). *Research with Hispanic Populations*. Newbury Park, CA: Sage.

Mason, H. R. C., Marks, G., Simoni, J. M., Ruiz, M. S., and Richardson, J. L. (1995). Culturally sanctioned secrets? Latino men's nondisclosure of HIV infection to family, friends, and lovers. *Health Psychology*, *14*(1), 6-12.

Mays, V. M. and Cochran, S. D. (1988). Issues in the perception of AIDS risk and risk reduction activities by black and Hispanic/Latina women. *American Psychologist*, *43*(11), 949-957.

Merson, M. (1993). Slowing the spread of HIV: Agenda for the 1990s. *Science*, *260*, 1266-1268.

Mikawa, J. K., Morones, P. A., Gomez, A., Case, H. L., Olsen, D., and Gonzalez-Huss, M. J. (1992). Cultural practices of Hispanics: Implications for the prevention of AIDS. *Hispanic Journal of Behavioral Sciences*, *14*(4), 421-433.

Mitchell, R. E. and Hodson, C. A. (1983). Coping with domestic violence: Social support and psychological health among battered women. *Psychoanalytic Review*, *71*(2), 305-317.

Moore, J. S., Harrison, J. S., and Doll, L. S. (1994). Interventions for sexually active, heterosexual women in the United States. In R. J. Clemente and J. L. Peterson (Eds.), *Preventing Aids: Theories and Methods of Behavioral Interventions*. New York: Plenum Press.

Negy, C. and Woods, D.J. (1995). The importance of acculturation in understanding research with Hispanic Americans. *Hispanic Journal of Behavioral Sciences, 14*(2), 224-247.

Nyamathi, A., Bennett, C., Leake, B., Lewis, C., and Flaskerud, J. (1993). AIDS-related knowledge, perceptions, and behaviors among impoverished minority women. *American Journal of Public Health, 83*(1), 65-71.

Nyamathi, A. M., Flaskerud, J., Bennett, C., Leake, B., and Lewis, C. (1994). Evaluation of two AIDS education programs for impoverished Latina women. *AIDS Education and Prevention, 6*(4), 296-309.

Nyamathi, A. M., Lewis, C., Leake, B., Flaskerud, J., and Bennett, C. (1995). Barriers to condom use and needle cleaning among impoverished minority female injection drug users and partners of injection drug users. *Public Health Reports, 110*(2), 167-172.

Nyamathi, A., Stein, J. A., and Brecht, M. (1995). Psychosocial predictors of AIDS-risk behavior and drug use behavior in homeless and drug addicted women of color. *Health Psychology, 14*(3), 265-273.

Nyamathi, A. and Vasquez, R. (1989). Impact of poverty, homelessness, and drugs on Hispanic women at risk for HIV infection. *Hispanic Journal of Behavioral Sciences, 11*(4), 299-314.

O'Donnell, L., San Doval, A., Vornfett, R., and DeJong, W. (1994). Reducing AIDS and other STDs among inner-city Hispanics: The use of qualitative research in the development of video-based patient education. *AIDS Education and Prevention, 6*(2), 140-153.

O'Donnell, L., San Doval, A., Vornfett, R., and O'Donnell, C. R. (1994). STD prevention and the challenge of gender and cultural diversity: Knowledge, attitudes, and risk behaviors among black and Hispanic inner-city STD patients. *Sexually Transmitted Diseases, 21*(3), 137-148.

O'Leary, A. and Jemmott, L.S. (1995). General issues in the prevention of AIDS in women. In A. O'Leary and L. S. Jemmott (Eds.), *Women at Risk: Issues in the Primary Prevention of Aids*, 1-12. New York: Plenum Press.

O'Leary, A., Jemmott, L. S., Suarez-Al-Adam, M., Fernandez, I., and AlRoy, C. (1993). Women and AIDS. In S. Matteo (Ed.), *American Women in the 1990s: Today's Critical Issues*, 173-192. Boston: Northeastern University Press.

Padilla, A. M. (1980). Acculturation as varieties of adaptation. In A. M. Padilla (Ed.), *Acculturation: Theory, Models, and Some New Findings*, 9-25. Boulder: Westview.

Panitz, D. R., McConchie, R. D., Saubev, S. R., and Fonseca, J. A. (1983). The role of machismo and the Hispanic family in the etiology and treatment of alcoholism in Hispanic American males. *American Journal of Family Therapy, 11*(1), 31-44.

Parker, R. and Carballo, M. (1990). Qualitative research on homosexual and bisexual behavior relevant to HIV/AIDS. *Journal of Sex Research, 27*, 497-525.

Powell, D.R. (1995). Including Latino fathers in parent education and support programs. In R. E. Zambrana (Ed.), *Understanding Latino Families: Scholarship, Policy, and Practice,* 85-106. Thousand Oaks, CA: Sage.

Quinn, T. C. and Cates, W. (1992). Epidemiology of sexually transmitted diseases in the 1990s. In T. C. Quinn (Ed.), *Sexually Transmitted Diseases,* 1-37. New York: Raven.

Ramirez, J., Suarez, E., Rosa, G., Castro, M. A., and Zimmerman, M. A. (1994). AIDS knowledge and sexual behavior among Mexican gay and bisexual men. *AIDS Education and Prevention, 6*(2), 163-174.

Rapkin, A. J. and Erickson, P. I. (1990). Differences in knowledge of and risk factors for AIDS between Hispanic and non-Hispanic women attending an urban family planning clinic. *AIDS, 4*(9), 889-899.

Reiss, I. L. and Leik, R. K. (1989). Evaluating strategies to avoid AIDS: Number of partners vs. use of condoms. *Journal of Sex Research, 26*(4), 411-433.

Remez, L. (1993). Consistent condom use is rare among never-married American women, 1988 survey shows. *Family Planning Perspectives, 25*(6), 283-284.

Robey, B., Rutstein, S. O., Morris, L., and Blackburn, R. (1992). The Reproductive Revolution: New Survey Findings, *Population Reports, Series M, No. 11.* Baltimore: Johns Hopkins University, Population Information Program.

Sabogal, F., Perez-Stable, E. J., Otero-Sabogal, R., and Hiatt, R. A. (1995). Gender, ethnic, and acculturation differences in sexual behavior: Hispanic and non-Hispanic white adults. *Hispanic Journal of Behavioral Sciences, 17*(2), 139-159.

San Doval, A., Duran, R., O'Donnell, L., and O'Donnell, C. (1995). Barriers to condom use in primary and nonprimary relationships among Hispanic STD clinic patients. *Hispanic Journal of Behavioral Sciences, 17*(3), 385-397.

Schilling, R. F., El-Bassel, N., Schinke, S. P., Gordon, K., and Nichols, S. (1991). Building skills of recovering women drug users to reduce heterosexual AIDS transmission. *Public Health Reports, 106*(3), 297-304.

Sikkema, K. J., Heckman, T. G., Kelly, J. A., Anderson, E. S., Winett, R. A., Solomon, L. J., Wagstaff, D. A., Roffman, R. A., Perry, M. J., Cargill, V., Crumble, D. A., Fuqua, R. W., Norman, A. D., and Mercer, M. B. (1996). Prevalence and Predictors of HIV Risk Behaviors Among Women Living in Low-Income, Inner-City Housing Developments. *American Journal of Public Health, 86*(8), 1123-1128.

Silvestre, A. J., Kingsley, L. A., Wehman, P., Dappen, R., Ho, M., and Rinaldo, C. R. (1993). Changes in HIV rates and sexual behavior among homosexual men, 1984 to 1988/92. *American Journal of Public Health, 83,* 578-580.

Singer, M., Flores, C., Davison, L., Burke, G., Castillo, Z., Scanlon, K., and Rivera, M. (1990). SIDA: The economic, social, and cultural context of AIDS among Latinos. *Medical Anthropology Quarterly, 4*(1), 72-114.

Solomon, M. Z. and DeJong, W. (1989). Preventing AIDS and other STDs through condom promotion: A patient education intervention. *American Journal of Public Health, 79*(4), 453-458.

Stall, R., Coates, T. J., and Hoff, C. (1988). Behavioral risk reduction for HIV infection among gay and bisexual men: A review of results from the United States. *American Psychologist, 43*, 878-885.

Stein, Z. (1990). HIV prevention: The need for methods women can use. *American Journal of Public Health, 80*, 460-462.

Stewart, M. (1993). Minorities, women who lack influence on partner often fail to use condoms. *Family Planning Perspectives, 25*(3), 143-144.

Straus, M. (1983). Societal morphogenesis and intrafamily violence in cross-cultural perspective. In R. J. Gelles and C. P. Cornell (Eds.), *International Perspectives on Family Violence*, (pp. 27-43). Lexington, MA: Lexington.

Straus, M. A. and Smith, C. (1990). *Physical violence in American families*. New Brunswick, NJ: Transaction.

Suarez, M. (1995). *The Impact of Psychological and Physical Abuse and Hypermasculinity on the Ability of Hispanic Women to Negotiate Safer Sex*. Unpublished Master's Thesis, Rutgers University, New Brunswick, NJ.

Suarez, M., Raffaelli, M., and O'Leary, A. (1995). *Physical and Psychological Abuse in an Inner-City Hispanic Population*. Paper presented at the Society of Behavioral Medicine, San Diego, CA.

Thompson, W. N. (1991). Machismo: Manifestations of a cultural value in the Latin-American casino. *Journal of Gambling Studies, 7*(2), 143-164.

Torres, S. (1991). A comparison of wife abuse between two cultures: Perceptions, attitudes, nature, and extent. *Issues in Mental Health Nursing, 12*(1), 113-131.

U.S. Bureau of the Census. (1995). *Residence Population Estimate for 1995*. Washington: U.S. Bureau of the Census.

Vega, W. and Miranda, M. R. (1985). *Stress and Hispanic mental health: Relating Research to Service Delivery*. Rockville, MD: U.S. Department of Health and Human Services, National Institute of Mental Health, Public Health Service.

Wagstaff, D. A., Kelly, J. A., Perry, M. J., Sikkema, K. J., Solomon, L. J., Heckman, T. G., Anderson, E. S., Roffman, R. A., Cargill, V., Norman et al (1995). Multiple partners, risky partners, and HIV risk among low-income urban women. *Family Planning Perspectives, 27*(6), 241-245.

Weeks, M. R., Schensul, J. J., Williams, S. S., Singer, M., and Grier, M. (1995). AIDS prevention for African-American and Latina women: Building culturally and gender-appropriate intervention. *AIDS Education and Prevention, 7*(3), 251-263.

Weiss, E. and Gupta, G. R. (1993). Women facing the challenge of AIDS. In G. Young, V. Samarasinghe, and K. Kusterer (Eds.), *Women at the Center: Development Issues and Practices for the 1990s*, 168-181. West Hartford: Kumarian Press.

Wiest, R. E. (1983). Male migration machismo and conjugal roles: Implications for fertility control in a Mexican municipio. *Journal of Comparative Family Studies, 14*(2), 167-181.

World Health Organization. (1992). *The global AIDS strategy* (WHO AIDS Series 11). Geneva: World Health Organization.

Winkelstein, W., Samuel, M., Padian, N. S., Wiley, J. A., Lang, W., Anderson, R. E., and Levy, J. A. (1987). The San Francisco Men's Health Study: III. Reduction in Human Immunodeficiency Virus transmission among homosexual/bisexual men, 1982-1986. *American Journal of Public Health*, *76*, 685-689.

Worth, D. (1989). Sexual decision making and AIDS: Why condom promotion among vulnerable women is likely to fail. *Studies in Family Planning*, *20*(6), 297-307.

Wurzman, I. (1982-1983). Cultural values of Puerto Rican opiate addicts: An exploratory study. *American Journal of Drug and Alcohol Abuse*, *9*(2), 141-153.

Wyatt, G. E. (1994). The sociocultural relevance of sex research: Challenges for the 1990s and beyond. *American Psychologist*, *49*(8), 748-754.

Chapter 2

Understanding Safer Sex Negotiation in a Group of Low-Income African-American Women

Gina Ann Margillo
T. Todd Imahori

As we approach the third decade of the AIDS pandemic, women, especially African-American women, have become the largest and fastest growing infected group. The Centers for Disease Control's statistics (CDC National AIDS Clearinghouse, 1995) show that African-American women are 16 times more likely to get AIDS than Euro-American women and that over 54 percent of HIV-positive women in the United States are of African-American heritage. There are currently 35,372 African-American women with AIDS in the United States, in contrast to 15,570 Euro-American women and 13,293 Latina women. Bear in mind, these are reported cases, not actual cases (which is no doubt, a greater number). Thirty-four percent of these African-American women have been infected through heterosexual contact, making it the second most common mode of transmission (CDC National AIDS Clearinghouse, 1995). These statistics highlight the need for an investigation of the relationships and communication patterns of African-American women and their male partners, an area in which relatively few studies have concentrated.

The authors would like to express sincere appreciation for valuable suggestions and guidance provided by Dr. Edith Folb, Professor of Speech and Communication studies, San Francisco State University, and Carla Dillard Smith, the Research Directors at the California Prevention and Education Project on the original thesis study.

Of greatest concern is the identification of factors which affect safer sex communication between men and women and the examination of ways in which African-American women are successful in getting their partners to practice safer sex. Another mandate is to understand these issues within the context of the African-American community. The study discussed in this chapter examines sociocultural, relational, and individual factors that help or hinder the practice of safer sex, including the women's financial conditions, attitudes toward condoms, issues of trust and gender roles within relationships, and compliance-gaining strategies.

LITERATURE REVIEW

Safer sex practices of low-income, African-American women cannot be understood without first taking into consideration the cultural, social, and economic contexts of their everyday lives. Literature presented here will discuss factors that affect African-American women's safer sex practices and compliance-gaining strategies they may use in safer sex communication.

Factors Affecting Safer Sex Practices

Safer sex practices are part of overall sexual behaviors that are exercised in a relationship between sexual partners. Individual sexual behaviors are best understood as sexual scripts, and sexual scripts exist at three levels: cultural, interpersonal, and intrapsychic (Simon and Gagnon, 1973, 1987). Sexual behaviors and negotiations are influenced by sociocultural images of sexual behaviors at the cultural level, what is appropriate within in the cultural and relational context at the interpersonal level, and finally, the individual, personal perceptions of sexual behaviors at the intrapsychic level (Yep, 1995). African-American women's safer sex practices are thus best understood by considering the cultural/social, relational (interpersonal), and individual (intrapsychic) factors.

Today, the most significant social factors affecting African-American women's risk for contracting the disease are economic conditions (Kane, 1990) and racism (Weeks et al., 1995). The state of poverty found in some inner-city African-American communities is accompanied by stress, depression, low self-esteem, lack of medical insurance and/or access to health care facilities, and lack of social support; African-American women living in these communities are more vulnerable to the disease (Gilliam, Scott, and Troup, 1989). In addition, African-American women have been found to weigh other concerns for survival over their risk for contracting the HIV virus (Nyamathi et al., 1993). Researchers also cite the use of drugs as a societal factor contributing to the high-risk status of African-American women (Fullilove et al., 1990; Kane, 1990; Nyamathi et al., 1993). Forty percent of African-American women with AIDS were infected through the use of intravenous drugs (CDC National AIDS Clearinghouse, 1995).

Within this social context of poverty and addiction, African-American women, more than women of other ethnicities, are generally found to engage in high-risk sexual activities such as sex work, "survival sex," or the exchange of sex for drugs (Nyamathi et al., 1993). Thirty to 50 percent of female I.V.D.U.s (Intravenous drug users) have engaged in sex work as a means of supporting their drug habit (Shayne and Kaplan, 1991). Also, in a crack culture, there exists a "sex for drugs" bartering system differing from sex work (Fullilove, Lown, and Fullilove, 1992).

"Survival sex" is usually exchanged for goods such as payment of rent or grocery bills (Nyamathi et al., 1993) between a woman and an acquaintance or friend. It is distinguished from sex work by the nature of the relationship between a woman and her sexual partner. Whereas the relationship between a client and a sex worker is mostly less personal and more "business oriented," the relationship between a woman engaging in survival sex and her partner may include some level of intimacy or emotional involvement. Therefore, safer sex negotiations in survival sex may be more complex than those in sex work.

Relational factors affecting safer sex practices among impoverished African-American women consist of women's gender roles and the amount of power they have to make safe sex decisions (Fullilove et al., 1990; Peterson and Marin, 1988). Some literature argues that African-American women's roles have historically included power and authority (Middleton and Putney, 1960) and financial responsibility (Malson, 1983) in the family. In recent years, the impact of racism has resulted in poverty and addiction in African-American communities, which in turn, has led to a severe increase in the unemployment rate and a decrease in the number of available black men. This scarcity of men is tied to an increasing imbalance between the number of available, marriageable male partners (heterosexual, employed, not incarcerated) and the number of marriageable women (Sampson, 1987). These recent changes have altered women's roles, resulted in more economic independence (Fullilove et al., 1990), affected gendered power relations (Kane, 1990; Kline, Kline, and Oken, 1992), and estranged the women from African-American men (Fullilove et al., 1990). All of these arguments point to a greater self-sufficiency among African-American women and less dependence on relationships with men.

On the other hand, there is literature suggesting the opposite trend. According to Weeks et al. (1995), racism "directly reduces African-American men's economic power" (p. 254). Fullilove et al. (1990) argue that the men tend to react to this reduced power by increasing dominance over women. In addition, some literature suggests that African-American women's gender roles pressure them to uphold the male status and provide emotional support (Kavenaugh et al., 1992) at the expense of compromising the true scope of their power (Whatt and Rowe, 1990). In terms of safer sex negotiation specifically, Wingood, Hunter-Gamble, and DiClementi (1993) argue that African-American women's gender roles impede a woman's ability to negotiate safer sex, and Fullilove et al. (1990) found that "good girl/bad girl" roles influenced the use of condoms with main partners by inhibiting discussion of condoms for fear of seeming too aggressive and/or compromising female respectability. These studies suggest that gender roles and the power of African-American women become barriers to safer sex negotiations, whereas the other studies reviewed above paint images of African-American women who are self-sufficient and able to initiate and gain safer sex negotiations. In our study, we found evidence of both of these seemingly contradictory positions.

Finally, the individual factor of women's desire for childbearing further affects safer sex negotiation. According to Weeks et al. (1995), African-American women gain a sense of self-worth and social support when they bear children. In this light, safer sex may not be valued unless when the risk of contracting the HIV virus is weighted more heavily than the social value gained by the women through childbearing.

In summary, the previous literature seems to overwhelmingly suggest that there are many social, relational, and individual factors that hamper African-American women's safer sex negotiation despite an observed increase in women's power. Particularly significant factors included lack of African-American men, changing gendered power relations, emotional and intimacy dependence on the relationship, and childbearing issues.

Compliance-Gaining Strategies

The complexity of factors affecting African-American women's safer sex negotiations has been well documented. However, safer sex negotiations must also be understood in terms of specific strategies for gaining compliance from partners in condom use. Previous studies provide contradictory evidence regarding African-American women's safer sex negotiation strategies. On one hand, Kline, Kline, and Oken (1992) found that both Hispanic and African-American HIV-positive women were effective in sexual negotiations with men through their use of a variety of strategies such as applying condoms with or without men's compliance, withholding sex, manipulating through sexual arousal, and reasoning about the importance of HIV risks. Wingood et al. (1993), on the other hand, reported that most African-American women exhibited nonassertive styles in their safer sex negotiation.

These studies may not have been conclusive because they did not examine safer sex negotiation via a prior set of compliance-gaining strategies. Therefore, this study attempts to investigate types of compliance-gaining strategies used by the African-American women based on the prior typology devised by Howard, Blumstein, and Schwartz (1986). Their typology was tested for its cultural fit in a pilot study (See Method—later in this chapter).

The typology includes six types of compliance-gaining strategies: autocracy, bargaining, bullying, disengagement, manipulation, and supplication. Autocracy includes asserting authority, claiming greater knowledge, making self-centered statements, or flatly insisting. Bargaining involves use of reasoning or compromise. Bullying uses threats, insults, ultimatums, or violence. Disengagement relies on indirect methods such as sulking, making the other feel guilty, or removing oneself from the situation (i.e., flight). Manipulation utilizes flattery, seduction, hints, or any practice which is secretive. Finally, supplication includes pleading or acting ill or helpless.

Literature on both the factors affecting safer sex negotiations and compliance-gaining strategies provided contradictory or insufficient evidence. This study thus attempts to augment the literature by conducting a more in-depth exploration of the factors affecting safer sex practices of African-American women and the specific safer sex communication strategies they may use. To accomplish this purpose, we conducted a qualitative study of African-American women in the Bay Area of California, as outlined below.

METHOD

Our main purpose for this study was to obtain an in-depth understanding of our target population: African-American women between the ages of 15 and 30 who were economically impoverished and who used condoms inconsistently. These women were chosen because the literature suggests that they are disporportionately represented among HIV-infected women. In addition, we focused mainly on safer sex negotiation with main partners because studies show that the greatest HIV risk a woman faces is from having unprotected sex with her main partner, a man with whom she is having a steady relationship (Mays and Cochran, 1988).

We collected data with personal interviews. The reasons for this are threefold. First, the complex nature of our topic demanded close attention to each subject's life story, and personal interviews are well-suited to gathering such rich data the woman's own words. Second, the highly personal aspects of our study (e.g., drug use, sex work, and sexual practices) mandated a small sample size, as few women would agree to reveal sensitive information, and thus qualitative data obtained from interviews were better suited for our study. Finally, the primary investigator of this study established rapport and trust with the target population in the Bay Area through her prior work with the California Prevention and Education Project

(CAL-PEP), a nonprofit AIDS education organization solely for African-American communities. Her personal connection with the women enhanced our ability to obtain candid, rich data.

Interview Schedule

All personal interviews were conducted following a semistructured interview schedule.[1] The interview schedule was constructed based on the literature review and a pilot study.[2] The pilot study revealed information regarding factors associated with not practicing safer sex and types of compliance-gaining strategies used by the African-American women to convince partners to use condoms. The information obtained was then incorporated into the interview schedule. Also, these and additional pilot study findings[3] were useful in guiding the analysis of the interview transcripts.

Interview Sample

Between June 10 and July 30, 1994, 47 African-American women were approached in locations such as "ho strolls" (outdoor areas where sex workers solicit customers), laundromats, parks, residential areas, check cashing lines, nail salons, and grocery stores within a ten-block radius of a low-income housing project in the Bay Area of California. Of the 47 women approached, 32 agreed to answer prescreening questions.[4] Twenty-one subjects fit our sample criteria of economically disadvantaged, sexually active, African-American women between the ages of 15 and 30. This particular age group was chosen because the pilot study aimed at this age group and also because women in this age group are (on average) sexually active. Each woman was paid 15 dollars for her time.[5]

Age distribution included six women (29 percent) between 15 and 18, 11 (52 percent) in their twenties, and four (19 percent) at 30 years of age. Nineteen (84 percent) of the 21 women had primary relationships at the time of the interview; the remaining two had primary relationships within six months prior to the interview.

Sixteen (84 percent) of the 19 women who had current relationships had outside relationships as well. Men in these outside relationships were either sex-work clients or were men married to other women. Five (24 percent) of the 21 women were involved with men who were over ten years older than themselves. Three (14 percent) of the 21 women were involved with married men. These statistics may reflect the lack of available, unmarried, not incarcerated men in the community who are close to our subjects' ages.

In terms of marital status, nineteen women (90 percent) were never married, one was divorced, and one was separated. Twenty (95 percent) of the 21 women were single mothers.

In contrast to what the previous literature has suggested, drug use was not a main factor in our sample. Only seven (33 percent) were drug users; two used marijuana occasionally, and the other five used cocaine in powder or freebase form. However, our finding may be affected by underreporting of drug use by the women.

The women had various sources of income: AFDC (monthly checks from Aid to Families with Dependent Children), baby-sitting jobs, contributions from family, hair styling out of the home, selling cans, stealing and reselling clothes, selling sex, and prostituting other women. Four women's (19 percent) incomes came solely from sex work. Twelve women (57 percent) in our study did not label themselves as sex workers though they engaged in survival sex or sex for drugs or money.

FINDINGS

All personal interviews were tape recorded and then transcribed. Transcripts were then analyzed by the primary investigator (a Euro-American female) and an independent reader (a Latina) for emergent and repetitive themes regarding: (1) factors that affected the women's safer sex practices; and (2) compliance-gaining strategies used to convince their partners to use condoms. In order to ensure that the findings would reflect African-American perspectives, an African-American research team from CAL-PEP joined in the analysis.

Factors Affecting Women's Safer Sex Practices

All 21 women used condoms inconsistently, and both relational and nonrelational factors appeared to influence their safer sex practices. Relational factors were those that were directly or indirectly influenced by the nature of relationships the women had with their main men, such as abilities or willingness to communicate about safer sex, issues of trust and/or mistrust, and emotional independence/dependence. Nonrelational factors were those that were independent from their relationships, including financial need, low-risk perception, and alcohol use.

Relational Factors

The inability to negotiate safer sex practices was the most common reason why women did not practice safer sex within their relationships, with eight women (38 percent) reporting this factor. There appeared to be several reasons why women had problems negotiating for safer sex. Eight women reported difficulty finding effective verbal "comebacks" when their compliance-gaining attempts were met by partners who strongly disliked condoms and flatly refused to use them. Two women gave examples of how safer sex communication was often thwarted:

> What happened was neither one of us didn't have one. Cause when we started out I was like, "You got a condom?" He was like, "No." And then I was like, "Well we can't do it." He kept on trying, kept on trying until it just happened. I just finally gave it to him. (Woman #18)

> He told me no. I say, "Oh well, we ain't doin' it then." [He said] "Come on, come on." I was like, "Uh,uh." "Baby, just come on then." I say, "Nope." Then we finally did it anyway. (Woman #11)

The second reason for negotiation failures was related to issues of trust. Six women (29 percent) described situations in which they attempted to negotiate, but lost their resolve when their partners challenged their trust in them. Some women were concerned that suggesting condom use would make their partners think that they were unfaithful while others worried that their partners might think they were accusing their men of cheating as in these examples:

> He said I should have more faith in him. But I tell him, "Look at the females you have sex with," 'cause he used to sell drugs;

he used to be out there with those females who tradin' themselves for drugs. He said, "You need to have more faith in me."
It tears it (the relationship) up. 'Cause like I say, he has walked
out. And he cursed, "You crazy, I not using something." Then
he try to turn it around, "Oh you must be doin somethin'."
(Woman #2)

He be like, "You don't believe me. You don't trust me?" and
this and that. And I be like, "Yea, in a way I do, but then again,
I don't," Then he start hollerin'. That's why most of the time I
don't ask him. (Woman #21)

These findings support the literature's suggestion that some women
were more concerned about the maintenance of their relationships
than the practice of safer sex.

Whereas some women did not want to undermine trust in their
relationships, the majority of the women outwardly acknowledged
lack of trust in their men. Seventeen (80 percent) of the 20 women
who talked about main partners either knew or suspected that their
partners had other sex partners. This example illustrates how many
women directly acknowledged the nonmonogamy of their partners,
but tended to overlook and accept it:

I don't care what to do, just as long as I know he be there, ya
know, want to be with me. . . . Like I told you, he got a wife. I
don't trip on that. (Woman #8)
**Interviewer: Do you trust that he doesn't have any other
woman in his life?**
He probably do. I don't know.
Interviewer: Does it matter to you if he does?
No. As long as he uses condoms, I ain't tripping. (Woman
#11)

While the women were aware of their men having multiple sexual
partners, they themselves were just as polygamous. Thirteen (68 percent) of the 19 women with primary male partners either knew or
suspected that their partners were not monogamous, yet, that knowledge was not enough reason for a breakup. The fact that 16 (84
percent) of the 19 women asked the question (see Note 1, # 48)
reported having their own extrarelational affairs suggests that "cheat-

ing" (in their own words) cut both ways. The following examples seemed to be the norm among the 21 women interviewed:

> We been together for a while, ya know, but then he does probably cheated on me, ya know, cheated on me several times. But then I messed around, you know, once or twice probably on him. (Woman #3)
> **Interviewer: Do you trust that he's not going out with anyone else?**
> No, 'cause I know he ain't going to be stuck just to one girl. 'Cause I know I ain't goin to be stuck to just one boy. He tells me that I'm his woman and I tell him that I love him, that he's my main man, but I know that he ain't going to be faithful. I just know that. Ain't no boy going to be faithful. (Woman #21)

In general, women seemed to believe that men could not be monogamous. Women in this sample expressed belief that they had very little control over the faithfulness of their men. The women were also nonmonogamous. This situation seemed to be the norm.

Five (24 percent) of the 21 women reported not using condoms because they completely trusted that their primary male partners were monogamous or that their partners had not been exposed to the HIV virus. These were primarily women who had long-standing relationships with older men or women who had married partners whom the women knew would not have the time to be nonmonogamous. Some women who did not use condoms at the start of their relationships adopted safer sex behaviors after losing trust in their partners later on in the relationship.

Even though most of the women were not able to carry the negotiation process to a successful conclusion, they exhibited important forms of communication power. For example, nine (64 percent) of the 14 women asked (see Note 1, # 38) said that they have initiated and would continue to initiate new sexual practices with their men. All 21 women said they have initiated safer sex talk, and 11 (58 percent) of the 19 asked (see Note 1, # 37) said they have directly discussed their personal sexual satisfaction with their partners. Women in the sample demonstrated power by initiating communication, but safer sex was not practiced consistently. This could be in part because a woman may not use her communication power if she is afraid of breaching trust in the relationship, if she lacks the skills to do so, or if she does not think she is at risk.

The ability of the women in our sample to successfully negotiate safer sex may have been undermined by emotional vulnerability which created a dependence on the relationship. In this sample, evidence of emotional vulnerability appeared in many forms. For example, eight (38 percent) of the women described situations in which they remained with a partner long after realizing that the relationship was not fulfilling or healthy, as in this example:

> [We've been together] six years. I don't know why we stay together. He's alright. He acts like he don't trust me, but, huh, it's not me, I don't trust him. 'Cause he lies a lot. I catch him. . . . But I feel secure with him. We have two children together. (Woman #9)

Nine (43 percent) of the women's partners were the fathers of their children and this may lead to greater emotional ties despite dissatisfaction (i.e., these men often were polygamous, financially dependent on the women, or dependent on drugs). Women countered this lack of satisfaction by not living with their partners. Only two of the women lived with their primary male partners.

Twenty-four percent of the women's primary partners were married to other women. The women in this study did not seem to be concerned about sharing the men with other women, which may be a function of lack of available men in the community:

> He's the type of man I always looked for, even though he's got a family of his own. . . . I have nothin' to do with that. . . . I'd rather be with him because he makes me happy—we have fun together, we laugh together. All the rest of the mens I been with, I been through ups and downs with them. With him, I don't have to go through that. (Woman #16)

In this sample, women reported high rates of loneliness and depression. Twelve (57 percent) of the women reported lack of a support system, feelings of alienation, depression, and thoughts of suicide. Such emotional vulnerability could be related to decisions to remain in unsatisfying relationships.

> All the time I do [feel lonely]. I think about suicide and better ways, leaving. All the time I do. 'Cause it's hard livin' out here, struggling. It's hard to find a good paying job. (Woman #1)

> [I'm lonely and depressed] a whole lot. 'Cause like I said, eight kids is not easy. My older ones is giving me problems that I just can't deal with. . . . Don't nobody understand what I'm going through. (Woman #2)

The relationships of the women in this study with their male partners appeared to serve an emotional support function which countered their loneliness. This is seen in the following examples:

> He takes care of me and the kids . . . he's like a friend, you know. If he's not around, I'm lonely and stuff. (Woman #13)

> I communicate with him 'cause none other people I can talk to . . . he have to be there for me when I need him, he be there for me. Or my kids, he help me with my kids. (Woman #5)

Although findings show evidence of a woman's need for companionship, our data show that women had a sense of independence and a need and ability to provide for themselves without relying on a male. For example, 13 (68 percent) of the 19 women with primary male partners did not want to get married, remain married, or live in the same house as their partners. This example sums it up:

> I ain't never been married. It's like a common law marriage, but I ain't got married. . . . 'Cause I don't have time for that. 'Cause when I want to leave, I go. I don't got to worry about no divorce, and all that. Now like, I can just say, "Get out of my house; it's my house." (Woman #13)

Nonrelational Factors

Eight (38 percent) of the 21 women reported nonrelational factors which affected the safer sex communication process. Even though much current literature suggests financial dependence as a significant nonrelational factor contributing to the practice of unprotected sex by an African-American woman, financial dependency was not an important relational factor for this sample. All of the women reported having a little financial help from men, but their sexual practices were not influenced by this.

However, it did emerge as a nonrelational factor for some women who engaged in various forms of sex work. The response from a self-identified sex worker below shows how the reliance upon that income caused women to sometimes decide against condom usage:

> **Interviewer: Have you ever met any guy that would pay you more money not to use a condom?**
>
> A few, that I charge him, I say I need $180. And he was like, "I only got $50." And I was like, "I ain't goin' home with you." And he was like, "I got $10 more and I just gave this man a 20 and I'll go back and get it, and I'll give you $80, then I'll give you $100 tomorrow." And I was like, "Hell no, and you know you got to use a condom." And he was like, "Well I don't get excited with a condom. I don't ejaculate." I was like, "So?" He was like, "OK, I give you the whole $180 right now if you just . . ." I was like, "OK." (Woman #1)

Other than the financial reasons, women also compromised safer sex because they perceived "pleasure" over risk as in the following example:

> **Interviewer: What are the different things that keep you from practicing safe sex?**
>
> If I see a boy and I think he's sexy, and just, 'cause I don't poke nobody that don't have no money. If I fuck 'um, they have to be, like, havin' some cash or something. I be like, if you don't use a condom, then it's better. You feel the flow of juices, and then it's fun and I get paid. So if I like them, and like their body and stuff like that, and I know they have cash and are going to take care of me, then I won't use it. (Woman #1)

Two (24 percent) of the eight women who reported nonrelational reasons appeared to have other types of low-risk perceptions. Some women had unprotected sex because they did not have condoms on them, they did not push the safer sex issue upon their partners, or they got caught up in the moment, as seen here:

Yea, I was scared he had a disease or something like that. I was afraid, you know, I didn't feel safe. (But) I didn't have one at the time. (Woman #5)

He had been waiting. He was like, "Can I have some?" I said, "Yea, I'll give you some in a minute." I sat there, finished drinking my drink. And the next thing you know, he was all over me. And that's . . . we didn't get to use a condom. . . . Rush job. I was like, "You can't get one?" He was like, "No." So we did it anyway. (Woman #13)

In some cases, even when risk was perceived, it was not weighed as heavily as the need for intimacy.

I guess if everything is goin' all right, if I kind of like him, if the mood is right, and to me it's not like fucking or having sex, it is more than that. Then at the time—'cause there's times when it seems like more than that. It's nice, you know, how he's treatin' me—real soft—then I probably wouldn't wear one. (Woman # 12)

Like, what they say or what they do, or the way they talk to me, and it hasn't happened too many times, but when it has happened, I guess the way they treat me takes my mind off it and makes me forget about it (condoms) and, which I really shouldn't. But I don't think about it, and it happens. Then afterwards, I go, "Oh God, I got to make that appointment." . . . I get worried. (Woman #9)

For three women, heavy drinking clouded their judgment and prevented them from using condoms. An example of one response sums it up:

Interviewer: Think back to a time when you didn't use a condom with him. Why didn't you use one?

Because I was drunk, and he was also. I always slip when I start drinking. Alls the time. Always. . . . I'm going to stop drinking because like I say, I think the alcohol just drives me— my sex drive. So I'm going to stop drinking. (Woman #2)

Finally, it cannot be overlooked that two (24 percent) of the eight women, both with high levels of AIDS awareness, were careless in ways that seemed to mirror the reality of their lives:

> **Interviewer: In general, what would you say are the main reasons why you don't use condoms?**
>
> Self-destruction. Self-destruction. That's the only way I can really explain it, because I don't know. I don't really have nowhere. I don't have an outlet to vent my anger. I feel that I'm out here by myself, taking care of my son. And the daily life here, to me, is real, real hard. And you come upon a problem, you don't know how to handle it . . . and it's not like I can talk to someone else about it. . . . That's pretty frustrating. (Woman #12)

In summary, it appears that the practice of safer sex is most often thwarted by a woman's inability to fully negotiate safer sex practices. Women's negotiation processes were often complicated by the issue of undermined trust, a lack verbal comebacks, or the lack of alternative options to unprotected intercourse. Women said they would "just give up" eventually and have sex without a condom after engaging in drawn-out negotiations with their insistent partners. This finding suggests two possibilities. First, women are concerned with maintaining their relationships and/or experiencing intimacy over safer sex. Second, women lack the skills to successfully negotiate safer sex.

Compliance-Gaining Strategies

The above findings indicate that there is a need to understand how African-American women succeed in negotiating for safer sex. Therefore, this section will examine only those compliance-gaining strategies that lead to *successful* negotiations. As the literature review suggested, African-American women were expected to use some of the six strategies defined earlier (Howard, Blumstein, and Schwartz, 1986).

The most widely used compliance gaining strategy was bargaining with 15 (71 percent) of the women reporting use of this strategy.

Although this strategy is characterized by reasoning, offering a trade-off, and/or compromising, most of the women employed reasoning as their method of choice and none used compromise. In this example, the woman used the bargaining/reasoning strategy with her partner by providing a reason for her condom request:

> I asked him, I said, "Are you going to use a rubber?" He said, "No, why should I?" I said, "For both of us." He said he didn't need a rubber and wasn't going to use one. [I said] "Get bent, go on, bye. You don't have to have something to use it, it's just to protect yourself." (Woman #7)

The method of bullying was the second most widely used with 14 (66 percent) of the women employing this strategy, as in the following example where threats were used toward the end:

> He would not use a condom. I would ask him to. Later on in the second year [when] I found out he was messin' around, a couple of times I made him. He would say, "No, I don't like it," and I really didn't push the issue. But then later on, I pushed the issue and said, "If you don't, you ain't gettin' none." And then he would use it. (Woman #19)

The autocratic method, used by 13 (62 percent) of the women, was the third most widely used. This method is exemplified in the following self-centered statement of "I don't want no more kids":

> He didn't used to like them. But I told him, I said, "We got to use them cause there ain't no tellin' what you did in the past, or who you had sex with. Ain't no tellin' what I did and who I had sex with. So we just got to be more careful. I love you, you love me. And I don't want no more kids. (Woman #13)

Three (14 percent) of the women used the strategy of manipulation to get their men to wear condoms.

> Putting them in your mouth, hiding them. I been a hooker for 11 years, I'm good at that, very good at that. They wouldn't even know it. It would be too late. (Woman #16).

Only two (10 percent) women employed the strategy of disengagement. In both cases, the women walked out of the room when the men did not want to use condoms. One women unsuccessfully used the supplication strategy by begging her boyfriend to use a condom.

Overwhelmingly, women employed compliance-gaining strategies of bargaining/reasoning, bullying, and autocracy in their attempts to convince their partners to practice safer sex. These strategies, as exemplified in the actual accounts recalled by the African-American women in this study, reflect their resourcefulness and independence when they were successful at negotiating for safer sex.

DISCUSSION

In our attempt to augment the previous literature, we believe that our in-depth qualitative approach with inclusion of the African-American perspectives and local community knowledge helps provide new findings. Before we interpret these findings below, it is imperative to first acknowledge some of the limitations of our study.

First, it is important to remember that this study was based on a small sample taken from a particular geographic area and focused on certain types of African-American women. In different economic, geographical, and social conditions, African-American women may face completely different issues; thus, their safer sex negotiations may be quite different those reported here. Second, this study did not examine the perspectives of the African-American males. Considering that negotiation, sex, power, and other significant issues affecting safer sex are relational, future studies are encouraged to incorporate both partners' perspectives. Finally, even though the study included African-American females in its analysis phase, absence of an African-American female in the authorship of this chapter may hinder it from being Afrocentric. Future research studies, particularly those by African Americans, are encouraged to rely on larger numbers of interviews that will allow both quantitative and qualitative analyses of African-American women's safer sex negotiations.

Interpretations of Findings

Our findings challenge past assumptions about the status, role, and risk factors of African-American women and appear to indicate a shift in African-American women's behaviors. The most prevalent emerging attitude was that men could not be counted on or trusted, which in turn may be leading to the women's self-sufficiency (e.g., having multiple partners to satisfy emotional needs and earning from multiple financial resources) as the norm in this particular sample.

As suggested by Kane (1990) and Kline, Kline, and Oken (1992), the traumas of poverty, addiction, and loneliness have pushed women out of prescribed roles such as worrying about "good girl" or "bad girl" images or holding back communication about safer sex and/or sexual satisfaction, and this has had an enormous impact on their behavior. Contrary to findings by Fullilove et al. (1990), our study did not find the double standard of behavior which allowed men to be polygamous and required good girls to passively accept this. Instead, having multiple sexual partners, which was once considered a "bad girl" behavior, was the accepted practice in this sample of women. By seeking other relationships for satisfaction, women attempted to compensate for their inability to find emotional, financial, and/or relational stabilities in their primary relationships with their main men. Women in our sample tended to compensate by dating men who were much older than they were or to have extended relationships with married men.

In terms of relational factors, intimacy and trust appeared to be the strongest factors accounting for the inconsistent safer sex practices by the women. The majority of safer sex negotiations examined in our study were initiated and then blocked by a woman's fear of undermining trust, or a lack of effective verbal comebacks after facing resistance from her partner. In some cases, condoms were rejected because they were viewed as barriers to intimacy and closeness.

Nonrelational reasons for lack of condom usage appeared to be primarily a function of HIV risk not being weighed as heavily as other factors. In addition, women expressed feelings of disillusionment, frustration, isolation and lack of support. Their sense of fatalism and/or resignation about their lives often prevented them from internalizing the importance of consistent condom use.

Finally, when the African-American women were successful in gaining compliance for condom use from their men, they mostly used the compliance-gaining strategies of bargaining, bullying, and autocratic methods. These strategies reflect a departure from the traditional "good girl/bad girl" fear of being viewed as sexually experienced or too demanding (Fullilove et al., 1990). Furthermore, many women used multiple compliance-gaining strategies in their successful safer sex negotiations.

Our finding poses a contradictory picture of safer sex negotiation dynamics between African-American women and their men. On one hand, we found that their overall emotional vulnerability, lack of available men, and desire for intimacy influenced them to compromise safer sex. In terms of communication behaviors, however, we found that the African-American women in our sample were able to use successful compliance-gaining strategies. This leads to the most significant finding in our study: African-American women were able to achieve safer sex negotiation sporadically but not consistently.

This finding implies that there is a need to investigate safer sex negotiation both at episodic level, i.e., a particular safer sex negotiation in a given safer sex communication situation, and at the relational and societal levels, i.e., the overall safer sex negotiation dynamics between the women and men. Weeks et al. (1995) explain the pressure of successfully negotiating for safer sex at each episode or encounter for a consistent use of condoms:

> For a woman to insist on condoms with a reluctant male partner requires discussion *at each sexual encounter*, often demanding that a woman have influence over a man in a setting that is highly emotionally charged and fraught with social meaning. Women may have few resources at their disposal to enforce an activity that many men perceive as limiting their sexual pleasure and possibly even their sexual abilities. Condoms themselves have implicit meaning, such as mistrust, infidelity, lack of intimacy . . . and, particularly in this context, accusation of the partner as diseased. (p. 253; an emphasis added)

To understand this dynamic of safer sex negotiations at a communication episode level and relational level, it is critical to consider the cultural, relational (interpersonal), and individual (intrapsyhic) levels of sexual scripts (Simon and Gagnon, 1987; Yep, 1995). In addition to sexual scripts, power relations must be considered within a context of relationship because power is a relational construct (Thibaut and Kelly, 1959). Thibaut and Kelly posit that a person who finds more resources in the relationship holds less power, as s/he is dependent on the relational resources. Specifically in romantic relationships, what Waller and Hill (1951) called the "Principle of Least Interest" applies: the partner who is less interested in the relationship holds more power. Conversely, Blau (1964) suggests that one way to gain power in a relationship is to facilitate one's social independence from the relationship through finding an alternative resource.

In this regard, the cultural sexual script that exists in the African-American community we studied suggests that the relatively greater levels of power are held by men who, by virtue of decreasing number, have more alternatives in sexual relationships. This was indeed reflected in our sample where most of the African-American women in our study were aware that their main men were involved in multiple relationships. Therefore, even though the women may be successful at negotiating for safer sex at times, the extent to which they desire the relationship does not allow them enough power to successfully negotiate safer sex on a consistent basis. Perhaps, the African-American women in our study sought alternative resources for intimacy, trust, and financial support through asserting their own power and independence. In order to confirm our speculation, it is necessary to examine African-American men and their perceptions of intimacy, emotional dependence, and availability of female partners.

Our findings also suggested that women lack the communication ability to use effective verbal comebacks in response to males who wish to have sex without condoms. Even though effective verbal comebacks may be useful in attaining compliance for condom use, comebacks will only lead to an episodic level success. Supporting this observation are our findings that the African-American women in our study had the communication power to bring up safer sex talk or discussions about sexual satisfaction but were unable to maintain safer sex practice. This suggests that research must account for the relational and cultural level factors that affect the overall safer sex negotiation dynamics as well as the communication and relational factors.

In applying our findings into the context of AIDS education, we thus find that AIDS prevention programs that rely on negotiation tactics alone may not be sufficient since they ignore the multitude of social, relational, and individual factors at play in any given safer sex communication encounter. Instead, an AIDS education program needs to consider the following two factors: (1) gender roles and power of African-American women directly affect the overall relational level dynamic for safer sex negotiations, which in turn, influence the episodic level negotiations at each sexual talk opportunity; and (2) condoms are perceived as a barrier to intimacy and trust between the African-American women and their men in this study, and these factors are often perceived as more important than are risks of contracting HIV. Therefore, the programs must not only educate both women and men of the risks but also facilitate the relational processes in which intimacy and trust can be established between them. In other words, safer sex negotiation cannot be taught without considering its larger context, relational negotiations, i.e., negotiating for more monogamous, satisfying, trustworthy relationships.

EPILOGUE

The study reported here shed light on the complex societal conditions in an African-American women's community where day-to-day survival is a main priority. In that community, one thing consistently affected the women's safer sex negotiation: The desire for a relationship. Contrary to the literature, it was not the financial desperation or gender roles. Instead, the women in our study emphasized relationships with their primary men and the social conditions which made it difficult to find marriageable, faithful men with whom they could develop a sense of intimacy, trust, and even self-worth. On one hand, in fear of losing the relationships they had, the women compromised safer sex practices with their primary men; on the other hand, they behaved independently, were economically self-sufficient, and were nonmonogamous. Perhaps, the following song by TLC captures their life stories most eloquently:

> I look him in his eyes but all he
> Tells me is lies to keep me near
> I'll never leave him down though
> I might mess around it's only
> 'Cause I need some affection oh
> (Austin, 1994).

As researchers and practitioners, we need to always remember to respect and account for the nature of women's lives when we design prevention programs or study safer sex practices.

NOTES

1. This was a semistructured interview because not all questions listed below were asked to all the subjects. Depending on the interviewed woman's situation, willingness to respond, and time constraints, the interviewer (the primary investigator) asked different sets of questions.

I. DEMOGRAPHIC INFORMATION

1. What is your name?
2. Your age?
3. Do you have any children?
4. What are all the ways you make money?
5. Drug use?
6. How many friends do you have that you feel close to? How many family members?
7. Do you ever feel lonely?

II. RELATIONSHIP WITH MAIN PARTNER

8. Are you in love?
9. How long have you and your main partner been together?
10. How would you describe your relationship?
11. Are you happy in your relationship? Why or why not?
12. How would your life be different if he was not in it?
13. Do you feel secure in the relationship?
14. Have you ever been physically abused by your partner?
15. If you could change anything about your partner/relationship, what would you change?

III. TRUST

16. How important is trust to you in your relationship?
17. Do you have trust in him that he will be there for you when you need him?
18. Do you have trust in him that he doesn't have other women in his life?

IV. ROLES

19. What part does he play in the relationship?
20. What part do you play in the relationship?
21. What does it mean to be a good woman to your man?
22. What does it mean to be a good man to your woman? Is he a good man to you?

V. INDEPENDENCE/DEPENDENCE

23. Do you depend on each other? How?
24. What does he do for you? What are his responsibilities to you?
25. What do you do for him?
26. What are your responsibilities to him?
27. Does he work? Do you work?
28. Who pays your bills?
29. What are some of the things he does for you that you couldn't do for yourself?

VI. COMMUNICATION POWER/SEX ROLES

30. Do you talk about feelings to each other?
31. Does he have a bad temper?
32. Do you argue with each other?
33. Have you ever been afraid of him?
34. Who initiates sex?
35. Do you tell him what you like in bed?
36. Do you talk about sex? Safe Sex?
37. If he didn't please you sexually would you feel comfortable telling him?
38. If you wanted to try something new like a new position or a sex toy, would you feel comfortable telling him? Showing it to him?
39. How do you feel about condoms?
40. Who buys the condoms?

VII. SAFE SEX NEGOTIATION AND COMPLIANCE-GAINING STRATEGIES WITH MAIN PARTNERS

41. What stops you from having safe sex with your main partner?
42. How would he feel if (what would he do) if you told him you wanted to use a condom?
43. If you suggested he use condoms, would he think you did not trust him?

44. How important is his reaction to you when your thinking about using condoms?
45. Have you ever had sex without a condom when you really wanted him to use one? Can you describe the situation?
46. Have you ever tried to get him to use a condom? What did you say to persuade him?
47. Have you ever decided not to use a condom as a way of doing something nice for your man?

VIII. RELATIONSHIPS WITH OTHER PARTNERS

48. Do you have any sex partners other than your main man?
49. How often do you use condoms with your other partners? Would you say never, sometimes, most of the time, or all the time?
50. Who usually buys the condoms?
51. Are these other partners sometimes people you know? Are they sometimes strangers?
52. What prevents you from practicing safe sex with your other partners?
53. Have you ever had sex with someone other than your main partner without a condom when you really wanted to use one? Describe the situation.
54. Do you talk to your other partner(s) about safe sex?

IX. SAFE SEX NEGOTIATION/COMPLIANCE-GAINING STRATEGIES WITH OTHER PARTNERS

55. How do you react if they do not want to use condoms? What strategies do you use to get them to·wear a condom (practice safe sex)?
56. Describe what happened the last time a guy did not want to practice safe sex? What did you say?

2. The primary investigator conducted the pilot study in 1992 and 1993 in conjunction with the CAL-PEP. Focus group interviews were conducted with 45 African-American women between ages 15 and 30 in the Bay Area.

3. Some of the additional pilot study findings that guided our analysis were: the women's definition of a "main man"; their general feelings about using condoms; the levels and types of resistance from their partners about using condoms; stories about survival sex and prostitution; and their levels of independence or dependence in their relationships with main partners. For a detailed report, see Margillo (1995).

4. Prescreening Questions

1. How old are you? (15–30)
2. When is your birthday? (born between 1964–1979).
3. Do you have a main or steady male sex partner?
4. Where do you live?
5. Have you ever used condoms with your partner?
6. Would you say you use them sometimes, all the time, most of the time, or never?

7. Do you go out (have sex) with others guys besides your main partner?

5. Women in the area expected monetary reward for participating in the study, as it is an usual procedure for them to be paid by participating in other studies conducted in the area by the CAL-PEP and the Center for Disease Control.

REFERENCES

Austin, D. (1994). *Creep*. EMI Apple Music Inc., Darp Music (ASCAP).

Blau, P. M. (1964). *Exchange and Power in Social Life*. New York: John Wiley.

CDC National AIDS Clearinghouse. (1995). Female..AIDS cases by exposure..race, HIV/AIDS surveillance tables 6/95. *NAC FAX* Document #005.

Fullilove, M. T., Fullilove, R., Haynes, K., and Gross, S. (1990). Black women and AIDS prevention: A view towards understanding the gender roles. *The Journal of Sex Research*, *27*, 47-64.

Fullilove, M. T., Lown, A., and Fullilove, R. E. (1992). Crack hos and skeezers: Traumatic experiences of women crack users. *The Journal of Sex Research*, *29*, 275-287.

Gagnon, J. H. and Simon, W. (1973). *Sexual Conduct: The Social Sources of Human Sexuality*. Chicago: Aldine.

Gilliam, A., Scott, M., and Troup, J. (1989). AIDS education and risk reduction for homeless women and children: Implications for health education. *Health Education*, *20*, 44-47.

Howard, J., Blumstein, P., and Swartz, P. (1986). Sex, power, and influence tactics in intimate relationships. *Journal of Personality and Social Psychology*, *51*, 102-109.

Kane, S. (1990). AIDS, addiction, and condom use: Sources of sexual risk for heterosexual women. *The Journal of Sex Research*, *27*, 427-444.

Kavenaugh, K. H., Harris, R., Hetherington, S. E., and Scott, D. (1992). Collaboration as a strategy for Acquired Immunodeficiency Syndrome prevention. *Archives of Psychiatric Nursing*, *6*, 331-339.

Kline, A., Kline, E., and Oken, E. (1992). Minority women and sexual choice in the age of AIDS. *Social Science Medicine*, *34*, 447-457.

Malson, M. R. (1983). Black women's sex roles: The social context for a new ideology. *Journal of Social Issues*, *39*, 103-113.

Mays, V. M. and Cochran, S. D. (1988). Issues in the perception of AIDS risk and risk reduction activities by Black and Hispanic/Latina women. *American Psychology*, *43*, 949-956.

Middleton, R. and Putney, S. (1960). Dominance in decisions in the family: Race and class differences. In C. V. Willie (Ed.), *The Family Life of Black People*, 16-22. Columbus, OH: Charles E. Merrill.

Nyamathi, A., Bennett, C., Leake, B., Lewis, C., and Flaskerud, J. (1993). AIDS related knowledge, perceptions, and behaviors among impoverished minority women. *American Journal of Public Health*, *83*, 65-71.

Peterson, J. L. and Marin, G. (1988). Issues in the prevention of AIDS among black and Hispanic men. *American Psychologist, 43*, 871-877.

Sampson, R. J. (1987). Urban black violence: The effect of male joblessness and family disruption. *American Journal of Sociology, 93*, 348-382.

Shayne, V. T. and Kaplan, B. J. (1991). Double victims: Poor women and AIDS. *Women and Health, 17*, 21-34.

Simon, W. and Gagnon, J. H. (1987). A sexual scripts approach. In J. H. Geer and W. T. O'Donohue (Eds.), *Theories of Human Sexuality.* New York: Plenum.

Thibaut, J. W. and Kelley, H. H. (1959). *The Social Psychology of Groups.* New York: John Wiley.

Waller, W. and Hill, R. (1951). *The Family: A Dynamic Interpretation.* New York: Dryden.

Weeks, M. R., Schensul, J. J., Williams, S. S., Singer, M., and Grier, M. (1995). AIDS prevention for African-American and Latina women: Building culturally and gender-appropriate intervention. *AIDS Education and Prevention, 7*, 251-263.

Whatt E. and Rowe, S. (1990). African-American women's sexual satisfaction as a dimension of their sex roles. *Sex Roles, 22*, 509-525.

Wingood, G. M., Hunter-Gamble, D., and DiClementi, R. J. (1993). A pilot study of sexual communication and negotiation among young African-American women: Implications for HIV prevention. *Journal of Black Psychology, 19*, 193-203.

Yep, G. A. (1995). Healthy desires/unhealthy practices: Interpersonal influence strategies for the prevention of HIV/AIDS among Hispanics. In L. K. Fuller and L. M. Shilling (Eds.), *Communicating About Communicable Diseases,* 139-154. Amherst, MA: HRD Press.

Chapter 3

HIV-Related Communication and Power in Women Injecting Drug Users

Deborah L. Brimlow
Michael W. Ross

The issue of injecting drug use, women, and HIV disease cannot be broached without identifying the central role of communication and power. Mann, Tarantola, and Netter (1992) have argued that until women have a status equal to that of men, prevention of HIV transmission to and from women will be hampered. In contexts where women do not have the power to request safe sexual intercourse or drug use, information, education, and motivation to remain safe will be of minimal use and indeed, attempts to ensure safer sex or drug use may put the woman at significantly increased risk of violence or rejection. This is particularly the case with injecting drug use. Women who are at risk of HIV transmission do not just include those women who inject drugs, but to a larger extent, those who are sexual partners of injecting drug users (IDUs).

Ross et al. (1993) carried out a study of the sexual partners of IDUs, and from a sample of over 1,200 in Australia, ascertained the details of the sexual partner for the last and second-last sexual encounter. For IDU women, the sexual partner was, in 75 percent of the cases, an IDU male. The corresponding figure for IDU men was 59 percent, with these proportions being stable between last and second-last sexual contact. These data suggest that while it is likely for IDU women to have an IDU male sexual partner, the converse of IDU men having an IDU woman partner was less likely, with

Correspondence should be addressed to Dr. Brimlow.

about half of IDU men having a non-IDU female partner. However, the ratio of male to female injectors may have some bearing on this. In most developed country sites such as New York City, Des Jarlais et al. (1992) found that the ratio was 2:1, although where there is less equality between the sexes, such as in Bangkok, the ratio is 19:1. In such a situation, the probability of the female partner of a male IDU being a noninjector is significantly higher.

Epidemiologically, the possibility of such partners acting as a bridge for transmission to the noninjecting heterosexual population is high. However, the central point to note is that women are more likely to be at risk due to the injecting behavior of their male partners than by reason of their own injecting behavior.

There is a relationship between noninjected drug use and risk as well, usually in the interaction between drug use and sexual behavior. When individuals are intoxicated during sex, they are significantly less likely to have safe or safer sex. Ross et al. (1994), in a study of injecting drug users, found that half of their subjects were intoxicated during sex, and that heroin, marijuana, and alcohol were the most common drugs on which there was intoxication during sex (of which only heroin was injected). Thus, drug use is likely to put people at sexual risk, even when those drugs are not injected. Avoidance of sexual risk, however, has no necessary implication for avoidance of risk from drug injecting, as Wodak et al. (1994) report: they found no significant relationship between sexual risk behaviors in IDUs and injecting risk behaviors. Friedman et al. (1993) note, however, that injecting behavior is easier to change than sexual behavior.

Risk perception is not related to actual risk: Crisp et al. (1993) found that there was no relationship between gender and risk perception, and that risk perception was not based on injecting or sexual behaviors, previous sexually transmissible disease (STD) history, age, or number of previous HIV tests. Kelaher and Ross (1992) did, however, find that personal perception of risk was related to estimates of the baseline rate of infection in the population (although they also note that those in the highest risk group based on their reported behaviors were most likely to underestimate their level of risk). These latter data suggest that denial may be one defense mechanism operating to reduce perception of risk. Denial is most likely to be used as a form of internal communication where there is limited chance of changing the behavior which places the individual at risk.

The implications of these data are that the central issue in the avoidance of risk is communication of the probability of risk. Even where that probability is salient, power differentials may make any alteration to the risk situation difficult or impossible. In this chapter, we explore the communication and power issues in the negotiation of safe and safer sex and injecting practices among women intravenous drug users.

Comparison of the actual risk of men and women intravenous drug users illustrates the magnitude of the gender differential and the central role of communication. Dwyer et al. (1994) compared HIV risks between men and women and confirm earlier findings that women who inject drugs are more at risk than men of HIV infection. Women were more likely to have shared needles and syringes (especially with sex partners) and to have shared injecting equipment with someone they later found out to be infected with HIV. They were also twice as likely to report that they had shared injection equipment because they could not use needles and syringes on their own and injected more frequently with others present. Sharing with lovers was the primary reason given by women for sharing equipment, and these findings are consistent with the suggestion that sharing with lovers may be a way of communicating trust and intimacy. Dependency of women (such as needing to rely on males to inject them) could also be a significant constraint on ability to negotiate safer injecting practices. Of further interest was the finding that the women started to inject at a significantly younger age than males, and thus are less likely to have the social and assertiveness skills necessary to enable them to negotiate safer injecting. If the male is the main drugwinner, then he is likely to go first and in situations where sterile equipment is not available, the risk increases as the person is lower on the injecting chain.

Dwyer et al. (1994) also found that sexual behaviors in IDU women differed, with less condom use reported by women (particularly with casual partners as compared with commercial partners when respondents were commercial sex workers). This compounds the higher risk associated with vaginal sex to the female partner (Shayne and Kaplan, 1991). The data of Ross, Wodak, and Gold

(1992) which show that woman IDUs who are commercial sex
workers are significantly more likely to use condoms with commercial partners compared with noncommercial and regular partners
are similar to the data of Shayne and Kaplan insofar as this difference is consistent. This pattern of condom use may be a strategy for
discriminating between men one loves and men with whom one is
just doing business. It might also be argued that some women in
commercial sex work (particularly those in more control of their
environment or those who are better organized) might have more
power to insist on condom use in a commercial relationship
compared with a personal relationship, although this is speculative. It
would be a mistake, however, to see this simply as a communications
issue in the narrow sense.

Richardson (1989) points out that it is not just a lack of social
skills or assertiveness which could put womens' lives at risk. Variations in levels of power and autonomy in the negotiation of sexual
and drug-taking behaviors also contributes to unsafe behavior among
women IDUs, and may be exacerbated by the generally more salient
role and power differences between men and women in some lower
socioeconomic contexts. Many women at risk of HIV infection lack
the economic and social power to protect themselves and colleagues
from infection. Drug use, Dwyer and colleagues note, leads to a
narrowing of employment and educational opportunities and the
effects of this are often more severe for women who already face
reduced access to employment and education in society. Women may
also have to resort to prostitution for survival or drugs, thus adding to
the number of interactions which may increase risk of HIV infection.

Further, Dwyer et al. (1994) note that women are far less likely to
use inpatient drug rehabilitation—one of the barriers to therapeutic
communities for women is that very few accept children, and thus
there are fewer services accessible, which in turn increases the risk
of women remaining IDUs. Removal from risk environments is
thus probably more difficult for women than men.

COMMUNICATION SKILL

In the health psychology literature, communication skill has been
studied in a number of settings. Gibson, Catania, and Peterson

(1991) discuss communication skill and its importance in settings where others are involved in behaviors affecting personal health. The ability to engage others in discussion of the behaviors in question may be critical. In the area of sexual behavior, several studies have linked communication with success in changing behavior such as introduction of condom use into a sexual relationship (Schinke, Gilchrist, and Small, 1979; Polit-O'Hara and Kahn, 1985). Currently, the literature reflects the attempts by researchers to teach women how to "negotiate" safer sex or condom use because as Wermuth, Ham, and Robbins (1991) entitled their article, "Women Don't Wear Condoms."

The release of the female condom has altered some of this discussion. Acceptability studies in the literature suggest that the female condom may be accepted among a number of women in the United States, Latin America, Africa, and Europe (Bounds, Guillebaud, and Newman, 1992; Hernandez-Avila, 1992; Colimoro, 1993; Ford and Mathie, 1993; Liskin, 1993; Bassett et al., 1993). There are no studies specific to drug using women or the sexual partners of drug using men. When condom use is discussed here, only male condoms are being considered.

Looking at studies of condom use among injection drug users, Magura et al. (1990) reported that condom use was associated with greater personal acceptance of condoms and greater partner receptivity to sexual protection. In Choi, Wermuth, and Sorensen (1990), discussion of condom use and the man's positive condom attitudes were shown as predictors of condom use of male IDUs with women sexual partners. For many women, it is problematic to discuss sexual matters with male partners; when condom use is initiated by women, it has the potential to cause distrust, termination of the relationship, and violence (Mays and Cochran 1988; Worth, 1989; Wermuth, Ham, and Robbins, 1991).

The subject of teaching women to negotiate condom use with male partners is difficult. Drug-using women and the sexual partners of IDUs may differ from other women in some crucial ways which influence education programs. For example, the discussion of sexual and physical violence against women has received scant attention in the HIV/AIDS literature until recently. For women who have a history of abuse, there are issues around boundaries, sexuality, and power that strongly influence such loaded issues as introducing condoms into the relationship. Weissman and Brown (1995) report on several studies that are addressing the issues of violence and abuse in the lives of drug-using women. Initial data from the National Institute of Drug Abuse (NIDA) funded Non-traditional Supports for Drug Using Women project show that a significant percentage of the women report that they have been sexually or physically abused. Childhood, adolescent, and adult sexual and/or physical abuse is reported; the authors suggest that the reports are probably underestimated.

Weissman and Brown (1995) also report preliminary results from the NIDA-funded Women Helping to Empower and Enhance Lives (WHEEL) project. Looking at almost 2,800 female sex partners of IDUs (many of whom are non-IDUs), the data shows that more than a third of the women report childhood sexual abuse, more than a third report teenage sexual abuse, almost half report adult physical violence, and almost a third report forced sex by a main partner. For many drug using women and women who are sexual partners of drug users, violence and abuse are often ongoing. Introducing condoms into an abusive relationship may pose a more immediate threat to these women than the risk of becoming HIV infected. Weissman and Brown (1995) bluntly advise that telling women who are currently in abusive relationships that they should learn how to "negotiate" with their partners is neither sensitive nor relevant advice. In Perez, Kennedy, and Fullilove (1995), the authors discuss their psychoeducational intervention aimed at women in recovery from substance abuse. For women who have been victims of child-hood sexual abuse, this traumatic past may shape the woman's style in choice of safe partners, adoption of safe sexual behaviors, and recognition and treatment of sexually transmitted diseases (STDs). The authors' intervention is centered around a curriculum designed to improve the women's assessment of their need to use condoms and other types of barrier protection. Their work addresses a number of ways that trauma and past sexual abuse are important for HIV prevention and treatment.

Often, it seems that communication in the HIV/AIDS risk-reduction literature is viewed as one way. Health care providers and researchers speak as if information is given to the patient or subject with no feedback loop. More interactive communication patterns can be created with different approaches. One suggested strategy is the adoption of "harm reduction" based approaches to changing both sexual behavior and drug use. Originally, the Harm Reduction Model was developed in Mersey, England in the mid 1980s for use in HIV/AIDS prevention efforts with drug users (Newcombe and Parry, 1988). The basic philosophy is to reduce the harm that HIV/AIDS and drug use can bring to the individual and to the public health.

Springer (1991) provides an excellent discussion of the Harm Reduction Model. The harm reduction approach is centered around nonjudgmental, user friendly services, and meeting clients' needs. Basically, it offers a new way of communicating and working with drug users. A nonjudgmental stance on the part of providers is critical to the success of this approach. Abstinence from drug use is not the goal at the top of the hierarchy. Instead, the approach is to work with the client to determine ways to make drug use safer, whether that is teaching someone how to inject safely, how to reduce needle sharing, how to use bleach to clean needles and syringes, or how to use the drug in a safer way (e.g., smoking versus injecting).

Harm reduction is not just restricted to drug users; it can be adapted to different groups, especially some who have been viewed as being hard to reach. Cohen and Alexander (1995) discuss the ways that prostitutes and other sex workers in Western, industrialized countries, began to adopt a harm-reduction approach to their work. Elimination of prostitution was not the goal, but efforts were made to reduce the harm that HIV/AIDS brought to the work. For example, sex workers looked at the need to change their practices, whether this was to insist on condom use or other barriers in the workplace. The authors caution that rapid change must not be expected. For female sex workers, it often takes approximately a year before they completely shift to safer sex practices, including condom use and lower-risk practices. These women also experience problems in getting regular clients as well as lovers/spouses to use condoms.

In addition to the harm reduction approach to communicating and working with drug-using women and the sexual partners of

IDUs, it is important to involve the women themselves in designing and carrying out programs. Promoting peer education programs is one way to actively engage women in HIV/AIDS prevention efforts. This approach can also be used to provide more skills than just condom negotiation for vulnerable women.

How we communicate and what we communicate as researchers, educators, and clinicians to drug-using women and sexual partners of IDUs is critical to the success of HIV/AIDS prevention efforts. The literature has painted a picture of these women as vulnerable to economic and social power imbalances. Often, they lead lives filled with violence and abuse. Daily struggles with shelter, food, drugs, children, and partners leave them with little energy to cope with the possibility of contracting HIV. For women who are already HIV positive, the situation is complicated by their roles as caretakers for HIV-infected partners and children. Programs that dictate a rigid, unrealistic approach to emotionally charged issues such as sexual behavior and drug use are doomed to fail. If not, they may provoke negative reactions ranging from abandonment to violence. It is critical that programs be designed that take into account the context of women's lives. A twofold approach is suggested: (1) the adoption of a harm reduction approach acts to open up the communication between provider and client; and (2) a more general approach to improving the communication skills of women rather than simply teaching condom negotiation is recommended. With some adaptation, health care providers and researchers can develop an approach that works for both sexual and drug-using behaviors in IDUs.

REFERENCES

Bassett, M., Ray, C.S., Nicolette, J., and Managazna, P. (1993). Acceptability of the female condom among CSWs. Eighth International Conference on AIDS in Africa (abstract TOP29), Marrakesh, Morocco.

Bounds, W., Guillebaud, J., and Newman, G.B. (1992). Female condom (Femidom): A clinical study of its use-effectiveness and patient acceptability. *British Journal of Family Planning*, *18*, 36-41.

Choi, K.H., Wermuth, L.A., and Sorensen, J.L. (1990). Predictors of condom use among women sexual partners of intravenous drug users. Poster presented at the Sixth International Conference on AIDS, San Francisco.

Cohen, J.B. and Alexander, P. (1995). Female sex workers: Scapegoats in the AIDS epidemic. In A. O'Leary and L.S. Jemmott (Eds.), *Women at Risk: Issues in the Primary Prevention of AIDS*, 195-215. New York: Plenum Press.

Colimoro, C. (1993). El condon feminino. Presentation at the Fourth National Congress on AIDS, Mexico City.

Crisp, B.R., Barber, J.G., Ross, M.W., Wodak, A., Gold, J., and Miller, M.E. (1993). Injecting drug users and HIV/AIDS: Predictors of risk behaviors. *Drug and Alcohol Dependence*, *33*, 73-80.

Des Jarlais, D.C., Choopanya, K.,Wenston, J., Vanichseni, S., Sotheran, J.L., Plangsringarm, K., Friedman, P., Sonchai, W., Carballo, M., and Friedman, S.R. (1992). Risk reduction and stabilization of seroprevalence among drug injectors in New York City and Bangkok, Thailand. In Rossi, G.B., Beth-Giraldo, E., Checo-Bianchi, L., Dianzani, F., Giraldo, G., and Verani, P. (Eds.), *Proceedings of the VII International Conference on AIDS*, Florence, Italy, 1991, 207-213. Kargher: Basel.

Dwyer, R., Richardson, D., Ross, M.W., Wodak, A., Miller, M.E., and Gold, J. (1994). Gender differences in HIV risks among injecting drug users. *AIDS Education and Prevention*, *6*, 379-389.

Ford, N. and Mathie, E. (1993). The acceptability and experience of the female condom, Femidom, among family planning clinic attenders. *British Journal of Family Planning*, *19*, 187-192.

Friedman, S.R., Des Jarlais, D.C., Ward, T.P., Jose, B., Neaigus, A., and Goldstein, M. (1993). Drug injectors and heterosexual AIDS. In L. Sherr (Ed.), *AIDS And The Heterosexual Population*, 41-65. Chur, Switzerland: Harwood Academic.

Gibson, D.R., Catania, J.A., and Peterson, J.L. (1991). Theoretical background. In J.L. Sorensen, L.A. Wermuth, D.R. Gibson, K.H. Choi, J.R. Guydish, and S.L. Batki (Eds.), *Preventing AIDS in Drug Users and Their Sexual Partners*, 62-74. New York: The Guilford Press.

Hernandez-Avila, M. (1992). Acceptability of female condoms among female prostitutes in Mexico City: Preliminary findings. Report to the Wisconsin Pharmaceutical Company.

Kelaher, M. and Ross, M.W. (1992). Sources of bias in HIV/AIDS risk perception in injecting drug users. *Psychological Reports*, *70*, 771-774.

Liskin, L. (1993). Using the female condom for AIDS prevention: Promises and problems (abstract TOP28). Eighth International Conference on AIDS in Africa, Marrakesh, Morocco.

Magura, S., Shapiro, J.L., Siddiqi, Q., and Lipton, D.S. (1990). Variables influencing condom use among intravenous drug users. *American Journal of Public Health*, *80*, 82-84.

Mann, J., Tarantola, D.J.M., Netter, T.W. (Eds.). (1992). *AIDS in the World*. Cambridge, MA: Harvard University Press.

Mays, V.M. and Cochran, S.D. (1988). Issues in the perception of AIDS risk and risk education activities by black and Hispanic/Latina women. *American Psychologist*, *43*, 949-957.

Newcombe, R. and Parry, A. (1988). The Mersey harm-reduction model: A strategy for dealing with drug users. Presentation at the International Conference on Drug Policy Reform, Bethesda, Maryland.

Perez, B., Kennedy. G., and Fullilove, M.T. (1995). Childhood sexual abuse and AIDS: Issues and interventions. In A. O'Leary and L.S. Jemmott (Eds.), *Women at Risk: Issues in the Primary Prevention of AIDS,* 85-100. New York: Plenum Press.

Polit-O'Hara, D. and Kahn, J. (1985). Communication and contraceptive practices in adolescent couples. *Adolescence, 20,* 33-42.

Richardson, D. (1989). *Women and the AIDS Crisis,* Second Edition. London: Pandera.

Ross, M.W., Kelaher, M., Wodak, A., and Gold, J. (1994). Predictors of intoxicated sex in injecting drug users. *Journal of Addictive Diseases, 12,*

Ross, M.W., Wodak, A., and Gold, J. (1992). Sexual behavior in injecting drug users. *Journal of Psychology and Human Sexuality, 5,* 89-104.

Ross, M.W., Wodak. A., Miller, M.E., and Gold, J. (1993). Sexual partner choice in injecting drug users from a "critical incident" measure: Its implications for estimating HIV spread. *Sexological Review, 1,* 77-92.

Schinke, S.P., Gilchrist, L.D., and Small, R.W. (1979). Preventing unwanted pregnancy: A cognitive-behavioral approach. *American Journal of Orthopsychiatry, 49,* 8188.

Shayne, V.T. and Kaplan, B.J. (1991). Double victims: Poor women and AIDS. *Women and Health, 17,* 21-37.

Springer, E. (1991). Effective AIDS prevention with active drug users: The harm reduction model. In M. Shernoff (Ed.), *Counseling Chemically Dependent People with HIV Illness,* 141-156. New York: Harrington Park Press.

Weissman, G. and Brown, V. (1995). Drug-using women and HIV: Risk reduction and prevention issues. In A. O'Leary and L.S. Jemmott (Eds.), *Women at Risk: Issues in the Primary Prevention of AIDS,* 175-190. New York: Plenum Press.

Wermuth, L.A., Ham, J., and Robbins, R.L. (1991). Women don't wear condoms: AIDS risk among sexual partners of IV drug users. In J. Huber and B.E. Schneider (Eds.), *The Social Context of AIDS,* 72-94. Newbury Park: Sage.

Wodak, A., Stowe, A., Ross, M.W., Gold, J., Miller, M.E. (1995). HIV risk exposure of injecting drug users in Sydney. *Drug and Alcohol Review, 14,* 213-222.

Worth, D. (1989). Sexual decision making and AIDS: Why condom promotion among vulnerable women is likely to fail. *Studies in Family Planning, 20,* 297-307.

Chapter 4

Safer Sex Negotiation in Cross-Cultural Romantic Dyads: An Extension of Ting-Toomey's Face Negotiation Theory

Gust A. Yep

We live in a "global village" (Barnlund, 1975; McLuhan, 1962). As cultures learn to coexist with one another in the same geographical area, intercultural dating and marriage are steadily increasing (Hormann, 1982; Kitano et al., 1984; Labor and Jacobs, 1986). Kitano and associates (1984) reported that Asian Americans date or marry out of their group more than any other ethnic group in this country. In addition, researchers (Kitano and Chai, 1982; Kitano et al., 1984; Lee and Yamanaka, 1990) observed that Asian-American women are likely to become romantically involved with non-Asian-American men. In Los Angeles County, for example, there have been almost twice as many Asian-American women involved in outmarriages, including Chinese, Japanese, Korean, and Vietnamese, than their male counterparts in the last two decades (Kitano and Daniels, 1988). Further, the majority of such outmarriages by Asian-American women are to Euro-American men (Kitano et al., 1984). East-West romance appears to be rapidly becoming the phenomenon of the decade. The purpose of this chapter is to explore intimate communication processes in cross-cultural romantic dyads. In particular, this chapter examines safer sex negotiation in East-West romantic dyads using Ting-Toomey's (1988) theory of face negotiation.[1]

Communication is the lifeblood of interpersonal relationships (Knapp and Vangelisti, 1992). It is through communication that people initiate, develop, maintain, and change their personal relationships (Millar and Rogers, 1976; Taylor and Altman, 1987). To emphasize the importance of communication in relationships, Millar and Rogers (1976) stated, "People do not relate and then talk, but they simultaneously relate *in* talk" (p. 89).

Through mutual communication, individuals define their relationships. Morton, Alexander, and Altman (1976) identified five universal themes associated with personal relationships. First, every relationship requires mutuality of control between interactants in which interpersonal communication is the primary vehicle for relationship definition; such definition requires consensus. In other words, for two individuals to have a relationship, they must communicate and perceive some degree of control over definition of the nature of their relationship; e.g., both parties must mutually agree to see each other as boyfriend/girlfriend. Second, every relationship is defined using multimodal—for example, verbal and nonverbal—and multilevel—for example, various degrees of intimacy and levels of self-disclosure—communication, for example, revealing personal information about oneself to the partner. Third, as relationships develop, expansion (i.e., the development of greater domains of interactions) and diversification (i.e., increase in variety of forms of interaction) of modes of exchange occur. In other words, communication becomes richer and more efficient as the relationship escalates, e.g., partners knowing what the other is thinking without uttering a word. Fourth, relationship crises are associated with nonmutuality of relationship definition. A crisis, in this instance, is a transitional process associated with changes in the relationship; it requires that interactants renegotiate their perceptions of the relationship. For example, an individual may no longer accept the other as boyfriend/girlfriend without the prospect of a greater future commitment. Finally, consensus about relationship influence potential—i.e., the degree of perceived rewards and costs associated with the relationship—defines the level of intimacy and intensity of the relationship.

Because of cultural differences, communication between constituents of Eastern and Western cultures can often be difficult (Lampe, 1988; Scollon and Scollon, 1994). Although a number of studies (e.g., Gao, 1991; Gudykunst et al., 1991; Gudykunst and Nishida,

1983, 1986; Sudweeks et al., 1990) have examined communication patterns in East-West relationships, research on communication about intimate behavior in such relationships is nonexistent. With the advent of HIV/AIDS, intimate communication is critical for satisfying relationships (Cupach and Comstock, 1990; Masters, Johnson, and Kolodny, 1986; Metts and Cupach, 1989) and for individual physical survival (Bowen and Michal-Johnson, 1989; Edgar and Fitzpatrick, 1988; Yep, 1995). To address this need in the literature, this chapter examines intimate communication between East-West romantic dyads using Ting-Toomey's (1988) face negotiation theory.[1]

INTIMATE COMMUNICATION
AND SAFER SEX NEGOTIATION

Communication about sexual intimacy is crucial in romantic relationships. Metts and Cupach (1989) elaborated further: "Communication is integral to the development, understanding, and consummation of human sexuality" (p. 139). Disclosure of sexual wishes, predispositions, preferences, apprehensions, standards, vocabularies, and personal idioms promotes acquisition of sexual knowledge (Sarver and Murry, 1981), increases feelings of closeness in the relationship (Bell, Buerkel-Rothfuss, and Gore, 1987; Cornog, 1986), and enhances sexual satisfaction (Cupach and Comstock, 1990; Masters and Johnson, 1979; Masters, Johnson, and Kolodny, 1986). Sexual communication satisfaction is also associated with relational growth and relational satisfaction (Banmen and Vogel, 1985; Cupach and Comstock, 1990; Wheeless, Wheeless, and Baus, 1984). During sexual encounters, communication is typically characterized by a heightened sense of emotional and physiological charge. Edgar and Fitzpatrick (1990) observed, "a sexual episode presents individuals with an extraordinary situation that is arguably more vulnerable and volatile than almost any other interaction context" (p. 107).

Because of the potential vulnerability and emotional volatility of sexual interaction, talking about sex and persuading a partner to practice safer sex are different from other compliance-gaining situations. Edgar and Fitzpatrick (1988) identified three important differences. First, the potential consequences of noncompliance to safer sex guidelines in intimate interactions can be, quite literally, deadly. Because a single exposure to HIV can result in infection, failure to use the proper health protective measures can be fatal. Second, the degree of emotional vulnerability and the potential for loss of face, rejection, embarrassment, shame, and frustration are much greater during a sexual episode than most other interpersonal influence situations cited in compliance-gaining research. Finally, the process of persuading a partner to engage in safer sex implicitly contains an element of negotiation. More specifically, the act of requesting a partner to "play safe" usually follows an action from the other to initiate or engage in sexual activity, i.e., the request to practice safer sex usually comes after the request to have sex. In this negotiation situation, conflict may arise threatening individuals' sense of relationship potential (e.g., the potential future of the romance), mutuality of control (e.g., the degree to which partners exercise power in the relationship), and personal identities (e.g., the potential loss of face during intimate negotiation).

FACE NEGOTIATION THEORY

The concept of "face" exists in all cultures (Brown and Levinson, 1978; Goffman, 1959, 1967, 1971; Gudykunst and Ting-Toomey, 1988; Hill et al. 1986; Hu, 1944; Ide et al., 1986; Katriel, 1986; Okabe, 1983; Ting-Toomey, 1985, 1988). Although it is not exclusive to Chinese culture, this notion of face stems back to fourth century B.C. in China (Hu, 1944). There are two types of face, according to Hu (1944): (a) *mien-tzu*, or accumulated reputation and prestige based on personal efforts, ostentation, and success; and (b) *lien*, or others' respect for the individual because of character, reputation, and personal integrity. Current conceptions of face are more consistent with *lien*. For example, in his work on interaction rituals, Goffman (1967) conceptualizes face as the positive social value an individual has in terms of society's approved image of him/her. More recently, Ting-Toomey (1988) defines face as "an identity that is conjointly defined by the participants in a setting" (p. 215). Taken together, face is the public self-image that all members of society want to claim and maintain for themselves and such image is negotiated through communication during social interaction.

Based on the work of Goffman (1967) and Brown and Levinson (1978), Ting-Toomey (1988) proposed a theory of face negotiation in the context of intercultural interactions. It has been applied to conflict situations between individualistic (e.g., United States) and collectivistic (e.g., Taiwan) cultures (Trubisky, Ting-Toomey, and Lin, 1991) and intergroup diplomatic communication using the Cuban Missile Crisis as a case study (Ting-Toomey and Cole, 1990). Ting-Toomey (1988) argued that: (a) The theory is applicable to any intercultural encounter where interactants experience difficulties (e.g., discussion of sexuality) that entail facework negotiation strategies (e.g., maintaining a good image with one's intimate partner); (b) the theory can be applied to communication encounters involving high degree of threat (e.g., shame, embarrassment) or uncertainty (e.g., unsure of a partner's responses to one's communication attempt) to the face of the interactants; (c) the theory can be applied to situations requiring high levels of politeness between interactants (e.g., the sensitive nature of intimate talk); (d) the theory can be utilized with other communicative acts (e.g., requesting safer sex with an intimate partner); and (e) the theory can be examined in relationship to other communication variables (e.g., sexual compliance-gaining, resisting unsafe sexual requests). Given the sensitive and emotional nature of intimate communication, face negotiation appears to be especially applicable to this context.

The concept of face consists of two related components: (a) positive face, and (b) negative face (Brown and Levinson, 1978). Positive face is an individual's basic assertion of his/her public self-image to be appreciated, included, respected, and approved by others. Positive facework are communication behaviors related to positive face or the need for association (e.g., self-disclosure, compliment giving, etc.). Negative face is the individual's assertion of his/her public self-image to have rights to space, territory, freedom, and personal autonomy. Negative facework are communication behaviors related to negative face or the need for dissociation (e.g., apology for imposition, compliance resisting message tactics).

Brown and Levinson (1978) identified five levels of communication behaviors that potentially threaten either the interactant's need for association (positive face) or dissociation (negative face) by acting contrary to the face wants of the individuals involved. Such behaviors are labeled face-threatening acts (FTA). There are two FTAs to positive face: (a) communication behaviors that indicate the speaker's negative evaluation of some aspect of the hearer's positive face; e.g., disapproval, criticism, contempt, ridicule, complaints, accusations, insults, contradictions, disagreements, challenges, and (b) communication behaviors that indicate that the speaker is indifferent toward the hearer's positive face; e.g., discussion of topics that are taboo or embarrassing to the hearer, expression of violent emotions such as extreme anger and frustration, blatant refusal to cooperate with the hearer. In addition, there are three FTAs to negative face: (a) communication behaviors that predicate some future act of the hearer, and in so doing, put some pressure on the hearer to engage in, or refrain from doing, the specified act; e.g., direct request, order, suggestion, advice, reminder, threat, warning, etc.; (b) communication behaviors that predicate some favorable future action of the speaker toward the hearer, and in so doing, put some pressure on the hearer to receive or refuse them, and possibly feel an obligation to return something in kind; e.g., offer, promise, pledge, proposition, etc.; and (c) communication behaviors that predicate some desire of the speaker toward the hearer (including the hearer's ideas and possessions), and in so doing, put pressure on the hearer to give the object of the speaker's desire to the speaker or to protect it from the speaker; e.g., compliments, expressions of envy and admiration, expressions of strong emotions such as anger and lust.

Based on her work on verbal expression of emotions, disclosure of affect, and request compliance with married couples, Shimanoff (1985, 1987) extended Brown and Levinson's (1978) FTA typology by identifying four additional types of strategies. Such strategies are defined on the basis of the degree of respect or threat to the interactants' face in problematic situations. They are: (a) face-honoring, i.e., disclosure of pleasant emotions (such as love) toward the hearer; (b) face-compensating, i.e., expressions of regrets for infringing on the hearer's space; (c) face-neutral, i.e., disclosure of strong emotions—either positive or negative—toward absent others; and

(d) face-threatening, i.e., disclosures of vulnerability or hostilities toward the hearer. Shimanoff (1985) reported that married couples engage in and have a preference for face-honoring, face-compensating, and face-neutral emotional disclosures than face-threatening ones. Later, Shimanoff (1987) found that disclosure of all unpleasant emotions are not equally negative.

Although both positive and negative facework are present in all cultures, Ting-Toomey (1988) pointed out that

> The value orientations of a culture will influence cultural members' attitudes toward pursuing one set of facework more actively than others in a face-negotiation situation. Facework then, is viewed as a symbolic front that members in all cultures strive to maintain and uphold; while modes and styles of expressing and negotiating face-need would vary from one culture to the next. (pp. 216–217)

In the case of East-West romantic dyads, two distinct cultural orientations might be present (see, for example, Gudykunst, 1989; Hall, 1976, 1983). For example, Eastern and Western cultures have different conceptualizations of selfhood and interpersonal relationships.

In terms of interpersonal relations, Triandis (1978) identified four universal dimensions that appear to exist in all cultures. They are: (a) association-dissociation; (b) superordination-subordination; (c) intimacy-formality; and (d) overt-covert. Association behaviors are cooperative actions, e.g., being helpful and supportive, while dissociation behaviors are uncooperative, e.g., being confrontational or avoidant. Superordination behaviors involve the exercise of power, e.g., criticizing others, while subordination is the opposite, e.g., help-seeking behaviors, agreement. The intimacy-formality continuum refers to how private social relationships are within the culture, e.g., degree of emotional expression, self-disclosure. The final dimension, overt-covert, indicates how visible one's behaviors are to others, i.e., the degree of openness in expressing one's likes and dislikes. These dimensions have been substantiated in crosscultural research (Lonner, 1980).

While Triandis' (1978) dimensions of social relations may be present in all cultures, differences in interpersonal communication, interpersonal relationships, and value orientations vary across cultures. In the East-West dyadic context, it appears that there are differences in sex role orientation and cultural variability including Hall's (1976) notion of low- and high-context cultures and Hofstede's (1984) individualism-collectivism dimension of culture.

Context and Face Negotiation

In *Beyond Culture*, Hall (1976) argued that cultures may be differentiated on the basis of their modes of communication by introducing the low-high context continuum. A low-context communication message is one in which most of the information is directly and explicitly stated in the verbalized message, e.g., a direct request for a romantic date. On the other hand, a high-context communication message is one in which most of the information is either implied in the social and physical context or internalized in the person leaving little information in the verbalized message, e.g., a woman hinting that she is free to go out instead of asking her hearer to go on a date because, in her culture, it is inappropriate for her to request a date. Kohls (1978) identified a list of 12 cultures on a continuum from low-context to high-context: Swiss-German, German, Scandinavian, American, French, English, Italian, Spanish, Greek, Arab, Chinese, and Japanese. Based on this classification, it appears that most Western cultures belong toward the low-context end, while most Eastern cultures fall on the high-context end of the continuum.

Context affects all aspects of communication within a culture including language (both written and spoken), patterns of social organization, and conflict resolution. More specifically, Hall (1976) stated:

> High-context cultures make greater distinctions between insiders and outsiders than low-context cultures do. People raised in high-context systems expect more of others than do participants in low-context systems. When talking about something that they have on their minds, a high-context individual will expect his [or her] interlocutor to know what's bothering him [or her], so that he [or she] doesn't have to be specific. The result is that he [or she] will talk around and around the point,

in effect putting all the pieces in place except the crucial one. Placing it properly—this keystone—is the role of his [or her] interlocutor. To do this for him [or her] is an insult . . . (p. 98)

Given these differences, Ting-Toomey (1985, 1988) discussed several specific communication applications of context and culture.

First, communicators from low-context cultures tend to separate the issue from the person while interactants from high-context cultures tend to do just the opposite, the person and the issue are inseparable; e.g., a mild disagreement may be perceived as an attack or face threatening. Such perceived attacks, from the high-context communicator perspective, need smoothing, therefore, the motivation to save face is generally very strong in Eastern cultures. In the intimate communication arena, discussion of sexual matters for East-West dyads is perhaps more face threatening than for Western dyads because: (a) Sexuality is a taboo topic in a number of Eastern cultures (Gock, 1994; Yep, 1993a, in press-a, b); and (b) A disagreement about sexual practices can be perceived as a personal attack (Yep, 1993a).

Second, members from low-context cultures have lower tolerance for uncertainty. In contrast, interactants from high-context systems are comfortable with ambiguity. Such tolerance for ambiguity may be manifested in the form of silence. In terms of intimate communication, it is not surprising that individuals from high-context societies (e.g., Eastern cultures) may use silence in discussion of intimate behavior (e.g., sexuality) which may produce a great deal of discomfort for the low-context partner.

Third, members of low-context societies use a very direct style of communication while high-context communicators utilize more indirect modes of expression. Such distinct styles of communication have important implications for intimate communication; for example, low-context partners prefer direct discussion of sexual issues while high-context individuals prefer talk around the issue of intimacy without ever getting to addressing sexuality between them (Yep, 1993a, 1997).

Fourth, members of low-context cultures tend to seek interpersonal data based on personal and individual characteristics of the partner as opposed to social and group information. High-context interactants prefer the opposite; they prefer to seek information about their partners through understanding the partner's social and group memberships, e.g., the family (Jue, 1987; Yep, 1993a, in press, 1997). In intimate situations, low-context communicators appear verbose, self-disclosing, and open, while their high-context counterparts seem more reserved, cautious, and withholding.

Fifth, negotiation styles between members of low- and high-context cultures differ. Low-context communicators tend to use linear logic in their bargaining style (e.g., a problem-solution approach). In contrast, high-context communicators use a more feeling and intuitive style of negotiation (e.g., a smoothing approach).

These differences in communication behavior between members of low- and high-context cultures—as exemplified in East-West dyadic interaction—can be difficult. Intimate communication and sexual compliance gaining are difficult challenges for intracultural dyads (Edgar and Fitzpatrick, 1990). For intercultural couples, this situation is further complicated by differences in styles of interaction. For example, Okabe (1983) argued that verbal skills are more highly valued in low-context cultures than in high-context societies. Conversely, nonverbal communication skills and nonverbal sensitivity are considered more important in high-context cultures.

Because communication between East-West romantic dyads is, in many ways, parallel to low- and high-context interactional styles, the discussion so far has focused on this dimension of cultural variability. Ting-Toomey (1988) also argued that another important schema for understanding interpersonal communication and face negotiation is Hofstede's (1984) individualism-collectivism dimension (see also Dion and Dion, 1988).

Individualism-Collectivism and Face Negotiation

Individualism-collectivism is a bipolar continuum that appears to characterize Western and Eastern cultures, respectively. Individualistic cultures such as the United States focus on the importance of the individual and highlight the "I" identity of the communicator. In contrast, collectivistic cultures, such as many Asian countries, emphasize the goals, needs, and perceptions of the group rather than the individual, therefore, focusing on the "we" identity. This dimension of cultural variability also has important implications for face negotiation processes.

In collectivistic cultures, the self is situationally and relationally defined; that is, the presentation of oneself is contingent upon the nature of the context, situation, and the relationship with the interactant. For example, it is difficult for an Asian woman to discuss sexuality or request for safer sexual practices with her intimate partner given the nature of the situation—discussion of taboo or sensitive topics—and the relationship—one that is characterized by emotional vulnerability and, possibly, gender role distinctions. Tu (1985) discusses this notion of self in relationship to Confucian philosophy, "a distinctive feature of Confucian ritualization is an ever-deepening and broadening awareness of the *presence of the other* [italics mine] in one's self-cultivation" (p. 232). In most collectivistic cultures, the self is defined and maintained through a complex and dynamic interaction of social and personal relationships; the self is never free. This is in direct contrast with individualistic (e.g., Western) cultures in which the self is a perfectly free entity—autonomous and free to go after its own personal and unique wishes, needs, and desires. Facework, or the behaviors that people engage in in order to make their actions consistent with their face, varies across cultures. In Asian cultures, it is focused on supporting another person's face while at the same time not bringing shame to one's own self-face; in Western cultures, it is focused on the preservation of one's individuality, autonomy, and space while simultaneously respecting the other's need for autonomy and territory.

Gender and Face Negotiation

In her review of verbal and nonverbal communication research associated with intimate encounters, Prager (1995) noted that "gender differences have proved to offer an invaluable window onto the kinds of effects sociocultural norms can have on intimate interactions" (p. 216). Gender is a sociocultural construction; it focuses on the enactment of appropriate behaviors associated with biological sex within a cultural domain. In other words, gender and sex role systems are at the core of any culture.

Gender affects intimate behavior (Prager, 1995). In the U.S. cultural context, research has identified gender differences in motives for seeking intimate interactions (Prager, Fuller, and Gonzalez, 1989), verbal intimacy (Dindia and Allen, 1992), self-disclosure patterns (Caldwell and Peplau, 1982; Hendrick, 1981; Petronio and Martin, 1986; Sprecher, 1987), sexual influence strategies (Christopher and Frandsen, 1990; Yep, 1995), sexual resistance tactics (Grauerholz and Serpe, 1985; McCormick, 1979; Yep, 1993b), and safer sex talk and communication about HIV/AIDS (Cline, Freeman, and Johnson, 1990; Cline and McKenzie, 1994), among others.

In his research of 40 national cultures, Hofstede (1984) noted that "the predominant socialization pattern is for men to be more assertive and for women to be more nurturing" (p. 176). Although this conclusion appears to support simplistic gender stereotypes, it may also imply that there are gender differences in face needs. More specifically, Hofstede's (1984) finding can imply that men might be more concerned about preserving their own face and women to be more yielding and focused on the preservation of their partner's face while simultaneously maintaining their own face. Shimanoff's (1994) work seems to support this contention; for example, women may have a greater need for solidarity or fellowship face, that is, the need to be included. Although it appears that there are some gender differences in face negotiation, past research on gender and facework behavior is largely inconclusive partly because gender interacts with other sociological factors such as status, age, context, and degree of relational intimacy (Shimanoff, 1994).

Theoretical Propositions

Taken together, individualistic, low-context systems (e.g., Western cultures) and collectivistic, high-context systems (e.g., many Asian cultures) are expected to have distinct face-negotiation styles. In addition, gender influences facework behaviors. In the intimate context, such differences are expected to be manifested in how individuals address intimate topics such as sexuality, sexual behavior, and safer sexual practices. Based on Ting-Toomey's (1988) theory and some preliminary observations,[2] several propositions[3] can be derived for empirical testing in intimate communication scenarios involving East-West romantic dyads:

Akiko, a Japanese woman, has been in a romantic relationship with Wolfgang (not his real name), a Euro-American man, for over three years. Akiko reports that since she and Wolfgang started dating, she was always "worried about saying something that would embarrass him in front of his family . . . and co-workers." She appears to have more other-face concern—that is, her orientation toward attention for the other (Wolfgang) during interaction—than self-face concern—that is, her orientation toward attention for self during interaction. Proposition one may be stated as follows:

1. Women from collectivistic, high-context (C/HC) cultures are expected to express more other-face concern than men from individualistic, low-context (I/LC) cultures. In contrast, males from I/LC cultures are expected to express more self-face concern than their C/HC female counterparts.

Akiko also expressed her desire for "[Wolfgang] to show me that he cares about me . . . that he needs me . . ." Proposition two is presented as follows:

2. Women from C/HC cultures are expected to express more inclusion, association, and positive-face needs than men from I/LC groups. On the other hand, males from I/LC cultures are expected to express more autonomy, dissociation, and negative-face needs than their C/HC female counterparts.

In intimate situations, men from I/LC groups are expected to communicate in such a way that they will protect their needs for association (i.e., approval and appreciation by his partner) and dissociation (i.e., preservation of personal freedom and autonomy in his relationship) through maintaining the authenticity of the self; on the other hand, women from C/HC cultures are expected to protect the same needs by maintaining the self that is simultaneously defined by lending role support to the other's face and not bringing shame to their own self-face. To synthesize the above, proposition three may be stated as follows:

3. Men from I/LC cultures are expected to use self-concern positive-face and self-concern negative-face suprastrategies while

women from C/HC cultures are expected to use other-concern positive-face and other-concern negative-face suprastrategies.

Fei, a Chinese woman, has been married to Jon (not his real name), a Euro-American man, for five months. In terms of discussions of physical intimacy and sexuality, Fei says: "I'm very shy [about sex] . . . When I need to talk [about sex], I would hint hoping that he will get it . . . but I can never say it straight out like some of my American [women] friends can . . . I'm too ashamed to talk [about sex]." Propositions four to six are presented as follows:

4. In intimate communication, C/HC female partners are expected to use indirect modes of communication while I/LC male partners are expected to use direct modes of communication.
5. In intimate communication, women from C/HC groups are expected to use more obliging or avoiding and affective-oriented styles while men from I/LC cultures are expected to use more confrontational and solution-oriented styles.
6. In intimate negotiation, C/HC female partners are expected to use more collaborative communication strategies while I/LC male partners are expected to use more competitive communication strategies.

When asked about how she would persuade her husband Jon to use condoms when they have sexual intercourse, Fei laughed nervously. Then she said, "I would probably tell him that I heard about a store on Melrose Avenue [in Los Angeles] that sells condoms . . . maybe he will want to try them . . ." Proposition seven may be stated as follows:

7. In intimate negotiation, C/HC female partners are expected to use more indirect compliance-gaining message tactics while I/LC male partners are expected to use more direct compliance-gaining message strategies.

Both Akiko and Fei indicated that they show their love and affection for their partners by "doing nice things" for them rather than telling them directly. As a matter of fact, neither one of them indicated that they felt comfortable with saying "I love you" to their partners. Proposition eight is presented as follows:

8. In intimate negotiation, C/HC female partners are expected to use more indirect emotional expressions while I/LC male partners are expected to use more direct emotional expressions.

SUMMARY, CONCLUSIONS, AND FUTURE DIRECTIONS

This chapter explored intimate communication in intercultural romantic couples. More specifically, it examined safer sex negotiation processes in East-West romantic dyads. Given the sensitive nature of intimate communication and the potential cultural differences in intercultural interaction, this complex communication system—East-West dyads communicating about sexuality, safer sex, and intimacy—was examined using the concept of face. Based on the notion that face is universal and omnipresent in all cultures, face negotiation theory makes specific predictions about intimate communication and safer sex negotiation. In particular, eight theoretical propositions are derived from the theory and relevant dimensions of cultural variability, namely, low-high context and individualism-collectivism, to predict intimate communication behaviors between women and men in East-West romantic dyads.

It is apparent that much work remains to be done in this emerging area of intercultural intimate communication. At the theoretical and research levels, future work needs to: (a) examine how culture and gender come together to influence face needs and facework behavior in intimate relationships; and (b) test the above predictions in research to assess the potential utility of this intercultural theory in the intimate communication context. At the methodological level, there is a need to integrate both qualitative (e.g., use of in-depth interviews, personal narratives, and open-ended survey questions) and quantitative (e.g., use of standardized paper-and-pencil measures) techniques to develop a more complete understanding of this sensitive intercultural communication process. At the practical level, theory and research in this area may provide individuals involved in intercultural romance with tools for greater understanding and appreciation of differences and similarities in interactional styles as well as safer intimate behaviors.

NOTES

1. This project was partially supported by a Research, Scholarship, and Creative Activity Faculty Development Grant awarded by the California State University (1993). I wish to acknowledge Ramin Ramhormozi, my research assistant, for his assistance in library research. An earlier version of this chapter was presented to the 80th Annual Meeting of the Speech Communication Association, New Orleans, 1994.

2. These preliminary observations are based on personal interviews with two Asian women: Akiko (Japanese) and Fei (Chinese). Their names have been changed to preserve their anonymity. I want to express my appreciation for their cooperation and willingness to discuss such personal and intimate behaviors. I would like to caution the reader that the data reported here are preliminary and, in a very limited way, illustrative of some of the theoretical propositions advanced in this chapter. These anecdotes do not, by any means, constitute empirical testing of the theory.

3. These propositions have been derived to predict intimate communication patterns between Asian women and Euro-American men based on traditional gender role behaviors reported in their respective cultural systems. I recognize that communication acculturation and intercultural transformation take place in global communities and they must be controlled for in empirical research that attempts to test the validity of the above propositions.

REFERENCES

Banmen, J. and Vogel, N.A. (1985). The relationship between marital quality and interpersonal sexual communication. *Family Therapy, 12*, 45–58.

Barnlund, D.C. (1975). *Public and Private Self in Japan and the United States.* Tokyo: Simul Press.

Bell, R.A., Buerkel-Rothfuss, N.L., and Gore, K.E. (1987). "Did you bring the yarmulke for the cabbage patch kid?" The idiomatic communication of young lovers. *Human Communication Research, 14*, 47–67.

Bowen, S.P. and Michal-Johnson, P. (1989). The crisis of communicating in relationships: Confronting the threat of AIDS. *AIDS and Public Policy Journal, 4*, 10–19.

Brown, P. and Levinson, S. (1978). Universals in language usage: Politeness phenomenon. In E. Goody (Ed.), *Questions and Politeness: Strategies in Social Interaction,* 56-289. Cambridge: Cambridge University Press.

Caldwell, M.A. and Peplau, L.A. (1982). Sex differences in same-sex friendship. *Sex Roles, 8*, 721–732.

Christopher, F.S. and Frandsen, M.M. (1990). Strategies of influence in sex and dating. *Journal of Social and Personal Relationships, 7*, 89–105.

Cline, R.J.W., Freeman, K.E., and Johnson, S.J. (1990). Talk among sexual partners about AIDS: Factors differentiating those who talk from those who do not. *Communication Research, 17*, 792–808.

Cline, R.J.W. and McKenzie, N. (1994). Sex differences in communication and the construction of HIV/AIDS. *Journal of Applied Communication Research,* 22, 322–337.

Cornog, M. (1986). Naming sexual body parts: Preliminary patterns and implications. *Journal of Sex Research,* 22, 393–398.

Cupach, W.R. and Comstock, J. (1990). Satisfaction with sexual communication in marriage: Links to sexual satisfaction and dyadic adjustment. *Journal of Social and Personal Relationships,* 7, 179–186.

Dindia, K. and Allen, M. (1992). Sex differences in self-disclosure: A meta-analysis. *Psychological Bulletin,* 112, 106–124.

Dion, K.L. and Dion, K.K. (1988). Romantic love: Individual and cultural perspectives. In R. Sternberg and M. Barnes (Eds.), *The Psychology of Love.* New Haven, CT: Yale University Press.

Edgar, T. and Fitzpatrick, M.A. (1988). Compliance-gaining in relational interaction: When your life depends on it. *Southern Speech Communication Journal,* 53, 385–405.

Edgar, T. and Fitzpatrick, M.A. (1990). Communicating sexual desire: Message tactics for having and avoiding intercourse. In J.P. Dillard (Ed.), *Seeking Compliance: The Production of Interpersonal Influence Messages.* Scottsdale, AZ: Gorsuch Scarisbrick.

Gao, G. (1991). Stability in romantic relationships in China and the United States. In S. Ting-Toomey and F. Korzenny (Eds.), *Cross-Cultural Interpersonal Communication.* Newbury Park, CA: Sage.

Gock, T.S. (1994). Acquired immunodeficiency syndrome. In N.W.S. Zane, D.T. Takeuchi, and K.N.J. Young (Eds.), *Confronting Critical Health Issues of Asian and Pacific Islander Americans.* Newbury Park, CA: Sage.

Goffman, E. (1959). *The Presentation of Self in Everyday Life.* Garden City, NY: Doubleday.

Goffman, E. (1967). *Interaction Ritual: Essays on Face-To-Face Interaction.* Garden City, NY: Doubleday.

Goffman, E. (1971). *Relations in Public.* New York: Harper and Row.

Grauerholz, E. and Serpe, R.T. (1985). Initiation and response: The dynamics of sexual interaction. *Sex Roles,* 12, 1041–1059.

Gudykunst, W.B. (1989). Culture and the development of interpersonal relationships. In J. Anderson (Ed.), *Communication Yearbook 12.* Newbury Park, CA: Sage.

Gudykunst, W.B. and Nishida, T. (1983). Social penetration in Japanese and North American relationships. In R. Bostrom (Ed.), *Communication Yearbook 7.* Beverly Hills, CA: Sage.

Gudykunst, W.B. and Nishida, T. (1986). The influence of cultural variability on perceptions of communication behavior associated with relationship terms. *Human Communication Research,* 13, 147–166.

Gudykunst, W.B. and Ting-Toomey, S. (1988). *Culture and Interpersonal Communication.* Newbury Park, CA: Sage.

Gudykunst, W.B., Gao, G., Sudweeks, S., Ting-Toomey, S., and Nishida, T. (1991). Themes in opposite-sex Japanese-North American relationships. In

S. Ting-Toomey and F. Korzenny (Eds.), *Cross-Cultural Interpersonal Communication*, 230-256. Newbury Park, CA: Sage.

Hall, E.T. (1976). *Beyond Culture*. New York: Doubleday.

Hall, E.T. (1983). *The Dance of Life*. New York: Doubleday.

Hendrick, S.S. (1981). Self-disclosure and marital satisfaction. *Journal of Personality and Social Psychology, 40*, 1150–1159.

Hill, B., Ide, S., Ikuta, S., Kawasaki, A., and Ogino, T. (1986). Universals of linguistic politeness: Quantitative evidence for Japanese and American English. *Journal of Pragmatics, 10*, 347–371.

Hofstede, G. (1984). *Culture's Consequences: International Differences in Work-Related Values*. Newbury Park, CA: Sage.

Hormann, B.L. (1982). The mixing process. *Social Process in Hawaii, 29*, 116–129.

Hu, H.C. (1944). The Chinese concept of "face." *American Anthropologist, 46*, 45–64.

Ide, S., Hori, M., Kawasaki, A., Ikuta, S., and Haga, H. (1986). Sex differences and politeness in Japanese. *International Journal of the Sociology of Language, 58*, 25–36.

Jue, S. (1987). Identifying and meeting the needs of minority clients with AIDS. In C. Leukefeld and M. Fimbres (Eds.), *Responding to AIDS: Psychosocial Initiatives*, 65-79. Washington DC: National Association of Social Workers.

Katriel, T. (1986). *Talking straight: Dugri speech in Israeli Sabra culture*. Cambridge: Cambridge University Press.

Kitano, H. and Chai, L. (1982). Chinese interracial marriage. *Marriage and Family Review, 5*, 75–89.

Kitano, H. and Daniels, R. (1988). *Asian Americans: Emerging Minorities*. Englewood Cliffs, NJ: Prentice-Hall.

Kitano, H., Yeung, W., Chai, L., and Hatanaka, H. (1984). Asian-American interracial marriage. *Journal of Marriage and the Family, 46*, 179–190.

Knapp, M.L. and Vangelisti, A.L. (1992). *Interpersonal Communication and Human Relationships*. Boston: Allyn and Bacon.

Kohls, L. R. (1978). Basic concepts and models of intercultural communication. In M. Prosser (Ed.), *USIA Intercultural Communication Course: 1977 Proceedings*. Washington D.C.: United States Information Agency.

Labor, T. and Jacobs, J.A. (1986). Intermarriage in Hawaii, 1950–1983. *Journal of Marriage and the Family, 48*, 79–88.

Lampe, P.E. (1988). The problematic nature of interracial and interethnic communication. *The Social Studies, 79*(3), 116–120.

Lee, S. and Yamanaka, K. (1990). Patterns of Asian-American intermarriage and marital assimilation. *Journal of Comparative Family Studies, 21*, 287–305.

Lonner, W. (1980). The search for psychological universals. In H. Triandis and W. Lambert (Eds.), *Handbook of Cross-Cultural Psychology (Vol. 1)*. Boston: Allyn and Bacon.

Masters, W.H. and Johnson, V.E. (1979). *Homosexuality in Perspective*. Boston: Little, Brown.

Masters, W.H., Johnson, V.E., and Kolodny, R. (1986). *Sex And Human Loving.* Boston: Little, Brown.

McCormick, N.B. (1979). Come-ons and put-offs: Unmarried students' strategies for having and avoiding sexual intercourse. *Psychology of Women Quarterly, 4,* 194–211.

McLuhan, M. (1962). *The Gutenberg Galaxy.* New York: New American Library.

Metts, S. and Cupach, W.R. (1989). The role of communication in human sexuality. In K. McKinney and S. Sprecher (Eds.), *Human Sexuality: The Societal and Interpersonal Context,* 131-161. Norwood, NJ: Ablex.

Millar, F.E. and Rogers, L.E. (1976). A relational approach to interpersonal communication. In G.R. Miller (Ed.), *Explorations in Interpersonal Communication,* 105-125. Beverly Hills, CA: Sage.

Morton, T.L., Alexander, J.F., and Altman, I. (1976). Communication and relationship definition. In G.R. Miller (Ed.), *Explorations in Interpersonal Communication,* 125. Beverly Hills, CA: Sage.

Okabe, R. (1983). Cultural assumptions of East and West: Japan and the United States. In W.B. Gudykunst (Ed.), *Intercultural Communication Theory: Current Perspectives,* 21-44. Beverly Hills, CA: Sage.

Petronio, S. and Martin, J.N. (1986). Ramifications of revealing private information: A gender gap. *Journal of Clinical Psychology, 42,* 499–506.

Prager, K.J. (1995). *The Psychology of Intimacy.* New York: Guilford.

Prager, K.J., Fuller, D.O., and Gonzalez, A.S. (1989). The function of self-disclosure in social interaction. *Journal of Social Behavior and Personality, 4,* 563–580.

Sarver, J.M. and Murry, M.D. (1981). Knowledge of human sexuality among happily and unhappily married couples. *Journal of Sex Education and Therapy, 7,* 23–25.

Scollon, R. and Scollon, S.W. (1994). Face parameters in East-West discourse. In S. Ting-Toomey (Ed.), *The Challenge of Facework: Cross-Cultural and Interpersonal Issues,* 133-157 New York: SUNY.

Shimanoff, S.B. (1985). Rules governing the verbal expression of emotions between married couples. *Western Journal of Speech Communication, 49,* 147–165.

Shimanoff, S.B. (1987). Types of emotional disclosures and request compliance between spouses. *Communication Monographs, 54,* 85–100.

Shimanoff, S.B. (1994). Gender perspective on facework: Simplistic stereotypes vs. complex realities. In S. Ting-Toomey (Ed.), *The Challenge of Facework: Cross-Cultural and Interpersonal Issues,* 159-207. New York: SUNY.

Sprecher, S. (1987). The effects of self-disclosure given and received on affection for an intimate partner and stability of the relationship. *Journal of Social and Personal Relationships, 4,* 115–128.

Sudweeks, S., Gudykunst, W.B., Ting-Toomey, S., and Nishida, T. (1990). Developmental themes in Japanese-North American interpersonal relationships. *International Journal of Intercultural Relations, 14,* 207–233.

Taylor, D.A. and Altman, I. (1987). Communication in interpersonal relationships: Social penetration processes. In M.E. Roloff and G.R. Miller (Eds.), *Interpersonal Processes: New Directions in Communication Research,* 257-277. Newbury Park, CA: Sage.

Ting-Toomey, S. (1985). Toward a theory of conflict and culture. In W.B. Gudy-kunst, L. Stewart, and S. Ting-Toomey (Eds.), *Communication, Culture, and Organizational Processes*. Beverly Hills, CA: Sage.

Ting-Toomey, S. (1988). Intercultural conflict styles: A face-negotiation theory. In Y.Y. Kim and W.B. Gudykunst (Eds.), *Theories in Intercultural Communication*, 213-235. Newbury Park, CA: Sage.

Ting-Toomey, S. and Cole, M. (1990). Intergroup diplomatic communication: A face-negotiation perspective. In F. Korzenny and S. Ting-Toomey (Eds.), *Communicating for Peace: Diplomacy and Negotiation*. Newbury Park, CA: Sage.

Triandis, H.C. (1978). Some universals of social behavior. *Personality and Social Psychology Bulletin, 4,* 1–16.

Trubisky, P., Ting-Toomey, S., and Lin, S. (1991). The influence of individualism-collectivism and self-monitoring on conflict styles. *International Journal of Intercultural Relations, 15,* 65–84.

Tu, W.M. (1985). Selfhood and otherness in Confucian thought. In A. Marsella, G. DeVos, and F. Hsu (Eds.), *Culture and Self: Asian and Western Perspectives,* 231-251. New York: Tavistock.

Wheeless, L.R., Wheeless, V.E., and Baus, R. (1984). Sexual communication, communication satisfaction, and solidarity in the developmental stages of intimate relationships. *Western Journal of Speech Communication, 48,* 217–230.

Yep, G.A. (1993a). HIV/AIDS in Asian and Pacific Islander communities in the United States: A review, analysis, and integration. *International Quarterly of Community Health Education, 13,* 293–315.

Yep, G.A. (1993b). *Intimate Communication Between Hispanic Adults, Part Two: An Exploratory Study of Message Strategies Partners Use to Resist Unsafe Sex*. Paper presented to the 79th annual meeting of the Speech Communication Association, Miami, FL.

Yep, G.A. (1995). Healthy desires/unhealthy practices: Interpersonal influence strategies for the prevention of HIV/AIDS among Hispanics. In L.K. Fuller and L. McPherson Shilling (Eds.), *Communicating About Communicable Diseases*. Amherst, MA: Human Resource Development Press.

Yep, G.A. (1997). Overcoming barriers in HIV/AIDS education for Asian Americans: Toward more effective cultural communication. In D.C. Umeh (Ed.), *Confronting the AIDS Epidemic: Cross-Cultural Perspectives on HIV/AIDS Education*. Lawrenceville, NJ: Africa World Press.

Yep, G.A. (in press). "See no evil, hear no evil, speak no evil": Educating Asian Americans about HIV/AIDS through culture-specific health communication campaigns. In L.K. Fuller (Ed.), *Media-Mediated AIDS*. Amherst, MA: Human Resource Development Press.

Chapter 5

Navigating the Freedoms of College Life: Students Talk About Alcohol, Gender, and Sex

Deborah J. Cohen
Linda C. Lederman

INTRODUCTION

The "learning" that occurs in college is not limited to the classroom. A very important area of learning for students is shaped by the college environment itself, an environment which affords independence, the opportunity for experimentation, self-expression, and the development of new ideas, attitudes, belief, and behaviors. Alcohol and sexual practices are two areas where college students experiment. In a study conducted by the New Jersey College Consortium for Health in Education (Fisch-Lewis and Goodheart, 1995), 84 percent of the college students surveyed reported having had sexual intercourse. Of those, 79 percent of the men and 84 percent of the women reported having one partner, 19 percent of the men and 15 percent of the women reported having two to three partners, and 2 percent of the men and 1 percent of the women reported having four to five partners. Less then half of those unmarried, sexually active students said they used a condom the last time they had sexual intercourse (p. 10).

Mixing alcohol consumption and sexual intercourse may, at least in part, explain why the majority of undergraduates do not report using condoms. Whether this combination increases the likelihood of having sex without a condom (or other types of risky sex) is somewhat open to question. Several studies have found significant differences in the use of condoms among those who drink and those who do not drink prior to sexual intercourse (Cooper and Pierce, 1991; Robertson and Plant, 1988; Flannigan and Hitch, 1986). Other researchers, however, have found no difference (Leigh, 1990; Harvey and Beckman, 1986). As Cooper (1992) suggests, there are several plausible explanations for this discrepancy. First, there may be a difference in the role that alcohol plays with new sexual partners and ongoing sexual relationships. Both of the studies reporting null results sampled populations of individuals in more stable, ongoing relationships. Second, those studies reporting negative findings were conducted among older, adult populations where those studies with positive findings used adolescent and young adult populations. Third, these discrepancies may be indicative of the difficulty in measuring risky sexual behavior and alcohol use in single, sexual acts (p. 69). These findings lead us to believe that alcohol use and the increased incidence of having risky sex remains a considerable concern in college aged populations.

Risky sexual practices can have considerable health repercussions. If more than 50 percent of those undergraduates having sex are not consistently using condoms, contracting STDs, including the HIV/AIDS virus, becomes more likely. According to the Center for Substance Abuse (1992), the number of reported cases of AIDS among 13 to 24-year-olds has risen 43 percent in two years. Colleges and universities across the country have instituted prevention programs aimed at increasing undergraduates' knowledge about the HIV/AIDS virus and teaching students how to practice safer sex. However, even those students who have reported attending such programs, exhibited knowledge about HIV/AIDS, and knew how to practice safer sex often do not do so (Stinson et al., 1992). Health educators need to better understand the roles of alcohol consumption and sexual behaviors in the lives of undergraduates in order to develop programs that will not only increase students' awareness about HIV/AIDS, but change students' risky sexual behaviors.

In this project, we worked toward developing such an understanding by talking with undergraduates about these issues. From our data, two intertwined themes developed: First, students talked of the sense of freedom and independence experienced when first arriving at college. For many, this was the first time away from home; freedom from the constraints of parents, families, and friends was central to the college experience. In exploring this theme, we looked at how undergraduates perceived the role freedom played in alcohol consumption and sexual behavior. Students' accounts suggested that alcohol provided both the initial and ongoing experiences with others that forged a connection to this community.

The second theme emerging from the data concerned students' learning to act responsibly in regard to alcohol consumption and sexual behavior. Here, we focused on the relationship between sexual interactions and existing community sexual mores. These sexual standards differed for male and female students and shaped the role alcohol played in the sexual practices of each group.

We had two overarching goals. The first was to begin to understand, from the perspective of undergraduates, how freedom and learning to act responsibly were importantly and meaningfully interconnected with alcohol consumption and sexual experiences. To achieve this goal, we organized this chapter to showcase the "voices" and responses of the students to whom we spoke. Our second goal was to connect what we learned from students with the existing practical and theoretical work in this area. We devoted the final section of this chapter to an integration of experiential learning theory and past research on college students' alcohol and sexual practices in order to suggest how the findings of this current project were practically and theoretically relevant.

METHODOLOGY

The bulk of the data for this analysis were generated from eight focus group interviews conducted with four male and four female groups from 1989 through 1990 at a large university in the Northeastern section of the United States.[1] This research project was initially conducted in response to a 1987 survey of student drinking behavior.[2] Information regarding the genders, ages of the students, and the types of drinkers (abstainer, low-to-moderate risk drinker, and high-risk drinker) was obtained in a screening interview. Student drinking behavior was classified using the following criteria: Abstainers did not consume alcohol; low to moderate risk drinkers consumed alcohol from time to time and had consumed alcohol in the last month, but consume less then five drinks when they do consume alcohol; and high-risk drinkers consume alcohol frequently and consume five or more drinks at a time (Berkowitz and Perkins, 1986; Ratliff and Burkhart, 1984; Wechsler and McFadden, 1979; Engs, 1977). Students were placed in focus groups based on gender, age, and drinker type.

Focus groups were conducted by professional male and female group moderators (where male moderators conducted the male groups and female moderators conducted the female groups). Group discussions were guided by a Focus Group Guide, created by a team of researchers including alcohol preventionists, communication specialists, and health educators. Participation in the focus group involved responses written by students which were followed by a semistructured discussion session.

In addition, there were a total of 12 one-on-one interviews conducted with students in 1989 and in 1995, and 20 hours of ethnographic data collected at university area bars. The interviews conducted in 1995 indicated that students' attitudes, beliefs, and practices regarding alcohol consumption and sexuality have remained consistent over the last six years. All the data collect between 1989 and 1995 were transcribed and used in this current analysis.

The goal of this project in 1989, as well as the present, was to shed light on quantitative data generated in the student drinking survey conducted in 1987, as well as findings generated in other alcohol-related research. Our focus was on the "why" underlying students' behaviors. Group interviews were designed to find out from students in their own words what drinking and sex meant to them. Since it was the students' views and experiences in which we were interested, we selected a grounded theoretical approach for analysis that would permit the emergence of such perspectives from the data (Straus, 1987). The theories and themes generated by the students shaped the form and content of our theoretical perspective and analysis (Straus, 1987). It was not until we felt the students' ways of seeing, experiencing, and understanding their own and others' behaviors and attitudes were accounted for that we began to look for connections between the students' ways of seeing and experiencing alcohol consumption and sexuality in college, and those discussed by researchers in the field of communication, alcohol studies, and education theory.

It is significant to point out that it was not the intention of the researchers, in the initial study in 1989, to engage students in a discussion of sexual attitudes and practices. Sexuality, however, was a topic brought forth by students in all interviews and focus groups. For students, there was an important link between sexual practices and alcohol consumption; for this reason, we were compelled to concern ourselves with this topic.

DISCONNECTION FROM FAMILY AND FREEDOM FROM PARENTAL CONTROL: THE ROLE OF ALCOHOL IN THE DEVELOPMENT OF SHARED EXPERIENCES, SELF-PRESERVATION, AND CONNECTING TO A NEW COMMUNITY

Alcohol played an important social function in the lives of undergraduates. Having been disconnected from their previous communities and from parental control, students came to college looking to exercise this freedom and hoping to connect themselves to their new environment. Finding such a connection was often difficult. Students described themselves as feeling overwhelmed, nervous, afraid to be themselves, and afraid to initiate interaction with others. Alcohol was talked about as a means of overcoming this anxiety. Alcohol consumption also symbolized the exercise of freedom and served as a shared life experience that formulated an initial bond among first-year students. This common bond resulted in friendships which transcended the limitations of physical space and served to construct a community. Alcohol, for better or for worse, was one medium these students talked about as helpful in this process of building or connecting themselves to the college or university community.

Freedom—Out from Under Parental Control

Overwhelmingly, students' accounts suggested that alcohol consumption in college was related to alcohol being a controlled substance in this country, one which high-school-aged and most first-year college students were not free to consume. For instance, one student suggested:

> And a lot of people—like Stan[3] was saying—like there is alcohol and drugs in your high school and you can't do that much because you have to go home to your parents. And here, you don't have to go home to anybody. You can go home stumbling drunk and nobody is going to know because your roommate is going to help you get in and they are going to direct you to your bed.

Students described this lack of connection as a "totally different experience" of freedom or independence.

> I went from like a real strict . . . my parents were like real strict and always kept an eye on me to make sure I didn't drink. They didn't know, but I did, and I'd have to come home and chew gum and stuff like that. I came here and no one kept an eye on me; you could go out as late as you want. It was a totally different experience.

These new freedoms must naturally be tested in order to explore the limitations of the authority and the rules of this new environment:

> It seems that as I remember, when you are a freshman, you just want to test the authority. I mean, it's your first time out and you just want to test all the rules around you. I guess that is sort of natural.

What we heard from students was that their parents usually "policed" their alcohol consumption in high school. But parents were no longer connected to students' lives in a way that ensured that such rules were followed. At least initially, college students saw alcohol consumption as a symbolic act, one which meaningfully expressed this freedom. This was most clearly characterized as independence from parental control. Alcohol may be a substance legally monitored in our country, but for most students, parents monitored alcohol consumption. Parents checked students' breath after parties, told them they could not drink in their rooms and stay up all night, and disciplined them if they were so drunk they had to be walked home and put into bed after being sick. Students equated the absence of parental control with the feeling of freedom and independence in college.

Making These Unknown Faces Known and "Fitting in"— The Role of Alcohol in "Loosening up" or "Breaking Down the Walls" Between Yourself and Others and Developing a "Circle of Friends"

The need to connect to the college community accompanied the freedom or disconnection from parents that college students experienced. This connection was a component of freedom; students were now open to experience a wide range of new religious, cultural, and sexual beliefs and practices. As one male respondent, a fourth-year student, stated:

> You're just in a totally new environment . . . I think when you come to a place like [this university] it's just like culture . . . culture shock. You just think whoa, like different religions, different races, different sexual preferences . . ."

In this sea of diversity, college students spoke of the importance of finding one's friends or finding one's "niche" in this community. One third-year female student, when asked what advice she would give incoming students, responded in the following way:

> I would say that find your group of friends and make them very important in your life because it's a big school and you're not going to have anybody to turn to if you don't have your friends, even if you have friends far away. Watch yourself when you're out because it's going to be a totally different atmosphere than a high school party and there won't be 30 kids there and everyone you know. Watch what you do; make sure you're always with somebody.

Like these students, others we spoke with thought finding one's niche or circle of friends was essential to college survival. This meant having people who were important to him/her; they could go out together socially, talk casually about life, and share the responsibilities, trials, and tribulations associated with college life. Initially, finding these people and developing this niche was described as quite threatening. Living with 50 new people on a dormitory floor or, as the above excerpt suggested, going to a party with hundreds of unknown faces was an entirely new, different, and often difficult experience to navigate.

Students described the role of alcohol in navigating through all of these unknown faces. One female third-year student, when asked if freshmen went out with the intention of drinking to "oblivion" (a word she used to describe this behavior), explained:

> It makes . . . it makes you less self-conscious; I mean, coming out of high school and going into college and not knowing anybody and then you need . . . you feel like you need to, you know, fit in with other people in this social environment and to meet people. So if you don't know anybody when you go to these huge parties, you know, I guess if you know you're not drinking you're going to feel nervous and I think that it loosens you up.

A male second-year student recounted a similar feeling:

> I think it's more of a . . . I think it's more of not knowing the other people around you and I guess that leads to drinking so you feel that you can drink and you're going to be able to go outside of your group; you know, maybe talk to other people and you would approach it better than before.

Many of the students suggested that friends often drank in their dorm room or apartment before going out. When asked about this practice, students explained that it helped overcome shyness. As one student stated, he was "too shy to just go up to someone I don't know in a bar or at a party and just start talking to them." He then explained:

> I think it makes it easier. I think it definitely . . . I think there is a wall around you when you're not drinking and it's kind of . . .

it's a wall . . . that I don't know if it's self-disclosure, but you don't let people see part of yourself. You keep that in. And, then once you start drinking, it's kinda like the bricks you start bringing down and taking them off and you let people see more of who you are and there's a point when you're drinking, I think, that lets you bring out yourself . . . that lets you . . . relaxes everything and you just become yourself.

These passages highlight commonly held beliefs among college students regarding the "power" or usefulness of alcohol in social situations. For first-year students, most college parties (unlike the familiar high school parties) consisted of more than "30 kids and everyone you know." Individuals experienced the discomfort described above; they did not know anyone, and opening up and initiating conversation was difficult. Students were afraid they would not fit in and be liked by others in this community. For students, these feelings explained the increased and often overindulgent drinking that occurred. Students spoke of alcohol as a social lubricant. They believed alcohol alleviated nervousness by decreasing inhibitions which normally protected or preserved the "self" and separated them from other students. Reducing this fear of rejection helped students initiate interactions with unknown others in a threatening and overwhelming social circumstance.

Feeling Connected to Others in the Community—The Role of Drinking and "Drinking Stories"

While undergraduates believed that drinking facilitated interaction with others, participation in alcohol-related activities was also the basis for bonding. Drinking activities fostered group participation. These shared experiences, as well as the stories students told together about these experiences afterward, forged a common bond among undergraduates. It was this common bond that created lasting friendships and connected students to this community. For instance, in college dormitories, students' responses indicated that alcohol was one experience students shared. This was the basis for many friendships.

I lived in a freshman dorm on Riley campus. My whole floor was freshman and my Preceptor [Resident Advisor] didn't

control it at all, basically. So there was a lot of drinking and a
lot of staying up all hours and making noise. He didn't mind
that we never slept. He didn't care that we never slept. Most of
the floor failed out of what they had started as; we had a very
bad floor. We are still friends, the ones that are still here.

This student's dormitory was comprised of all first-year students.
Using "we" to refer to this group, the student indicated some bond
existed among these individuals. Additionally, the shared experience emphasized in this passage was the staying up late and drinking—"we never slept." In concluding, the respondent pointed out
that those individuals described as drinking and staying up late
together remained friends. This implied that drinking together was
one shared experience (important enough to mention) for developing a community where the friendships forged lasted beyond the
time spent living together.

One way these bonds were developed was through a process of
shared storytelling. After partaking in a drinking experience, students discussed telling and retelling stories, among friends, about
these encounters. For instance, one male student told a "drinking
story" he shared with some family members while in high school.
When asked if this was a story he continued to tell he replied:

Yeah, we joke about it, oh God yeah. I mean, I've gotten
birthday cards with like purple circles on it (reference to the
story) and it's just like an ongoing joke in my family . . . yeah.
But in college, huh God. Oh man. I'm kinda disappointed with
college . . . like my whole aspect of social life sucks here. Like
with, I think [this college] has a horrible social life; I think
because it's so spread out.

A female student, when asked the same question, laughed and
said, "Oh yeah, we laugh about it; we laughed about it for a while."
Both replies suggested that talking about such encounters or sharing
drinking stories with other participants occurred regularly. Note the
juxtaposition of the sharing of family-related drinking stories with
the first respondent's criticism of his social life at college. We were
told that his college social life "sucks," for it is too spread out. The
implication is that the closeness experienced with family members,

through sharing such stories, was not a part of this student's social experience in college. In fact, he was unable to recall a story he has continued to tell with college friends.

The accounts given by undergraduates suggested that alcohol-related activities, which, importantly, included the telling and retelling of "drinking stories," were a common thread binding undergraduates together. These drinking stories undergraduates shared were significant, for they were a way of communicating to those participating that the ways seeing events, relationships, and the world were shared. This built a common bond between students, constructed a community for them, and made them feel as though they fit in.

FREEDOM, SELF-PROTECTION, AND RESPONSIBILITY FOR ONE'S SELF: ADD ALCOHOL AND SEX AND STIR

Much like alcohol consumption, undergraduates talked about sexual practices as expressions or behaviors tightly monitored by parents. In this section, we will look at how gender, sexual behavior, and alcohol consumption were interwoven for students. As we pointed out in the previous section, students believed that alcohol reduced the fear and anxiety that inhibited conversation initiation. In addition to facilitating social interactions of both a sexual and nonsexual nature, alcohol played another important role in the sexual practices of undergraduates. Students spoke of alcohol as an "excuse" which could be used to deny responsibility for engaging in sexual practices deemed socially unacceptable in this community. This excuse making afforded students the freedom to experiment sexually while "saving face" or absolving themselves of the social ramifications that followed certain sexual interactions.

For students, these excuses were closely tied to the meaning of sex, and the gendered sexual roles men and women played in this community. For this reason, we need to first develop what sex or "hooking-up" meant to students. Then, we can begin to look at and understand the role of alcohol and excuse making.

Defining Hooking Up—Developing a Context for Understanding Excuse Making

Students called their sexual encounters "hook-ups."[4] When asked what constituted a "hook-up," both men and women initially provided a physical definition of the extent of sexual involvement. Both felt that a kiss does not constitute a hook-up. As one male stated:

> Well, it depends how much you're kissing. If you just get a kiss on the lips and that's it and you leave, that's not a hook-up. And there's gotta be some stuff involved—I mean a little roll around and smooching and doing all that. I mean . . . that . . . that I mean there's definitely a little bit more involved. But, I mean you don't have to have sex with the person to hook-up.

A female respondent defined hooking-up similarly:

> **Respondent:** Hooking up is . . . I guess it is anything other than kissing.
> **Interviewer:** Oh, okay. So kissing is not hooking up?
> **Respondent:** Nah, you can just kiss a guy (unclear). Hooking up is like anything that you do past . . . I would say . . . kissing.

The physical dimensions of hooking-up were quite similar for men and women—hooking-up required that one did more than kiss, though it was not necessary that the two have sexual intercourse.

Hooking-up also had a social dimension. One male student shared the following account:

> So, usually it was just that night . . . no big deal, but with my luck, I always saw them on campus the next week. God forbid. But it didn't last longer than that. It just goes on, you fool around with them and then move on . . . I guess some people expect a relationship from it. I certainly never did. Who would want to meet like that? You met in a drunken stupor, naked in the backyard of some fraternity in the snow. That's not the way to meet anybody.

There was little to suggest this respondent saw his behavior as not respectable. However, it was clear from this account that he would never develop a relationship with a woman with whom he hooked up. He implied this "one-night stand" was not entirely acceptable for women, but it was not problematic for him. Another male student felt similarly:

> I know some girl that drank me under the table. And one girl told me, she said, "If I go out, if my lipstick is still on at the end of the night, I consider it a failure." I don't know, but this isn't the kinda girl I'd want to date.

There are two points these account highlighted. First, hooking up is, for most students, a one-time encounter with someone they typically do not know. Second, these accounts suggested the existence of a double standard. It was not problematic for men to "hook-up," but women's engaging in this type of sexual behavior was socially unacceptable.

Women described this same double standard. One student described this in the following way:

> I've done a lot of talking with people about that, and they think that a drunk woman is really disgusting, but she's like an easy and quick lay. So that's what they see them as. So the people I know that are in fraternities that have girlfriends, they wouldn't tolerate their girlfriends being drunk that way. They don't want them to be sober, but to be in control of themselves and to be like clean.

Again, this student's account suggested a difference existed between those women who were "clean" and someone's "girlfriend" and those women who were "dirty" and hooked up with men to whom they were uncommitted. While social implications existed for women who hooked up, men who did the same were neither mentioned nor faulted in these accounts. Other women we spoke with did depict the behavior of some men as "disgusting." These men were said to "get women drunk and take advantage of them." While this did cast blame on the male who hooked up, the labels women received for hooking up (weak, passive, dirty, naive) seemed more severe.

There was, however, some evidence in the responses given by three of the participants that men and women who hook up should be viewed similarly. One male respondent suggested this when asked if men and women who hook up were viewed differently. He stated:

> I think if you're thinking sexually, I think I don't really hold that in high regards with anybody. I don't respect that at all in people. If you're going to have . . . I don't hold it against people, but I don't think of that person as any greater if they had sex with the person.

One female respondent said, "As far as I'm concerned, hooking up *should* be viewed equally for men and women." Another female respondent suggested that hooking up is just a game, one which both men and women can play.

> And you may think that that person . . . you may think that person likes you and they may like you, but you may be one of ten people. So that took a lot for me to get used to. So I just play the game.

Such statements indicted that while there was a double standard in this community, some saw it as unfair. These views, however, were marginally represented in this data set.

That Wasn't Me; It Was the Beer: Alcohol and Excuse Making

Within this context of gender and sexual practices, we can come to see how, after one engages in sexual encounters thought to be socially unacceptable, alcohol-related excuses function to defer responsibility from the individual to one's excessive consumption of alcohol.

Both men and women used alcohol as an excuse for the previous night's sexual behavior. When asked if alcohol was ever used as an excuse after hooking up, one male responded:

> Like, if they hook up with someone that they weren't inter-ested in, or you heard the term beer goggles, you see someone

that isn't attractive. You might regret doing something with someone and you'd be like, "Oh, I was drunk" and think it's just an excuse to make you feel better.

A female respondent responded similarly:

> **Respondent:** Um, well, if we do something really stupid, we'll say, "Oh my God, I was so drunk last night." I mean I don't think it's an excuse, but it's definitely a reason—it's definitely a reason. But I think when you're drunk . . . I think your true self comes out. I really do, because you say things to somebody that you normally wouldn't say to them. Not because you're not thinking it normally, but because you don't think that you can say it. Because of the social restraints on you, you would just . . . I know I just would go up to a guy and say, "You're so cute. Oh my gosh." But at a party, if you're talking to him, you know you might say, "I always thought you were so cute."
> **Interviewer:** And, so alcohol generally isn't used as an excuse? Like if I hooked up with him or her last night because I was drunk?
> **Respondent:** No, it's said. It's definitely said.

These responses indicated that both men and women used alcohol as an excuse for sexual behavior. Males, however, talked about alcohol as an excuse for "beer goggling"—hooking up with people who the person would not normally find attractive. On the other hand, the female respondents used alcohol as an excuse for engaging in behaviors, sexual or otherwise, that were typically socially restrained.

While women suggested alcohol was often an excuse for socially unacceptable sexual behavior, they did not go into detail about how and when they used excuses. Men, however, stated explicitly how such excuses were used. One male student suggested he would have "some explaining to do if the person is ugly or something." Another told us that "you might wake up in the morning or the next day and go, 'What the hell did I do?'" Men also discussed women's use of drinking excuses. For instance, these students told us:

Student 1: I think some girls use it as an excuse. I've seen like in bed, like one girl hook up and the next day she is like, "Oh my God, I was drunk," and the next time I see her, she does it again; it is "Oh my God, I was drunk." And they just do it and then they think just because they were drunk, it was okay. They make themselves feel better because they were drunk. In a sense, they know exactly what they were doing.

Interviewer: Why do you suppose that is?

Student 1: Guilt, because she doesn't want to look like a slut; so she gives an excuse like that.

Student 2: A lot of people take that to be. I guess it is as far as I figure, you would say it is socially unacceptable to sleep with a different person every night for an entire semester. It would be dangerous. I know women who do that—try to rationalize their behavior.

From the males' perspective, women either used alcohol as an excuse to engage in sexual behavior deemed socially unacceptable, to alleviate the feelings of guilt, or to avoid negative social labeling (e.g., "slut") that may result after engaging in socially unacceptable sexual behavior. The absence of this type of discussion among women respondents may suggest women were less inclined to publically discuss their sexual practices.[5]

According to undergraduates, alcohol was both a lubricant in initial interactions and an excuse for engaging in some forms of sexual activity. As an excuse, alcohol allowed students to experiment and engage in sexual activities while avoiding the social repercussions that might follow such behavior. What this community deemed sexually appropriate and inappropriate shaped students' feelings of "guilt" and thereby influenced the ways alcohol was used as an excuse for one's behavior.

LEARNING THE DOs AND DON'Ts OF COLLEGE DRINKING: STUDENTS' PERCEPTIONS OF THE NEGATIVE CONSEQUENCES OF DRINKING, AND LEARNING TO AVOID THESE CONSEQUENCES

Faced with the freedom and independence to act as they see fit, students described the process by which they learned to consume alcohol responsibly as a process of "growth" or maturation which occurred naturally through experience and mistake making. In developing an understanding of how students see this learning process occurring for themselves and others, we will begin by discussing how students viewed the negative social and sexual consequences of excessive consumption. Then, we will discuss how students talked about learning to avoid these negative consequences while still managing to fit into a community in which one's participation in alcohol-related events was, for many, a critical dimension of social acceptance.

Going Too Far—Talking About the Negative Consequences of Excessive Drinking

Students were aware of the negative consequences that can be associated with excessive alcohol consumption. In all cases, the negative consequences that students spoke of were associated with the loss of control over one's behavior. This loss of control was described as taking several forms. For some, the most serious implications of losing control were related to sexual interactions. Under the influence of alcohol, it was often more likely that students could be "taken advantage of" or "take advantage of others" sexually. Additionally, many students mentioned that people make more impulsive and less rational decisions in regard to sexual behavior when intoxicated.

For instance, one student suggested that under the influence of alcohol, men take advantage of women sexually:

> . . . a girl who lived on the floor that he went pretty far with that night, and when it comes down to it, he says that he has too much beer, he was drunk . . . It was just a chance to take advantage of somebody.

In another description of the same kind of problem resulting from excessive alcohol, a student said:

> The guys that are looking for a really drunk girl . . . you see a girl walk in that has had too much to drink and all of the sudden guys are looking at her, checking her out, and they

know that will probably have a better chance with her than somebody who is more sober.

These responses suggested students were aware that drinking influenced their sexual interactions. Those partaking in the encounter may lose control and be taken advantage of sexually (typically females) or take advantage of others (typically male behavior) in ways that would not normally occur without the excessive consumption of alcohol.

In addition, the impulsive decisions that students often talked about making in terms of sexual interactions, such as "hooking up too fast" resulted in a variety of relationship problems. As one student explained:

> . . . girls who have gotten up the next morning totally regretting what they did with some guy or somebody on the floor, and just didn't want to face them the next day. There are a lot of situations where if they hadn't have been drinking, they wouldn't have done the things they did.

Beyond regretting one's actions, students suggested that "hooking up too fast" was often unexpected. As one male respondent stated: ". . . there have been chicks I met at a party and you get along good and not that I wasn't ready, it was just like, I didn't expect to hook up after the first night or something." Also, another male student suggested that meeting while under the influence of alcohol was not the way to develop a relationship with a person:

> A girl that I like was drinking and I see her drinking to the point where she is totally gone and I'm like, "stop," because I would really rather develop a real relationship with her, than to have it alcohol-based or whatever.

Students also mentioned problems related to relationship fidelity. As one student stated: "Women usually try to pick up on other girls' boyfriends and stuff, and guys are usually drunk and usually go with them."

Students were aware of the sexual and relational ramifications associated with drinking to excess. Yet no one interviewed was advocating that these were reasons not to drink. Rather, these seemed to be, for some students, reason to avoid drinking to excess.

Students Learn from Their Own Experiences About Drinking

When asked about how students learned to avoid drinking to excess, students consistently explained that while some "rules" (e.g., not drinking on an empty stomach, not chugging, not doing shots, and drinking liquor before beer) were talked about, they felt that such rules simply had to be learned by doing. Through their own experiences with alcohol, students could come to know what they personally could and could not do in terms of their limits and capacity for alcohol consumption. For instance:

> The first time I got drunk, I puked and I got really sick and ugly. I realized that drinking a lot is not a whole lot of fun.

Drinking and learning to handle it was about students testing the limits of their newly found freedom and independence and learning from those experiments and experiences. As one student described a drinking experience:

> It was the worst experience of my life. I thought I was going to die; I wanted to die. I will never do it again, ever.

When students talked about their initial experiences with alcohol in college, they suggested at the end of these stories that they "grow out of" or "grow into" these new situations. For instance, one student explained:

> And even if people start exploiting that [alcohol] and after a while, you get tired of it, you start waking up on Saturday morning and you can't think because your head is pounding so bad; after a while, people just grow out of it; I don't need to do that anymore.

Another student recounted a similar experience:

> . . . Like I had beers or whatever when I came here, you know. I never yakked [vomited] in high school. When I came here, I

yakked. I don't think it has gotten to the point where I was one of those people who were restricted in high school and every night I was passed out. I mean . . . you know, I have gradually grown into it.

What we heard from students was that they saw their experiences with alcohol as learning experiences. Learning how to drink in a more responsible manner (which according to these students, would be defined as avoiding the hurtful, negative outcomes associated with overconsumption of alcohol, making sure one arrives home safely, and avoiding feeling physically ill the following day) is spoken about as a growing experience. This may be seen as a growth into the independence from parental control associated with being a college student. Thus, the freedom to consume alcohol as well as learning how to consume alcohol in a way that these students felt was responsible or unproblematic, was an important aspect of college life which, according to students, required experiencing things for oneself, experimenting, making mistakes, and learning from one's mistakes.

CONNECTING THE STUDENTS' VOICES WITH THE RESEARCH ON COLLEGE ALCOHOL CONSUMPTION, SEXUAL PRACTICE, AND EXPERIENTIAL LEARNING THEORY

Drinking has been and continues to be an important facet of college life (Maddox, 1970; Straus and Bacon, 1953). Research since the mid 1960s indicates that approximately 90 percent of college students report occasional alcohol use (Berkowitz and Perkins, 1989; Hughes and Dodder, 1983; Wechsler and McFadden, 1979.) For most undergraduates, patterns of alcohol consumption vary over the course of their college careers. Typically, students' alcohol consumption increases after arriving at college (Berkowitz and Perkins, 1989; Friend and Koushki, 1984). However, as Harford, Weschler, and Rohman (1983) suggest, at least for most women, frequent heavy drinking decreases as years in school increase. And, for both men and women, frequent light drinking is more likely as students progress through college.

While these findings suggest that drinking may be both frequent and heavy for some (particularly in the first year of college) the motivation for most college drinking is social (Montgomery, Benedicto, and Hammerlie, 1993). Additionally, most students do not report using alcohol to "drink their troubles away" but, rather, use alcohol to enhance positive emotions (Carey, 1993). While these findings suggest that the majority of college drinkers are not problem drinkers, it is important to note that even when the drinking itself is not problematic, students do still experience problems or negative consequences when drinking. However, these are negative consequences that students normally try to minimize and avoid (Werch and Gorman, 1988).

When it comes to alcohol and sexual behaviors, research suggests a sizable population of students take sexual risks when under the influence of alcohol. Students have one-night stands or hook up with people they do not know and engage in sexual relations under the influence of alcohol that they would typically avoid. And, students who know to protect themselves from STDs such as chlamydia, gonorrhea, genital herpes, and HIV and AIDS infections by using a condom, do not do so when they have been drinking prior to sexual intercourse (Cooper and Pierce, 1991; Robertson and Plant, 1988; Flannigan and Hitch, 1986).

Our findings are consistent with these studies. However, rather than focusing on a single aspect of students' experiences with alcohol and sex, we have attempted to forge connections and paint a larger picture. Our goal is to elucidate how undergraduates see and understand their own experiences and begin to explain *why* some college students drink and engage in risky sex. What seems to pull these pieces together into a coherent picture is echoed in the responses of the students to whom we spoke: Drinking and sexual practices are closely tied to students' struggles to balance the desire to exercise freedom and independence with the need to learn to control this newfound freedom. And, most students eventually develop ways of managing these new freedoms which they are initially eager to exploit.

Of importance is the social function alcohol plays in this community. Students recount feeling a great deal of anxiety when first arriving at college. Students spoke of two interrelated sources of anxiety. The first is associated with going away to college. Students are no longer attached to a community in which they are told how to act, as well as how to interpret the actions of others. Students were not sure where they fit into this community, and they were eager to forge a new connection by developing a "circle" or "niche" of friends. The process by which such a network of friends is developed is laced with the fear of rejection and not fitting in. This fear of rejection, students believe, can be managed by alcohol consumption. Alcohol eases social interactions and provides the basis for bonding with other students. Through activities that focus on alcohol consumption, initial contacts are made and deeper, stronger bonds developed.

Second, student discussions depict how alcohol consumption and sexual interaction are intimately interwoven. While on one hand, alcohol reduces one's fear of rejection and facilitates initial sexual interaction, such interaction can also be impeded and distorted by the consumption of alcohol. Individuals under the influence of alcohol often engage in sexual activities they later regret, and act in ways that are emotionally and physically hurtful to the person with whom they hook up. When such negative outcomes arise, alcohol can often be a useful excuse for deferring the blame away from the individual and onto the alcohol. While excuse making may defer blame, it can do little to eliminate the health risks associated with high-risk sexual practices.

Students did feel they learned important lessons about alcohol consumption and sexuality in college. However, the picture students paint does not suggest that they learned about drinking and sexuality from classroom lectures, workshops, books, or pamphlets, even when those were available to them. Rather, students spoke about learning from their own experiences and experiences shared with others. What students thought of those experiences and how they interpreted them greatly influenced the behaviors that followed later.

The learning process that students describe can be explained by applying experience-based learning theory. Beginning with the work of Dewey in the 1920s and continuing throughout the rest of the century with the work of Piaget in the 1930s and 1940s, Lewin's work in the 1950s and 1960s, and Kolb's work in the 1980s, the process involved in learning experientially has been articulated.

These insights, taken together, form a theory of experiential or experience-based learning (Kolb, 1984; Lederman, 1992) that provides a useful way of understanding how college students use their experiences with alcohol and sex to teach themselves and one another about drinking and sexuality.

While Dewey identifies the concept of the "impulse" which precedes all learning, it is in the work of Lewin in the 1960s that the processes involved in experiential learning may be most clearly modeled. Lewin (cited in Kolb, 1984) explains experiential learning processes as cyclical. The process begins with an experience. This experience is followed by the observation of that experience, the interpretation of what is observed, trial and error in applying what was learned, and new ways of dealing with these experiences. The cycle continues as initial actions inform future experiences. Kolb (1984) suggests that all knowledge is socially constructed. The process of learning through experience takes place in a social context, and the social context has a role in shaping the learner's experiences. This aspect of the model is critical for it provides a relational or social dimension to the learning process.

This theory of experiential learning may explain how students learn about alcohol and sex and why students do not necessarily learn what and when administrators and health educators would like them to. Students do talk about learning, but because college students live in a community in which the normative behaviors typically condone alcohol consumption and sexual experimentation, students do not learn to curtail their drinking behavior or take the necessary precautions prior to sexual intercourse from their peers. In fact, we see from this analysis that drinking behaviors are often reinforced by other students through group drinking activities and sharing of "drinking stories" afterward amongst friends.

Students do learn to avoid those consequences that are not accepted in their college community. Students talk about learning how to moderate or avoid drinking in ways that help them maintain control and avoid the negative consequences associated with drinking and hooking up—while still feeling as though they fit into a community in which there is a premium placed on alcohol consumption and social acceptance. They learn about moderation through harsh, personal experience. Most students are fortunate enough to avoid the most extreme consequences that may be associated with drinking and sexual experimentation. They talk about receiving bad grades, feeling ill after drinking, or feeling bad about themselves after hooking up as experiential moments when they realize they have to change their habits. Such experiences may change students' interpretations of their experiences, forcing self-reflection, and result in more reasonable drinking and sexual practices.

This, however, is not the case for all students. Not all students learn the same lessons from their experiences (Kolb, 1984). For some, a hangover can be an experience that catalyzes a change in drinking behavior; for others, a near-death experience may not result in any changes in behaviors. Most problematic in this college community is the interpretive spiral that may perpetuate these behaviors. It is virtually impossible for heavy drinkers and those who engage in risky sexual practices, who interact and have friends who do the same, to see the signs of problem drinking or the sexual risks they are taking. Behaviors which might be met with disapproval among other students are often met with reinforcement among a group of individuals who have similar patterns of behavior. The result is that students caught in such spirals may not have experiences from which to learn that their behavior is excessive and dangerous. When they do finally have such experiences it may be too late.

CONCLUSION

Our understanding of how students learn about excessive alcohol consumption and unsafe sexual behavior suggests that measures administrators and health educators are currently taking may ultimately not succeed. By instituting more rules which are meant to control underage drinking, institutions are increasing students' desire to exercise their freedom and rebel against authority. These rules also fail to address the unsafe sexual practices that threaten students' lives. In addition, lecture-like sessions, books, and pamphlets meant to inform students of the risks of drinking are likely to be unsuccessful, for students themselves suggest they learn from engaging in an active experience-based learning process, not one which is passive. These findings suggest that successful programs must facilitate active learning and allow students to make mistakes, while providing peer and professional assistance to help students to learn from their mistakes.

Most heavy drinkers left to learn from their own mistakes will learn, without doing harm to themselves or others, how to balance their freedom and social needs with the responsibility for their own well-being and academic work. However, allowing this learning process to occur naturally has some serious implications for alcoholics who are not yet aware that they have the disease, heavy drinkers whose behaviors are reinforced by peers, and those students who take sexual risks. For each of these groups, programs need to be developed that will simulate the natural learning process and help students feel they are learning from their own mistakes and experiences. Additional research should be conducted about how students learn about alcohol and sex and new educational programs that take students' learning processes into account should be developed.

There is still a great deal to be learned about the gender differences that arose in this analysis. While we assume that we live in an age where men and women are equal, and we hope that the academic community is one in which this equality is unquestioned, we see that there is a significant double standard which exists in terms of sexual practices for male and female undergraduates. What is socially acceptable in the college community for men, is not acceptable for women, particularly in terms of sexuality. We need to understand how women view their own sexuality in this community, and how they come to see themselves as sexual beings. Future research should explore these issues in greater detail and new educational programs should be developed that recognize the gendered nature of sexual experimentation.

This research project focused on the drinking and sexual behaviors of heterosexual college students of a single ethnic group. Future work should seek to understand such behaviors among members of a variety of ethnic groups, people who engage in same-sex sexual activity, and people of various ages, social classes, and educational levels. A research program with these foci would facilitate a broader understanding of the issues we have started to address in this project.

Colleges and universities provide protected environments within which students can experiment with new thoughts and ideas. Our research suggests that the challenge to health educators in college settings is to make the environments within which alcohol and sexual experimentation occur more protected by helping students to learn from their experiences and providing support for those who do not.

NOTES

1. FIPSE funded project from the U.S. Department of Education, 1989.

2. Rutgers University Health Service Anonymous Survey, 1987.

3. All of the names used are fictitious in order to protect the identities of participants.

4. "Hooking up" was a term I was familiar with prior to beginning this project for it was commonly used when I was in college. This suggests that it is a term that is a common part of the vocabulary at many colleges and universities; thus, it is not unique to this one university or to the students we interviewed.

5. While such a suggestion would be consistent with the findings of this analysis, such an explanation is not evidenced in our data. It might be worthwhile to conduct research that would focus on showcasing the voices of women in regard to such sexual behaviors.

REFERENCES

Berkowitz, A.D. and Perkins, H.W. (1986). Problem drinking among college students: A review of recent research. *Journal of American College Health, 35*, 21-28.

Carey, K.B. (1993) Situational determinants of heavy drinking among college students. *Journal of Counseling Psychology, 40*(2), 217-220.

Center for Substance Abuse. (1992). *Making the Link: Sex Under the Influence of Alcohol and Other Drugs.*

Cooper, M.L. (1992). Alcohol and increased behavioral risk for AIDS. *Alcohol and Health Research World, 16*(1), 64-72.

Cooper, M.L. and Pierce, R.S. (1991). Sex differences in alcohol use and sexual risk taking. Paper presented to the annual meeting of the American Psychological Association, San Francisco, CA.

Engs, R.C. (1977). Drinking patterns and drinking problems of college students. *Journal of Alcohol Studies, 38*(21), 2144-2156.

Fisch-Lewis, D. and Goodhart, F. (1995). A report of the New Jersey college health survey: Findings from a statewide youth risk behavior assessment. New Brunswick, NJ: NJCCHE, Willets Health Center, Rutgers University, and U.S. Public Health Services, Centers for Disease Control and Prevention.

Flannigan, B.J. and Hitch, M.A. (1986). Alcohol use, sexual intercourse, and contraceptives: An exploratory study. *Journal of Alcohol and Drug Education, 31*(3), 6-40.

Friend, K.E. and Koushki, P.A. (1984). Student substance use: Stability and change across college years. *International Journal of Addiction, 19,* 571-575.

Harford, T.C., Wechsler, H., and Rohman, M. (1983). The structural context of college drinking. *Journal of Studies on Alcohol, 44*(4), 722-731.

Harvey, S.M. and Beckman, L.J. (1986). Alcohol consumption, female sexual behavior, and contraceptive use. *Journal of Studies on Alcohol, 47*(4), 327-332.

Hughes, S.P. and Dodder, R.A. (1983). Alcohol consumption patterns among college populations. *Journal of College Student Perspectives, 24,* 257-264.

Kolb, D.A. (1984). *Experiential Learning: Experience as the Source of Learning and Development.* Englewood Cliffs, NJ: Prentice-Hall.

Lederman, L.C. (1992). *Communication Pedagogy: Approaches to Teaching Undergraduate Courses in Communication.* Norwood, NJ: Ablex.

Leigh, B.C. (1990). Alcohol and unsafe sex: An overview of research and theory. In D. Seminara, A. Pawlowski, and R. Watson (Eds.), *Alcohol, Immunomodulation, and AIDS,* 35-46. New York: Alan R. Liss.

Maddox, G.L. (Ed.). (1970). *The Domesticated Drug: Drinking Among Collegians.* New Haven: College and University Press.

Montgomery, R.L., Benedicto, J.A., and Haemmerlie, F.M. (1993). Personal versus social motivations of undergraduates for using alcohol. *Psychological Reports, 73,* 960-962.

Ratliff, K.G. and Burkhart, B.R. (1984). Sex difference in motivation for and effects of drinking among college students. *Journal of Studies in Alcohol, 45,* 26-32.

Robertson, J.A. and Plant, M.A. (1988). Alcohol, sex, and risks of HIV infection. *Drug and Alcohol Dependence, 22*(1), 75-78.

Stinson, F.S., DeBakey, S.F., Grant, B.F., and Dawson, D.A. (1992). Association of alcohol problems with risk for AIDS in the 1988 National Health Interview Survey. *Alcohol, Health, and Research World, 16*(3), 245-252.

Straus, A. (1987). *Qualitative Analysis for Social Scientists.* New York: Cambridge University Press.

Straus, R. and Bacon, S.D. (1953). *Drinking in College.* New Haven: Yale University Press.

Wechsler, H. and McFadden, M. (1979). Drinking among college students in New England. *Journal of Studies in Alcohol, 40,* 969-996.

Werch, C.E. and Gorman, D.R. (1988). Relationship between self-control and alcohol consumption patterns and problems of college students. *Journal of Studies on Alcohol, 49* (1), 30-36.

PART II:
NEGOTIATING CARE

Chapter 6

Communicating
an HIV-Positive Diagnosis

Lorraine D. Jackson
Michael J. Selby

The incidence of AIDS is increasing faster among women than men and is now the fourth leading cause of death among women aged 25 to 44 years (Horton, 1995, p. 531). As a result, more women are receiving an HIV-positive diagnosis than at any time in history. Yet because truthful disclosure and valuing patient autonomy have only recently become the norm, there is a paucity of research addressing the question of how to communicate a serious diagnosis in a manner that will best enable the patient to adjust.

The disclosure of a serious diagnosis to a patient is a critical communication event. Roth and Nelson (1996) also document the life-changing impact of an HIV-positive diagnosis. In the actual case reported below, a ten-minute segment of time was so vivid that it was etched in the individual's mind for the rest of her life.

Nothing was handled well as far as I'm concerned. On November 14, 1989 at 4 p.m., the doctor called me at home asking me to come in the next day. When I asked if she would tell me something, she just kept stating to come in the next day. I went crazy all night. The next day at 11 a.m., I was waiting in the exam room when the doctor came in and stood in front of me,

The authors wish to acknowledge Beth Breece (California School of Professional Psychology) and Laura Hernandez (California Department of Corrections) for their assistance with data collection.

avoiding eye contact and looking at her papers. She told me I was HIV positive. Needless to say, my whole world came falling in front of my eyes. I asked the doctor if I was going to die and she told me she did not have an answer. The doctor did tell me I needed to have all kinds of tests done right now, and she would refer me to another doctor to care for me. I was given a load of lab slips and a prescription for valium and sent on my way ten minutes later. I felt the doctor could have had more compassion and manners. I also feel the doctor could have given me some idea of what to expect. Just telling me and sending me off in that manner was cruel. I felt very alone. The doctor and the lab gave me a day that I will never forget.

Despite the profound impact of learning of a diagnosis, the consultations in which they are given have yet to receive adequate attention in the health communication literature. Very little is known about patients' perceptions of the delivery of a serious diagnosis *in general*; even less is known about the perceptions of incarcerated women receiving a diagnosis of being HIV positive. This chapter aims to shed light on women's perceptions by reporting both qualitative and quantitative data from incarcerated female patients, some of which have received an HIV-positive diagnosis while incarcerated. Others received their diagnosis prior to their incarceration. Specifically, this chapter will examine these patients' communication needs and the factors corresponding with negative versus positive experiences associated with their HIV-positive diagnosis. Our intention is to provide awareness and information that will help health care professionals to avoid the insensitive and inadequate interaction which often proves to be distressing for both patients and health care professionals.

DEATH, FEAR, AND STIGMA

A diagnosis of HIV (the virus causing AIDS) is devastating to the patient because of its association with death. AIDS is much more than a biomedical phenomenon; it is a socially constructed phenomenon as well. Perhaps more than any other disease in recent history, AIDS has instilled worldwide fear.

It is powerful . . . because it is associated with the perversion of both the vital fluids: Blood and semen are normally the source of life; infected with an AIDS virus, they become agents of death . . . However, ultimately the idea of AIDS is powerful because it is about sex and death together. In all cultures, these are primordial issues, heavy with ambiguity and the oppositions of good and evil . . . because AIDS is associated with sex and death in combination, it carries a double load of symbolic weight. (Wallman, 1988, p. 571)

Wallman (1988) notes the logo chosen by the World Health Organization in 1987 conveys AIDS by the combination of a heart and a skull, accepted representations of sex and death. Cline and Freeman (1988) report that AIDS and death are virtually synonymous in the minds of college students; thus, it is not surprising that in a 1987 poll, it was discovered AIDS is the most feared disease.

Persons with AIDS are stigmatized by this association with death, and are additionally stigmatized because of perceptions regarding intravenous (IV) drug use, prostitution, or homosexuality. Cline (1989) notes that communication typically directed toward the stigmatized is consistent with disconfirmation rather than confirmation. Confirmation/disconfirmation is a relational dimension that implies acceptance or rejection of a person. Disconfirmation includes behaviors such as ignoring the person, discouraging discussion and participation, disaffiliation or distancing, presenting ambiguous messages, and outright rejection in the form of disparaging communication.

In the case outlined earlier, the doctor's words and actions were disconfirming and caused the patient severe distress. In addition to the lack of time spent exploring the patient's feelings, the avoidance of eye contact likely served to heighten feelings of anxiety and isolation. Eye contact often demonstrates interest in another person and indicates receptivity to feedback (Thompson, 1986). The absence of eye contact during interpersonal communication in North America is generally considered deviant. In the case presented earlier, the lack of eye contact may have reflected the physician's fear of the patient's reaction. It was a nonverbal, perhaps unconscious means of evading feedback from the patient. Furthermore, the physician verbalized that she would be referring the patient to another doctor. Although this physician may have had the best intentions when referring the patient to someone else whom she felt was more experienced in the treatment of HIV, this verbal and behavioral disaffiliation tended to exacerbate feelings of abandonment and rejection.

Ideally, a continued presence and ongoing doctor-patient relationship can be a source of social support. However, if referral is necessary, it would be more appropriate to discuss the referral with the patient at a later meeting, and to allow the patient some sense of control by offering choices regarding care. In an initial diagnosis meeting, it is especially important that communication be characterized by confirming messages. However, without highly developed interpersonal communication skills, some health care providers may neglect this aspect of caregiving. In order to understand these issues surrounding caregiving and the candid disclosure of a serious diagnosis, it is first necessary to explore current and historical influences on the doctor-patient relationship.

COMMUNICATION WITH HEALTH CARE PROVIDERS

Physicians are not immune to the fear of death. In fact, the fear of death, fear of uncertainty, and stigma have had powerful effects on health care providers and their communication with patients. Feifel (1976) demonstrated that contrary to what the public might expect, medical students dread death more than other students, and physicians are even more fearful than medical students. Kastenbaum (1967) noted that health care providers often respond with some form of avoidance to dying patients' attempts to discuss their feelings. Avoidance may take the form of changing the subject, false reassurance, or evasion.

Prior to the mid 1960s, patients were routinely deceived about a grave diagnosis. Information was withheld for fear that the truth would harm the patient, and also because of health care providers' discomfort in confronting issues of death and dying (Brody, 1989, p. 79). Katz (1984) explains that this history of nondisclosure is a result of strong psychological forces, designed to protect both the patient and caregiver from the natural fear of uncertainty.

In a 1961 study reported in the *Journal of the American Medical Association*, 90 percent of cancer physicians favored nondisclosure of a cancer diagnosis (Oken, 1961). Interestingly, in a similar study 20 years later, a radical shift became apparent: over 90 percent of physicians favored full disclosure of a cancer diagnosis (Novack, 1979). As evidenced by changing perceptions in the medical community and society concerning *truthful disclosure*, or the delivery to a patient of bad news about a diagnosis, our society is moving away from a paternalistic approach in medicine. We are experiencing a paradigmatic shift whereby paternalism is being replaced by consumerism. There is now greater value placed on patient lucidity and autonomy—the rights of the patient to be fully informed, to participate in decisions about care, and to be self-governing.

Coinciding with these changes, there is a growing body of literature in the social sciences (particularly psychology and communication) in which patient satisfaction is an important outcome variable. Patient satisfaction is a multidimensional variable consisting of *affective*, *behavioral*, and *cognitive* components (Stiles et al., 1979). The *affective* dimension is concerned with such aspects of care as empathy, warmth, and trust. The *behavioral* dimension relates to such behaviors as whether a patient is kept waiting or whether the examination is rushed. The *cognitive* dimension relates to the transmission of information concerning the diagnosis, illness, and treatment. A female patient who is treated warmly, who trusts her doctor, but is given very little information may be satisfied with the affective dimension of care but dissatisfied with the cognitive dimension of care. Clearly, these dimensions overlap and interact with one another, influencing patients' evaluations of general satisfaction. Consequently, when measuring patient satisfaction, researchers need to consider the multidimensional nature of this variable.

Several researchers have described verbal and nonverbal communication behaviors which influence patient satisfaction. These variables include nonverbal immediacy (DiMatteo et al., 1980; Conlee, Olvera, and Vagim, 1993), nontechnical language (Ley, 1983; Jackson, 1992), listening skills (Harrington and Rosenthal, 1983), encouragement and empathy skills (Evans et al., 1989), managing turn taking, and interviewing logically (Novack, 1985).

Patient satisfaction appears to be associated with important outcomes. For example, a positive relationship between satisfaction,
patient compliance, and recovery has been reported in routine medical care (Burgoon et al., 1987; Bass et al., 1986).

While a growing body of research concerns communication variables associated with patient satisfaction, most of the research findings are based on typical medical encounters. As Kreps (1993)
explains, patient satisfaction research has focused primarily on
interpersonal communication patterns during medical interviews.
Although routine medical interviews share some similarities with
consultations in which a grave diagnosis is delivered, there is also
an important difference. A consultation regarding a grave diagnosis
presents a unique communication situation because of the salience
of emotion. A few notable articles discussing strong emotions during such consultations exist. Fallowfield's (1993) essay advises
physicians to prepare for giving sad news, to ensure the patient
understands the message, and to meet the patient's needs after the
consultation. Quill and Townsend (1991) analyze a transcript of one
physician/patient dialogue in which an HIV diagnosis is delivered,
and outline the nature of the patient's needs for information and
emotional support. Pergami and Catalan (1994) report that satisfaction with the manner in which an HIV-positive diagnosis is delivered is associated with the health care provider's attitude and the
amount and quality of the information given. The aforementioned
articles, with the exception of Pergami and Catalan (1994), base
their recommendations on clinical experience, stress intervention
literature and a case study. The present research aims to expand
upon these insights concerning diagnosis consultations. Specifically, there is a need for more data from the patients who receive the
diagnosis, and particularly from females.

Roth and Nelson (1996) observe that pre- and postdiagnosis
counseling for HIV-positive patients is universally advocated; however, data on patients at the time of the diagnosis are largely absent
in the literature. When the topic of truthful disclosure is explored in
the literature, it is often related to medical ethics. Many past medical scholars have spent a great deal of energy debating whether the
patient should be told. Few articles provide explicit, research-based
advice on *how* the patient should be told. Although physicians now

agree that disclosing the truth to a patient is important, many lack the information and skills necessary to deal with the psychosocial aspects of disclosing such news (Fallowfield, 1993). This is an important issue because the insensitive handling of a serious diagnosis may impair the patient's long-term adjustment to that illness. One study assessing anxiety and depression a year after breast cancer treatment found women who perceived that the "bad news" consultation was inappropriately handled were twice as anxious or depressed as those who were satisfied with the manner in which the consultation was handled (Fallowfield, Baum, and Maguire, 1986). In light of this, health professionals have a medical, as well as a social obligation, to attend carefully to patients' communication needs when delivering an HIV-positive diagnosis. Despite the fact that physicians and other health care providers deliver bad news on a regular basis, there is little medical literature about it and almost no formal training which addresses it (Quill and Townsend, 1991).

THE PRESENT RESEARCH PROJECT

This study was designed to provide health care professionals with information to help them identify those communication behaviors that are associated with negative versus positive experiences for women receiving an HIV-positive diagnosis. This research has future implications on how women should be told about their HIV-positive diagnosis.

Subjects and Method

In order to explore incarcerated women's perceptions of communication during HIV-positive diagnosis consultations, 32 females who had previously been diagnosed with HIV were recruited from a central California women's facility. Thirty-eight percent report contracting HIV from intravenous drug use, 44 percent report sexual behavior as the cause, and 18 percent indicated other causes. (Note: when asked to specify, "other" frequently meant "I don't know how I got it.") The women ranged in age from 21 to 56 years, with an average age of 35.5. Twenty of the subjects were black (62.5 percent), six were Hispanic (18.8 percent), four were white (12.5 percent), one was Asian (3.1 percent) and one was Native American (3.1 percent). Fifteen women (48.4 percent) had received their diagnosis from health professionals within the facility, 14 women (45.2 percent) received their diagnosis from health professionals outside of the correctional facility, and the remaining three women (9.3 percent) did not respond to this question.

Each participant completed a questionnaire; women with HIV were asked in Likert format whether their needs for (a) information, (b) emotional support, (c) time to process the information, (d) answers to questions, and (e) arrangements for follow-up and social support were met by their health professionals. Additionally, participants responded in an open-ended format to the following questions:

> Please think back to the time when you were first told you were HIV-positive. What aspects of the appointment were handled well? What aspects were not handled well? Describe in detail who said what. Do you have any advice about how the health professional could have handled this differently?

Women with HIV also completed the Mental Adjustment to HIV Scale, a validated scale consisting of five subscales measuring *Helplessness-Hopelessness*, *Fighting Spirit*, *Denial-Avoidance*, *Fatalism*, and *Belief in Influencing the Course of the Disease* (Ross et al., 1994). This scale was administered to determine the women's psychological adjustment to HIV. Psychological adjustment is important because depression and anxiety are associated with lowered immune system functioning (Bloom, 1988).

RESULTS

Trends in both the quantitative and qualitative data are examined in the analyses. The key variables investigated in relation to positive and negative consultation experiences include (a) the length of time spent with the patient, (b) compassion and attention to feelings, (c) the gender of the health care professional disclosing the diagnosis (d) information and answers given to questions, and (e) arrangements for follow up and social support. The data for each category are presented in the following paragraphs.

Time Spent

The amount of time reportedly spent during the diagnosis consultation ranged from as little as one minute to as much time as four hours, with an average time of 62 minutes. Ten of the subjects spent under 20 minutes with their health professional, and of these, six subjects reported having less than five minutes to discuss the diagnosis with their health professional. Eleven subjects reported having 30 minutes to one hour, nine subjects reported consultations ranging from two to four hours, and two subjects did not reply.

There was a strong correlation between the *amount of time spent* and *satisfaction with amount of time* (r = .62, *p* < .001). In other words, as the amount of time (in minutes) increased, satisfaction also increased. Additionally, the *amount of time* correlated strongly with perceived *amount of information given* (r = .67, p < .001), and *satisfaction with amount of information* (r = .55, p < .01). Correlations also existed between *amount of time* and *satisfaction with attention to feelings* (r = .49, p < .01), *satisfaction with communicating a plan for follow-up* (r = .48, p < .01), *satisfaction with the discussion of a support group* (r = .48, p < .01), and *satisfaction with answers to questions* (r = .42, p < .05).

Finally, the amount of time spent correlated with scores on the Mental Adjustment to HIV scale (MAHIV) (r = .41, p < .05). Women who reported having little time during the diagnosis consultation were not as psychologically well-adjusted to their illness. The importance of the time variable was reinforced in the women's narratives. For example, a 42-year-old African-American female who contracted HIV through drug use writes:

> I feel that every professional should take more time to talk to that person. As for myself, I really felt shoved out the door. I was mad and upset and didn't know what to do. They need to spend more time.

A 33-year-old African-American female who contracted HIV from rape writes:

> The health professional was just that—professional. She was quite compassionate and was willing to spend as much time as

necessary with me to ease the blow and help me understand the conditions involving and surrounding the virus.

Thus, the amount of time the health professional spent with the patient during the diagnosis consultation is a critical variable that has an impact on the patient's perceptions of the entire consultation.

Compassion and Attention to Feelings

When patients were asked whether or not they were satisfied with the health professionals' attention to their feelings, responses tended to polarize toward extreme satisfaction or extreme dissatisfaction; very few subjects were neutral. Approximately two-thirds of the sample (20 subjects) were dissatisfied, while the remaining one-third reported being satisfied with the attention to their feelings. A common theme which emerged in the narratives of the subjects who were dissatisfied depicted a "cold" professional detachment which caused patients considerable anguish. As in the introduction of this chapter, that case illustrated a health professional who focused solely on medical issues (e.g., arranging for lab tests, giving a prescription for valium) without first addressing the patient's psychological pain. This physician engaged in a form of avoidance. This failure to provide socially supportive communication caused the physician to be perceived as lacking in compassion.

Another example of a health care provider neglecting to provide social support can be seen in the following case. This health care provider avoided having to deal with the patient's reaction by first preventing one-on-one communication, and second, by leaving the room promptly. A 43-year-old white female explains:

> I was in _____ county jail. I signed up just to support a friend being tested. When the results came back, the physician called me in a room with my friend and he said to her, "You are negative" and said to me, "You are positive. Thank you, and someone will see you soon." And then he left. That's it! I don't think he even cared at all. They should sit down and at least talk it over and give a chance for the shock to wear off.

Another inappropriate method of delivering the diagnosis can be seen in this 29-year-old's case:

I found out I was HIV-positive in 1990. The health center called my house and told me and that was it.

Similarly, a 40-year-old African-American female who reported she was completely dissatisfied wrote:

I was in another jail and he just told me and I was sent back to my cell to deal with it alone.

Research has shown that the distant stance that was adopted by these physicians and health care professionals serves to protect *them*. Wortman and Lehman (1985) observed that communication about terminal illness may evoke feelings of emotional distress, insecurity, and uncertainty in *physicians and health care providers*. Avoidant behaviors protect these health care professionals from dealing with their own feelings. Additionally, it also prevents them from taking further time for the patient's feelings, and it reduces professional burnout caused by overidentification with the patient (Maguire, 1985).

Unfortunately, this protection is purchased at a price. As Cline (1989) explains, disconfirmation consists of explicit and implicit messages that negate the value of the other person (p. 41). The underlying message the patient receives is something akin to: "Your reaction and feelings are unimportant to me—they do not matter." On an unconscious level, may be perceived as, "You are unimportant—you do not matter." Patients who receive disconfirming messages experience more psychological pain. Facing both a serious diagnosis and feeling alone can be the source of great unnecessary suffering (Cassell, 1982).

In an effort to be compassionate and control the situation, some health professionals may rely on more positive statements than are warranted, thus denying the patient's immediate reality (Cline, 1989, p. 43). This, too, can be disconfirming. A 31-year-old female wrote:

For Mrs. _____ to tell me, "You are HIV-positive, but everything will be all right" wasn't enough. I was mute and frozen. I can't explain it. But I guess what else could she do. I don't know if there is an easy way to tell it.

Being compassionate and communicating in a confirming manner involves more than offering false reassurance or clichés. An HIV-positive diagnosis can pose a serious threat to an individual's self-concept. The patient's feelings should be legitimized and explored.

Women who report supportive experiences tend to have received confirming messages. For example, a 28-year-old Hispanic female writes:

> I feel everything was handled quite well. She spent two hours with me. She was very caring and listened to me when I cried. Later, she explained what we would do and told me about the resources I would need.

In the above case, as in other examples, satisfaction with the caring demeanor of this female health care professional is expressed. Trends concerning the health care provider's gender and satisfaction with attention to feelings were apparent in the women's narratives, and these are explored next.

The Gender of the Health Care Professional

In this sample, 18 of the subjects received their diagnosis from a male, and 14 subjects received their diagnosis from a female. In order to assess whether differences existed between those told by males (Group 1) and those told by females (Group 2), independent samples (*t* tests) were conducted. Patients in Group 1 and Group 2 were asked to indicate their satisfaction with the health professionals' attention to their feelings. A five-point scale was used which ranged from *completely dissatisfied* [1] to *very satisfied* [5]. Female health professional communicators yielded significantly higher satisfaction levels than did males. (Means and standard deviations for females and males were respectively: 3.7, SD = 1.1 and 2.6, SD = 1.4, with $t = -2.40$, $p < .05$). Comparably, significant results were also found for satisfaction with time spent. (Means and standard deviations for females and males were respectively: 3.7, SD = 1.5 and 2.5, SD = 1.3, with $t = -2.24$, $p < .05$.) On average, female health professionals spent more time with patients than males (an average of 20 minutes extra), and this resulted in greater patient satisfaction.

The findings associated with gender are reinforced in the women's narratives. For example, a 29-year-old African-American female who received her diagnosis inside the correctional facility explained:

> When I found out about HIV, I was very satisfied with it. I had a very good RN and she was really good to me. We spent two and a half hours talking it over. I understood everything and know what I have to do to take care of myself.

A 40-year-old African-American respondent who received her diagnosis from a physician outside of a correctional facility wrote:

> He abruptly with callous (sic) informed me of having HIV. He appointed me for follow-up. It seemed as though he was on the other side, pretending and then silently being dominantly macho in himself. Kind of like knowing, "I got her." I didn't appreciate him at all. He was the first doctor to tell me. I still hate him.

The clear differences between gender and patient *satisfaction with attention to feelings* were not paralleled in other findings; no significant gender differences were found between patients' perceptions of health professionals in terms of *satisfaction with answers to questions, amount of information given, satisfaction with the plan for follow-up,* or *satisfaction with discussion of joining a support group.* Nevertheless, each of these variables has a bearing on the quality of the diagnosis consultation.

Information and Answers Given to Questions

Subjects were asked to indicate the amount of information they were given about their illness on a five-point scale. The frequency of responses in each of the following categories is as follows: Nine subjects (28.1 percent) indicated *none,* seven subjects (21.9 percent) indicated *small amount,* nine subjects (28.1 percent) indicated *medium amount,* two subjects (6.3 percent) indicated *large amount,* and five subjects (15.6 percent) indicated *very large amount.* A strong positive correlation existed between the *amount of information given* and *satisfaction with information* ($r = .67$, $p < .001$). In

light of the previously reported correlation between the time variable and *amount of information given,* it is not surprising that
amount of information given correlates with *satisfaction with ability
to answers questions* (r = .50, p < .01), *satisfaction with follow-up*
(r = .40, p < .05), and *satisfaction with attention to feelings* (r = .59,
p < .001). Perhaps the most provocative correlation involves the
relationship between *amount of information given* and *Mental
Adjustment to HIV* scores. As the perceived *amount of information
given* increased, so did mental adjustment (r = .40, p < .05). Additionally, higher *satisfaction with amount of information given* is
associated with higher mental adjustment scores (r = .51, p < .01).

Subjects who spent more time with the health professional during
the diagnosis consultation, who received more information, and were
more satisfied with information tended to be better adjusted. A closer
examination of subfactor correlations revealed that *fighting spirit* and
belief in influencing the course of the disease were also implicated in
this relationship. Women who were reportedly given more information felt there were things they could do to improve their health. A
health professional who takes the time to discuss the difference
between HIV and AIDS, who explains that a person can remain
asymptomatic for years, and who gives information about the importance of maintaining a healthful lifestyle is likely to reduce uncertainty and anxiety for the patient, and to instill feelings of hope. On
the other hand, a patient who encounters a health professional who
does not give this information may view the HIV-positive diagnosis
as an immediate death sentence. The patient is likely to experience
more uncertainty, more anxiety, and possibly more depression. Consider the following narrative from a 41-year-old woman who
reported having a five-minute diagnosis consultation:

> I went to the doctor to get blood test results. He thought I
> might have mono. At any rate, he informed me that my HIV
> test was positive. I didn't know what to say. Basically, I was in
> shock. The doctor just stared at me and said nothing. I left in a
> depression. I don't think some doctors should be giving a
> diagnosis like HIV. It was a nightmare.

This diagnosis consultation is particularly troublesome because not
only was information about HIV lacking, but it appears that there

was no communication regarding a plan for follow-up care and social support.

Arrangements for Follow-Up and Social Support

Subjects were asked how satisfied they were with their health professionals' ability to communicate a plan for follow-up. Nine subjects (28.1 percent) were *completely dissatisfied*, five subjects (15.6 percent) were *somewhat dissatisfied*, six subjects (18.8 percent) were *neutral*, three subjects (9.4 percent) were *somewhat satisfied*, and eight subjects (25 percent) were *completely satisfied* (missing data = 1).

When asked if the health professional discussed joining a support group, 18 subjects (56.3 percent) reported yes and 14 subjects (43.8 percent) reported no. Despite the fact almost half the subjects did not receive the benefit of this discussion, many still found their way into a support group. Twenty-three subjects (72 percent) currently attend a support group and nine (28 percent) are not attending a support group. Support groups serve to provide outlets for the expression of emotions, enable members to gather information, and to reduce uncertainty. Support groups also offer a safe place for adjusting to a new role, and can provide forums to discuss AIDS-related social, political, and medical issues (Cawyer and Smith-Dupre, 1995; Cline and Boyd, 1993). Social support can increase longevity in patients with a serious illness (Weisman and Worden, 1975). The following narrative from a 32-year-old woman discusses the positive impact of social support:

> I've known about having the virus for three years. When first told, it was a great shock to me. But I'm a strong black woman that will live until it is my time to go elsewhere. I feel special having the virus. I enjoy my friends in my support group. I've never had so many friends to talk with me. And I enjoy being able to talk about the virus in hopes it does not happen to others.

DISCUSSION

The primary finding in this study is that women who reported receiving little time for their diagnosis consultation were not as psychologically well-adjusted to their illness. Spending an adequate amount of time appears to be a necessary but insufficient condition to ensure a positive experience during the diagnosis consultation. The willingness of health care professionals to spend time with the patient appears to be associated with the ability to demonstrate compassion and attend to the patient's needs. Because most patients have such strong emotional reactions, including shock, patients will likely have questions after the initial meeting, and should feel they will be given the opportunity for continued information and support. Balancing emotional and informational needs is a process that should continue over time. Quill and Townsend (1991) advise that a plan for how to inform and involve the patients' significant others should also be discussed. With such a plan, the health professionals reduce the patients' feelings of isolation.

The multidimensional nature of patient satisfaction, particularly the affective, behavioral, and cognitive elements, must be considered. In addition to wanting health care providers who take the time to provide emotional support, patients also want information. As Pergami and Catalan (1994) report, the quality of the information given and the attitude of the person giving the diagnosis are associated with satisfaction in this sample as well. Furthermore, appropriately giving information appears to have additional effects beyond satisfaction. Women who report having more information are also psychologically better adjusted and more likely to believe they can do things to improve their health. For these reasons, information and education about HIV should be delivered over time, and health professionals should maintain a patient-centered approach whereby information is tailored to the individual.

This study also was concerned with the differences regarding gender and patient satisfaction. A likely explanation for the observed differences concerning gender and patient satisfaction with attention to feelings involves gender role socialization. Thompson (1986) asserts, "Due to socialization differences, men and women frequently have different orientations toward people and problems" (p. 15). One possible area of difference concerns perceived empathy. To be empathetic involves the process of recalling past emotions, being a sensitive perceiver of cues offered by another person, having skill in interpretation, and having an ability to communicate this understanding (Pearson and Spitzberg, 1990). Several studies (e.g., Berman and Smith, 1984; Fugita, Harper, and Wiens, 1980) indicate females tend to be more sensitive perceivers of nonverbal cues than males. From an early age, females tend to be socialized toward caregiving and being other-directed. For example, most children's toys reinforce traditional gender roles, in particular, the nurturing role for females, and the action/adventure role for males. Pearson, West, and Turner (1995) note that girls are portrayed as kind, attentive, and serving in children's literature, while boys are portrayed as "strong." Throughout the life span, males and females continue to learn gender-appropriate emotional behavior through families, educational institutions, peers, and the media.

Providing social support to patients has both rewards and costs. The patient certainly benefits, and the health care provider may benefit from a satisfying feeling by caring for others. Yet time, energy, and emotional nurturance are not unlimited resources for providers. Belle (1982) suggests that women are particularly prone to the strain of caregiving, especially if their support is unrecognized and unreciprocated (perhaps through other sources). Thus, many health care providers may also need support.

It is noteworthy that biological sex does not guarantee or prohibit empathetic skills. Bem (1975) found that psychological gender is a better predictor of empathetic behavior than biological sex. This may explain why male nurses have greater empathy than males who are not nurses (MacDonald, 1977). Handling strong emotions, working empathetically with patients, and delivering information can be both learned and improved upon by utilizing certain techniques. These are outlined in the recommendations contained in the next section.

RECOMMENDATIONS

Based on this research, a number of recommendations can be made to health professionals who face the process of delivering an HIV-positive diagnosis to patients.

(1) Take the Time Necessary to Explain Things to Patients and to Minimize Their Isolation

Advance planning is needed. It may be necessary to schedule two hours or more for this initial meeting. If time constraints prevent this, find a health professional who does have the time (nurse, hospice worker, social worker, etc.) to be with the patient and explain the diagnosis. There is need to be available for follow-up. It is important to reduce the patient's feeling of isolation. Many patients view referrals at this stage as a form of abandonment; therefore, referrals should be explored in a subsequent meeting. At a later time, patients may wish to have a voice in deciding who is involved in their care.

(2) Adopt a Patient-Centered Approach

Realize that a health care provider's medical view of HIV is likely to be different from the patient's connotative understanding of the virus. Many patients view HIV as pronouncing an imminent death sentence. It may be appropriate for physicians to discuss at the time the blood is drawn how a positive diagnosis would be handled should one occur. By having earlier discussions, more knowledge of the patient's personal perceptions of HIV, the patient's values, personality, family, religion, and support networks can be understood and considered. Such information may give some indication of the patient's coping style, strengths, and weaknesses. This, in turn, will likely help health care providers to decide how to present the news.

(3) Be Prepared for Strong Emotions Such as Guilt, Remorse, Anger, Sadness, Fear, and Shock

One technique for handling strong emotions is called N.U.R.S. (*N*aming the emotion, *U*nderstanding/legitimizing it, *R*especting it, and *S*upporting it [Marshall, 1993]). For example, a physician using the N.U.R.S. technique might say, "You seem scared. I can understand how this diagnosis would be frightening to you." After listening to the patient's immediate concerns and addressing them, the physician could offer support: "You and I are going to work together on this problem. There are different treatment options and many people with HIV are able to maintain good health for a long time." Although emotional pain and anxiety is necessary when coming to terms with an HIV-positive diagnosis, it is possible for health care professionals to communicate in a manner that lessens a patient's emotional discomfort and provide confirmation.

(4) Reinforce Confirming Words with Appropriate Nonverbal Behavior

For example, it is important for health care providers to look patients in the eyes when speaking with them. There is a need to be mindful of one's nonverbal behavior and the message that it sends. It is also important to be attentive to the patients' nonverbal feedback. Simple gestures, such as appropriately providing a tissue to a crying patient can communicate caring through a nonverbal gesture.

(5) Be Aware of Gender Issues

If the health care provider is a man talking to a woman, there may be differences in the way he expresses or handles strong emotions. If he feels he has difficulty in expressing or responding to strong emotions, then he should enlist a supportive person in the beginning of the diagnosis process.

(6) Patients Have Informational Needs in Addition to Affective Needs

It is necessary to know as much as possible about HIV/AIDS and to be prepared to discuss the course of the disease with the patient. Information must be tailored to the patient's needs. Quill and Townsend (1991, p. 467) advise giving simple, focused information, and avoiding "information-laden soliloquies" which can alienate patients. Again, feedback from the patient is important. One must give patients a reason to hope for some quality of life in the immediate future. In doing so, one must avoid clichés that deny the reality of the situation (e.g., "You'll be okay."). Caregivers should be willing to talk about dying, but balance this discussion with the communication of a treatment plan for prolonging life.

(7) Discuss and Arrange a Plan

The communication of a treatment plan increases patients' perceived control. As part of this plan, be prepare to discuss how the patient will communicate this fact to loved ones. Furthermore, patients should learn about, and be encouraged to attend social support groups.

(8) Caregivers Should Be Aware that They May Also Have Needs for Support

This is particularly true in the case of ongoing doctor-patient relationships and especially when the patient's response is strong. Burnout among HIV/AIDS care providers is commonly a process involving interpersonal, organizational, and societal antecedents, and specific interventions are available for care providers (Roth, 1995).

CONCLUSION

From this research, it is apparent that incarcerated women encountered a range of experiences when they were first diagnosed as being HIV-positive. For instance, diagnosis consultations lasted anywhere from one minute to four hours. This variation makes it possible to comment upon associated trends and findings. It is clear that a short consultation was consistently dissatisfactory. A short visit tended to lack compassion, information, and discussion of follow-up plans and social support. Additionally, women who had less time to discuss their illness had less information, and also tended to have more difficulty adjusting to their illness. Psychological adjustment is a means toward extending the patient's life because depression and anxiety are associated with lowered immune system functioning. In light of this, attending carefully to patients' communication needs is a necessary part of any effective treatment plan.

Female health professionals spent more time with patients and were perceived to be more compassionate. It is important to note that empathy, skill in demonstrating compassion, and attention to feelings can be cultivated in both males and females. Perceived compassion appears to be the product of empathy and skill in communication. For this reason, health care providers need to be aware of the effects of their distancing tactics on patients. Communication patterns consistent with disconfirmation cause patients considerable distress and may influence their health outcomes. Confirming messages, such as spending more time with patients, legitimizing and exploring their emotions, and attending to both informational and support needs appear to help patients to begin to adjust to their HIV-positive diagnosis. Ultimately, the human spirit is remarkable and complex; we must not underestimate the therapeutic effects of skillful and compassionate communication, even upon those who are facing the inevitability of death. Although this study has been concerned with the communication of HIV-positive diagnoses, the results, recommendations, and conclusions might well be more broadly applicable to communication by health professionals of other grave diagnoses.

REFERENCES

Bass, M. J., Buck, C., Turner, L., Dickie, G., Pratt, G., and Robinson, H. C. (1986). The physician's actions and the outcome of illness in family practice. *The Journal of Family Practice, 23*(1), 43-47.

Belle, D. E. (1982). The stress of caring: Women as providers of social support. In L. Goldberger and S. Breznitz (Eds.), *Handbook of Stress,* 496-505. New York: Free Press.

Bem, S. (1975). Sex-role adaptability: One consequence of psychological androgyny. *Journal of Personality and Social Psychology, 31,* 634-643.

Berman, P. W. and Smith, V. L. (1984). Gender and situational differences in children's smiles, touch, and proxemics. *Sex Roles, 10,* 347-356.

Bloom, B. L. (1988). *Health Psychology.* Englewood Cliffs, NJ: Prentice-Hall.

Brody, H. (1989). The physician-patient relationship. In R. M. Veatch (Ed.), *Medical Ethics,* 65-91. Boston: Jones and Bartlett Publishers.

Burgoon, J. K., Pfau, M., Parrott, R., Birk, T., Coker, R., and Burgoon, M. (1987). Relational communication, satisfaction, compliance-gaining strategies, and compliance in communication between physicians and patients. *Communication Monographs, 54,* 307-324.

Cassell, E. J. (1982). The nature of suffering and the goals of medicine. *New England Journal of Medicine, 306,* 639-645.

Cawyer, C. S. and Smith-Dupre, A. (1995). Communicating social support: Identifying supportive episodes in an HIV/AIDS support group. *Communication Quarterly, 43*(3), 243-358.

Cline, R. J. W. (1989). Communication and death and dying: Implications for coping with AIDS. *AIDS & Public Policy*, *4*, 40-50.

Cline, R. J. W. and Freeman, K. E. (1988). *Asking the Right Questions: A Qualitative Analysis of AIDS in the Minds of Heterosexual College Students.* Paper presented at the meeting of the International Communication Association, New Orleans, LA.

Cline, R. J. W. and Boyd, M. F. (1993). Communication as threat and therapy: Stigma, social support, and coping with HIV infection. In E. B. Ray (Ed.), *Case Studies in Health Communication,* 131-147. Hillsdale, NJ: Lawrence Erlbaum.

Conlee, C. J., Olvera, J., and Vagim, N. N. (1993). The relationships among physician nonverbal immediacy and measures of patient satisfaction with physician care. *Communication Reports*, *6*(1), 25-33.

DiMatteo, M. R., Taranta, A., Friedman, H., and Prince, L. (1980). Predicting patient satisfaction from physicians' nonverbal communication skills. *Medical Care*, *18*, 376-386.

Evans, B. J., Stanley, R. O., Burrows, G. D., and Sweet, B. (1989). Lectures and skills workshops as teaching formats in a history-taking skills course for medical students. *Medical Education*, *23*, 364-370.

Fallowfield, L. (1993). Giving sad and bad news. *The Lancet*, *341*, 476-478.

Fallowfield, L., Baum, M., and Maguire, G. P. (1986). The effects of breast conservation on the psychological morbidity associated with the diagnosis and treatment of early breast cancer. *British Medical Journal*, *293*, 1331-1334.

Feifel, H. (1976). Toward death: A psychological perspective. In E. S. Schneidmen (Ed.), *Death: Current Perspectives.* Palo Alto, CA: Mayfield Publishing Co.

Fugita, B., Harper, R., and Wiens, A. (1980). Encoding and decoding of nonverbal emotional messages: Sex differences in spontaneous and enacted expressions. *Journal of Nonverbal Behavior*, *4*, 133-141.

Harrington, J. A. and Rosenthal, R. (1983). Physician's head and body positions as determinants of perceived rapport. *Journal of Applied Social Psychology*, *13*, 496-509.

Horton, R. (1995). Women as women with HIV. *The Lancet*, *345*, 531-532.

Jackson, L. D. (1992). Information complexity and medical communication: The effects of technical language and amount of information in a medical message. *Health Communication*, *4* (3), 197-210.

Kastenbaum, R. (1967). The mental life of dying geriatric patients. *Gerontologist*, *7*, 97-100.

Katz, J. (1984). *The Silent World of Doctor and Patient.* New York: Free Press.

Kreps, G. L. (1993). Relational communication in health care. In B. Thornton and G. Kreps (Eds.), *Perspectives on Health Communication,* 51-65. Prospect Heights, IL: Waveland Press, Inc.

Ley, P. (1983). Giving information to patients. In R. Eiser (Ed.), *Social Psychology and Behavioral Medicine,* 339-374. Chichester, England: Wiley.

MacDonald, M. R. (1977). How do men and women students rate in empathy? *American Journal of Nursing*, *77*, 998.

Maguire, P. (1985). Barriers to psychological care of the dying. *British Medical Journal, 291*, 1711-1713.

Marshall, A. A. (1993). Whose agenda is it anyway? Training medical residents in patient-centered interviewing techniques. In E. B. Ray (Ed.), *Case Studies in Health Communication*, 15-29. Hillsdale, NJ: Lawrence Erlbaum.

Novack, D. H. (1979). Changes in physicians' attitudes toward telling the cancer patient. *Journal of the American Medical Association, 241*, 897-900.

Novack, D. H. (1985). Beyond data gathering: Twelve functions of the medical history. *Hospital Practice, 20*, 11-12.

Oken, D. (1961). What to tell cancer patients. *Journal of the American Medical Association, 175*, 1120-1128.

Pearson, J. C. and Spitzberg, B. H. (1990). *Interpersonal Communication: Concepts, Components, and Contexts* (second edition). Dubuque, IA: William C. Brown Publishers.

Pearson, J. C., West, R. L., and Turner, L. H. (1995). *Gender and Communication* (third edition). Dubuque, IA: Brown and Benchmark Publishers.

Pergami, A. and Catalan, J. (1994). How should an AIDS diagnosis be given? [on-line]. *International Journal of Studies of AIDS, 5*, 21-24. Abstract from PAPERCHASE File: 94191066.

Quill, T. and Townsend, P. (1991). Bad news: Delivery, dialogue, and dilemmas. *Archives of Internal Medicine, 151*, 463-468.

Ross, M. W., Hunter, C. E., Condon, J., Collins, P., and Begley, K. (1994). The Mental Adjustment to HIV Scale: Measurement and dimensions of response to AIDS/HIV disease. *AIDS Care, 6* (4), 407-411.

Roth, N. L. (1995). Structuring burnout: Interactions among HIV/AIDS health workers, their clients, organizations, and society. In L. Bennett, D. Miller, and M. Ross (Eds.), *Health Workers and AIDS: Research, Intervention and Current Issues in Burnout and Response,* 73-91. Chur, Switzerland: Harwood Academic Publishers.

Roth, N. L. and M. S. Nelson (1996). *HIV Diagnosis Rituals and Identity Narratives.* Manuscript submitted for publication.

Stiles, W. B., Putnam, S. M., Wolf, M. H., and James, S. A. (1979). Interaction exchange structure and patient satisfaction with medical interviews. *Medical Care, 17*, 667-681.

Thompson, T. L. (1986). *Communication for Health Professionals.* New York: Harper & Row.

Wallman, S. (1988). Sex and death: The AIDS crisis in social and cultural context. *Journal of Acquired Immune Deficiency Syndromes, 1* (6), 571-578.

Weisman, A. and Worden, J. (1975). Psychosocial analysis of cancer deaths. *Omega, 6*, 61-75.

Wortman, C. B. and Lehman, D.R. (1985). Reactions to victims of life crises: Support attempts that fail. In I. G. Sarason and B. R. Sarason (Eds.), *Social Support: Theory, Research and Applications,* 463-489. Dordrecht, the Netherlands: Martinus Nijhoff.

Chapter 7

Affirming the Role of Women as Carers: The Social Construction of AIDS Through the Eyes of Mother, Friend, and Nurse

Diane M. Kimoto

The psychosocial impact of Human Immunodeficiency Virus (HIV) and Acquired Immune Deficiency Syndrome (AIDS) is experienced not only by people with the disease, but also by those who care for them (Committee on Substance Abuse and Mental Health, 1994). Based on United States national and central city probability samples of 2,673 and 8,263 subjects respectively, 3.2 percent of all adults aged 17 to 75 years have provided care to someone with AIDS (Turner, Catania, and Gagnon, 1994). Yet, the importance of formal and informal AIDS carers has not been adequately recognized in the health care system nor has it been researched (Miller, 1992; Turner, Catania, and Gagnon, 1994; Wardlaw, 1994). In particular, the "reality" of women as carers has virtually disappeared from the literature on AIDS (Brackley, 1994; McCann and Wadsworth, 1992; Schiller, 1993; Wilson, 1992). In this way, women are rendered socially invisible. In fact, any role that women play is normally subsumed under the rubric of "community care" (Aronson, 1992; Schiller, 1993).

The purpose of the chapter is twofold. First, the chapter seeks to explore women's association with AIDS caring. Second, social constructionist principles are presented in order to emphasize the part that gender-role explanations play in assigning meaning to caregiving. Therefore, the chapter (a) begins with a review of the current literature pertaining to AIDS caring, women as AIDS carers, and social constructionism; (b) proceeds to an explanation of methodology; (c) moves on to a discussion of important findings; and (d) concludes with a presentation of implications for future research. It is hoped that the chapter will provide the reader with a better understanding of how women as part of a family (e.g., mother, sister, or cousin) or as informal (e.g., friend or buddy) and/or formal (e.g., nurse, social worker, or doctor) carers construct their roles in relationship to HIV and AIDS.

LITERATURE REVIEW

AIDS Carers

As the AIDS virus diffuses into larger demographic populations, the range of individuals becoming both directly and indirectly affected by the epidemic will increase. It has been suggested that the simple act of "knowing someone with AIDS represents a minimum prerequisite for having the potential to give care" (Turner, Catania, and Gagnon, 1994, p. 1543). With a large portion of the population as potential caregivers for someone with AIDS, it is important to know who these individuals are and what they do.

The majority of AIDS carers in large cities are under the age of 40, particularly between 18 and 39 years of age, and white. Although most of these urban carers are gay or bisexual, heterosexual men and women have also been documented as providing care (Turner, Catania, and Gagnon, 1994; Wardlaw, 1994), with women being regarded as the primary providers of domestic tasks (shopping, cooking, housekeeping, etc.) and personal care tasks (bathing, dressing, giving medication) (Committee on Substance Abuse and Mental Health, 1994; Folkman et al., 1994; Turner, Catania, and Gagnon, 1994; Wardlaw, 1994).

With so many individuals becoming AIDS carers, it is imperative that we realize from the onset that AIDS care is quite different from other forms of health care. First, the stress associated with "the social climate of illness and death surrounding many AIDS carers is a remarkable deviation from the context in which most care is provided" (Wardlaw, 1994, p. 376). Many carers who have never before given physical care to someone who is seriously ill must now deal with constant death and morbidity (Committee on Substance Abuse and Mental Health, 1994; Dhooper, Royse, and Tron, 1987; Miller, 1991; Silverman, 1993; Wardlaw, 1994). Second, carers, even those directly involved with epidemiological investigations, are not equipped with the latest information regarding HIV and AIDS. As a consequence, many are still fearful of contracting the virus (Blumenfield et al., 1987; Rizzo, Marder, and Wilkie, 1990; Silverman, 1993; Wardlaw, 1994).

Third, the burden associated with caring often extends beyond physical and emotional health to include strains associated with interpersonal relations, social life, and financial status (Turner, Catania, and Gagnon, 1994). AIDS caring takes time away from an individual's opportunity to participate in activities leading toward an increase in income or standards of living (e.g., relationships, hobbies, or education).

Individuals from various walks of life provide care to those affected by HIV. As the preceding section suggests, maintaining the vitality of each carer is crucial in sustaining an effective AIDS caring system. Why, then, are the efforts of women, the largest group of AIDS carers across the country, especially in rural areas, not adequately supported in practice or recognized in the literature?

The Role of Women as AIDS Carers

"Historically determined" assumptions appear to be at the foundation of women's invisibility in the AIDS care literature (Wilson, 1992). History has mistakenly considered "women as carers" as a natural phenomenon rather than a social one (Hall, 1988; Schaffer, 1988; Schiller, 1993; Wilson, 1992). "On the basis of this presumed natural ability, the role of caring is overwhelmingly ascribed to women" (Wilson, 1992, p. 119). Thus, women's caring activities, much like other biological activities such as childbearing, are regarded as obligatory, unending, and effortless. This antiquated manner of defining women as carers imprisons them within highly prescriptive behaviors. It obliges them "to assume responsibility for others' needs, confines them to the private sphere, and constrains their access to resources and to independence" (Aronson, 1992, p. 9). Furthermore, it completely negates women's identity as a group of individuals who have interests of their own, and it plagues those who cannot fulfil their "supposed" natural caring responsibilities with feelings of inadequacy, guilt, and loss of identity. For women AIDS carers in rural environments, this situation is compounded. Here, a lack of public knowledge (i.e., fear of casual transmission) coupled with inadequate community support (i.e., homophobic attitudes) exacerbates the normative expectations surrounding gender and caring (Koch et al., 1991). Women are presumed to be the principal AIDS carers (a) in their family and social settings, where they carry the emotional and practical responsibilities of tending for loved ones with the virus; (b) in the community or in statutory settings, where they provide care as either low-waged support or as unpaid volunteers; and (c) in health and social services, where their skills are integral in halting the spread of HIV.

Still, the number of women providing AIDS care continues to grow. As concerned individuals, it is our responsibility to hallmark women's contributions to AIDS care rather than to limit and distort their expectations. As researchers, it is our responsibility to investigate the contexts, both private and public, where women feel comfortable to question historical definitions of the caring role (Chafetz, 1988).

Social Constructionism: Establishing the Visibility of Women AIDS Carers

In order to develop an understanding of the women's constructions, this chapter adopts a social constructionist perspective. In doing so, we accomplish two general goals. First, we emphasize a reality that is defined not so much by individual acts, but through "the contingent, indeterminate, and historical flow of continuous communicative activity between human beings" (Shotter and Gergen, 1994, p. 14). Second, we enhance our understanding of individuals' roles by perceiving the reality created and explained for them by their social group or community (Harre, 1979, 1984, and 1986).

In reference to this study, we examine the manner in which the women talk about themselves and their experiences to better understand them as a group of rural AIDS carers. As such, a social constructionist perspective enables us (a) to consider the women's protestations about the stresses and burdens of AIDS caring as signs of their departure from gendered notions of caring; and (b) to examine the women's constructions as tools which "create, sustain, and validate the attitudes and practices that render women and their work more visible" (Bohan, 1993, p. 75).

METHODOLOGY

Two focus groups were conducted as part of a larger needs assessment for a public health area composed of six counties in western Alabama. "Intensity sampling procedures" (Patton, 1990; Morse, 1994) were employed in order to select women who were experts and authorities about HIV/AIDS care from the area. A list of potential participants was drawn from the formal and informal agencies listed in the HIV/AIDS Directory of Alabama Education and Services Program (1992–1993) (Alabama Department of Public Health, 1992). In order to insure that the focus groups had an ample number of participants, 25 women were invited. From this number, 15 women agreed to participate in the focus group sessions that were conducted in July 1994 at the research facilities of a large southeastern university.

The focus group sessions, which were videotaped and transcribed, lasted approximately two hours. During this time, the participants were asked to discuss three topics that had been identified through survey materials as significant to those affected by HIV/AIDS: Basic Needs and Services, Medical Needs, and Counseling and Support Needs (see Appendix A for a more complete detail of the question and topic format). At the end of the sessions, the women were asked for final comments about their relationships with PWAs and their suggestions for implementation procedures for AIDS-related services (see Appendix B).

WOMEN AIDS CARERS: ESTABLISHING THEIR VISIBILITY

Since the underlying foundation for this chapter is based upon an inductive analysis, the categories, themes, and commonsense understandings used to discuss women AIDS carers originate in the data. The images constructed during the focus groups are supported through the use of direct and paraphrased passages. In addition, relevant aspects about the public health area and the group members are provided.

Experiential Background: A Common Reality

Data from the 1990 Census indicate that the population of the public health area, located in western Alabama, is approximately 231,627. The area is basically rural with a per capita income ranging from $8,564 to $11,406. The gender breakdown of the area reveals that 52.3 percent of the residents are women and 47.7 percent are men. The racial composition consists of 71.6 percent caucasian, 27.6 percent African American, and 0.8 percent other (e.g., Hispanic, Native American, Asian American, etc.). It is within this setting that the first case of AIDS was reported in 1982. At that time, only one individual had been diagnosed as having AIDS. A period of four years went by until consistent records were kept for both HIV and AIDS. As of July 1994, (a) the morbidity rates per 100,000 people ranged from as low as 5.57 to as high as 118.20 (Alabama Department of Public Health, 1994a) and (b) the greatest number of adults had been exposed to HIV through sexual relations and the injection of drugs. Thus, from January 1986 through July 1994, a total of 101 AIDS cases had been identified (Alabama Department of Public Health, 1994a).

The 15 women who volunteered to participate in the study were divided into two focus groups. The first group was composed of eight women, five formal and three informal AIDS carers, who identified themselves as: Vurlie (infectious disease coordinator), Jordan (psychiatric nurse), Doris (church volunteer), Lisa (nurse), Stephanie (lawyer), Patrice (student volunteer), Cindy (AIDS buddy), and Sherry (nurse). In the second group, there were five formal and two informal AIDS carers who identified themselves as: Charlotte (substance abuse coordinator), Shannon, (home health worker), Roberta (chaplain), Pat (AIDS clinic volunteer), Margaret (hospice worker), Leigh (nurse), and Scarlett (mother).

Constructing a New Reality

As mentioned earlier, AIDS care was quite different from other forms of health care. Interestingly, the women in this particular study employed their discussions to construct a common identity or culture. Consequently, the images that resulted from these discussions were reflective of the way the women identified themselves in their role as rural AIDS carers.

HIV/AIDS Caring: Constant Death and Morbidity

> One of the things with AIDS that's different from cancer is that it's an up-and-down roller coaster. Death could happen any day and you wouldn't necessarily be prepared. (Vurlie)

While many diseases such as cancer typically followed a very consistent pattern, the trajectory of HIV/AIDS was not so easily mapped. Sadly, AIDS carers found that they were unable to answer simple questions for PWAs such as why they felt so healthy one day and ill the next. As evidenced by the statement above, the only certainty about HIV/AIDS was the eventuality of death. Not so obvious, however, was the effect that this constancy of death had upon the AIDS carer.

In constructing their image as AIDS carers, the women stressed an inescapable association between their caring activities and death. Where death for the PWA meant the total consumption of life, death for the AIDS carer referred to a steady depletion of personal energies and resources. This depletion or exhaustion, which occurred on both an interpersonal and an intrapersonal level, served as a continual reminder to the women that their role as carers had drastically changed.

When referring to death on an interpersonal level, the women discussed their direct, hands-on treatment of PWAs. They distinguished HIV/AIDS caring from other forms of health care by the fact that they were so often required to bargain with the health care system (e.g., Medicaid, Social Security, insurance companies) just to provide palliative services for their patients and loved ones. Instead of being able to expend their energies toward the provision of immediate care, the women found themselves fighting the technicalities of a bureaucratic system.

> **Roberta:** But how do we get individuals into the system?
> **Margaret:** According to hospice requirements, a doctor has to say they have six months or less to live. It's the only requirement. We're really designed for the patient who's tried everything.
> **Scarlett:** My son did not have insurance. He did not have Medicaid. It looks as if you have to live on disability for two years before you can get on Medicaid. I really feel that if he'd had insurance, it would have helped. Someone ought to organize these programs.
> **Margaret:** Can't they waive the two-year waiting period? Dialysis is the only exception I know of. . . . Maybe if the doctor says you only have six months, then the Medicare should kick in.
> **Pat:** Look, we've got to do something first because the insurance companies and the government are just going to try and keep us ignorant. That's why its important that all service providers either know how to counsel PWAs or know where to send them for information about service benefits.

When referring to death on an intrapersonal level, the women commented on their exhaustion in providing HIV/AIDS care. Without breaks and respites, the women were close to burnout. Disheartened by the lack of community involvement and the litany of conditions required just to secure support, the women were eager to vent their frustrations.

> **Vurlie:** Sometimes, the patients get dementia and the family can't take care of them. That's when they turn to us.
> **Jordan:** But there's respite care, isn't there?
> **Vurlie:** Yes, but it has to be someone who's educated about AIDS that the patient and the family can trust. They need to know universal precautions. And it's only for five days.
> **Jordan:** It's time for the local agencies to go past education and start providing some services. We need two sets of services. One for a mental break from all this death and the other

for medical. Kind of like a buddy system. It's time *we* get some burnout services because we're the people doing this everyday.

Vurlie: You see death so much, you have to get to the point where you can talk about it.

Leigh: If something doesn't change soon, we're not going to make it.

As illustrated in the next example, the need for support programs, targeted specifically for women AIDS carers, was long overdue. The women felt taken for granted and unappreciated by PWAs who casually missed their appointments. AIDS carers considered the expenditure of their "free" or personal time in the rescheduling of appointments and the securing of duplicate services as lost opportunities. The women also felt taken for granted by a society which still imagined them as the all-giving, ever-present carers.

> **Vurlie:** Some of the patients don't care. The doctor's doing all he can and so do I. We take a lot of pain to set up their appointments and they don't even show.
>
> **Cindy:** It seems as if you're asking people to care more than the patient cares. That's the problem.
>
> **Vurlie:** It's really frustrating to us because we spend so much extra time trying to notify people and get them into the system. I don't understand.
>
> **Roberta:** I spend most of my spare time calling churches and nearby facilities. We've just about drained our churches for medical supplies.
>
> **Cindy:** It seems as if it's expected for us as women to organize these appointments and services over and over again. That might have been the way it was years ago, but not anymore.
>
> **Vurlie:** Are we supposed to take care of everyone all of the time? No way! It's about time that the community gets involved. And the community means men, women, and children!

As the primary, often the sole, carers for those affected by HIV/AIDS, these women found their energies and resources severely taxed. Instead of directing their energies toward patient care, the women were forced to fight the bureaucracy of federal programs or to spend time rescheduling casually missed appointments. However, the women persevered. In openly discussing their grievances about the state of AIDS caring in their communities, the women vented pent-up emotions and signaled their departure from traditional notions of caring.

Rural AIDS Caring: Fear of the Unknown

Even though it's not a gay disease anymore, people have such a stigma about AIDS. What people don't realize is that it's fast hitting the heterosexual population. Nonetheless, whether it's a stigma about death or a fear of contagion, once people hear you have it, they're going to stay away from you. (Leigh)

On a broad level, the statement above reflected the local viewpoint about AIDS caring. These fears, which originated from a lack of adequate educational and support programs, were typically expressed as acts of prejudice. In fact, many of the individuals affected by HIV/AIDS and their families felt isolated by their communities due to these misinformed fears. Likewise, the women carers commented on how they felt as if they were being stigmatized simply because of their association with PWAs.

As rural AIDS carers, the women dealt with the PWAs' concern for privacy and anonymity, often feeling like accomplices to the fantasies of their clients. In small, rural environments such as the one in Alabama, PWAs were worried about what their neighbors might do or say if they found out they had HIV/AIDS. In order to disguise the true nature of their illnesses, the PWAs asked the women carers (a) to park their hospice-identified vans around the corner instead of in their driveways; or (b) to refer to their medical appointments with infectious disease physicians as routine physicals instead of AIDS clinics. As suggested by the following example, the women's caring duties were compounded by the educational, emotional, and fraternal needs of PWAs.

Vurlie: There is a great need. Once a person has been diagnosed with AIDS . . . they really don't know that HIV is . . . that they can't catch it. I . . . this is a big area that needs to be worked on . . . that if I touch them, I'm not going to catch it.

Doris: And the first thing they tell you is that they're in a very small area. They'll say, "I don't want the neighbors to know what's wrong." Well, everybody knows. But it's like a fantasy they have that nobody knows what's wrong.
Cindy: But, when you're told you have AIDS . . . that's a death sentence. It's not like cancer; you might be cured from it. Everybody knows there's no cure.
Vurlie: Especially in a rural area, there's greater stigma. If you got it through transfusion, there's anger. If you got it through behavior, you feel guilt. It doesn't matter which way you got it. When you've got AIDS, people aren't around.

The women described a rural environment where PWAs such as Scarlett's son were often treated in an unprofessional manner. Whether this lack of professionalism was based on fear or prejudice, the results were the same: an impairment of individuals' abilities and desires to provide thorough care to PWAs. However, as indicated below, the women believed that their co-workers' fears could be allayed if only there was additional hands-on assistance.

Scarlett: There's the ear, nose, and throat ones. They still don't want to be known as AIDS doctors.
Pat: We're not prepared. People are just afraid.
Scarlett: That's right. We weren't treated as professionally as we could have been by the nurses. They said they were so busy with paperwork that my son couldn't get in.
Margaret: I've seen the fear with nurses though. It's like a "hot potato," passing around drawn blood.
Charlotte: And every year, they're saying that something new is coming out. They know it. It's a prejudice like any other prejudice.
Scarlett: Nurses envision an AIDS patient as being in a bed. They have no idea who has AIDS. They look just like you and me. But my son felt it wasn't honest not to tell doctors about himself.
Margaret: Education won't get it. We needs hands-on assistance, like respite services, a directory of companies that pro-

vide free or reduced cost medications, and networking to provide case management for the PWAs and their families.

When discussing the basic needs of PWAs (e.g., housing, transportation, job placement/benefits counseling, and other food, clothing, and childcare issues), another commonality amongst the women
was revealed: a federal prejudice toward rural AIDS caring. The
women attributed their inability to provide proper medical, educational, and emotional AIDS-related care to PWAs, in part, to federal
agencies that did not seem to consider their concerns a major issue.
According to Vurlie:

> If they're not poor enough to be on Medicaid . . . they're only
> going to get $10 worth of treatment. The PWA doesn't feel as
> if it's worth all the time and energy to fill out all those applica-
> tions and wait in all those lines. It seems as if you have to wait
> until 30 or more people die in an area before the government
> will do anything. Unfortunately, it's going to stay that way,
> too, because the government doesn't care what happens out
> here.

While the previous dialogues appeared quite indicative of AIDS
caring in rural Alabama, they illustrated the degree to which fear,
prejudice, and stigma influenced the women's perceptions. In turn,
the dialogues suggested that the parameters of rural AIDS caring
had challenged both the way the women thought of themselves and
the nature of their responsibilities.

Women as AIDS Carers: Summary

The construction of a culture for women AIDS carers in rural
Alabama was built upon shared expressions and common understandings of language and meaning. Images surrounding the notion
of AIDS caring were portrayed through the recurring theme of
death. Perceptions about rural AIDS caring focused upon the
themes of fear, prejudice, and stigma. Together, these constructed
images emphasized a reality where women's contributions to AIDS
caring were both identified and validated.

This newfound sense of reality was further illustrated amongst
the women carers through the sharing of common concerns about

the exhaustive burdens associated with the provision of rural AIDS care. Within the confines of same gender groups, the women felt comfortable in "letting their hair down." By the same token, this new reality signaled a departure from traditional notions of caring. Unlike their more conventional counterparts, the women proclaimed their identity by acknowledging their frustrations in being expected to function as the sole carers of those affected by HIV/AIDS. In this manner, a social rather than a biological division for caring was promoted.

Upon returning home, the women commented to the researcher on the importance of their new relationships, both personal and professional. Rather than considering the focus group sessions as a chance or singular encounter, the women used their group affiliation (a) to enhance their visibility as AIDS carers; and (b) to gain greater assistance for counseling, education, and hands-on training. Thus, the ability to elicit change within their communities confirmed the women's existence and significance as AIDS carers.

CONCLUSION

The goal of this chapter has been to better understand the role that women play in providing AIDS care. In addition, the chapter has utilized social constructionist principles to support the notion that women's social invisibility in the literature and in the community is promoted through the use of historically determined assumptions about gender roles. In light of present and future research concerns, the following implications are advanced. The conclusions indicate that the individual realities of women AIDS carers are inextricably connected to their identification as members of a group. The findings further suggest that the women's constructions of self are (a) underscored by their feelings toward AIDS care; and (b) heightened by the prejudices of their small, rural environments. However, through the group processes of construction making, the women are enabled to reject historically determined assumptions and to affirm their relevance as AIDS carers.

According to Aronson (1992), women have been "torn between adherence to prevailing cultural values about femininity, care, and family ties and the wish to enhance their own autonomy and interest"

(p. 25). Social constructionism facilitates our understanding of this dilemma by recognizing it as a "social artifact or product of historically situated interchanges among people" (Gergen, 1985, p. 267). Research of this type, then, which takes an integrative approach, becomes essential in promoting women's AIDS caring as a communication-based production of collective experiences.

In order to sustain the developments that women have made toward an equitable division of caring labor, future research needs to contribute to the integrations, practices, and policies that benefit rather than constrain women (Aronson, 1992). For example, it is important that we give women the opportunity to explain what it is that they do and what supportive services they feel are necessary in relieving stress and burnout (McCann and Wadsworth, 1992; Miller, 1992; Viney, Crooks, and Walker, 1995). In this manner, the needs of those who are just beginning to work with AIDS-related cases as well as those who are seeking to alleviate continuous feelings of discomfort, fear, and fatigue might both be addressed.

APPENDIX

Table A

MODERATOR'S GUIDE FOR NEEDS ASSESSMENT

First of all, I'd like to thank each of you very much for participating tonight. We are conducting this focus groups to help us understand your thoughts about the perceived needs of the HIV/AIDS infected and/or affected population.

What you say is very important to us, and we are recording this session with two video cameras and a tape recorder. A few of my associates and some representatives from the Needs Assessment Committee are behind a two-way mirror because they are especially interested in what you have to say.

This discussion is informal and there are no right or wrong answers. We only are interested in your perceptions. Everybody's viewpoint is important, and we hope that all of you will share your views with us.

We will be discussing three key service areas. First, we will discuss basic needs and services such as food and housing. Second, we will focus more specifically on medical needs. The third area we will discuss will be counseling and support needs, including patient education. For each of these areas we will discuss specific services. We are interested in: (1) what current services are available, (2) the current and future demand for such services, and (3) suggestions for what might be done to better meet the needs of both the clients and the service providers.

Why don't we begin with each of you introducing yourself. Tell us a little bit about your role in working with HIV-infected individuals. O.K., now the first area we will discuss is Basic Needs and Services.

BASIC NEEDS/SERVICES

Housing

1. What current assistance is available for housing those infected with HIV? AIDS?

    Prompts: What organizations are responsible for this?

    Direct assistance versus referrals?

2. What is the current demand for housing assistance?

    Prompts: How many individuals need help?

    What kind of help do they need (reduced rate, etc.)?

2a. How do you see this demand changing in the future?

    Prompts: Will the need increase suddenly (as more individuals get AIDS) or gradually?

3. What might be done to improve housing assistance?

    Prompts: Realistically, given time and budget constraints?

3a. Do you think that there is a lack of awareness? Do clients and other service providers know about the services currently available?

4. What might be done to assist organizations providing housing assistance?

    Prompts: Get other organizations involved/better communication?

    Training?

Transportation

1. What current assistance is available for transportation for individuals infected with HIV? AIDS?

    Prompts: What organizations are responsible for this?

    Direct assistance versus referrals?

2. What is the current demand for transportation assistance?

   Prompts: How many individuals need help?

   What kind of help do they need (reduced rate, etc.)?

2a. How do you see this demand changing in the future?

   Prompts: Will the need increase suddenly (as more individuals get AIDS) or gradually?

3. What might be done to improve transportation assistance?

   Prompts: Realistically, given time and budget constraints?

3a. Do you think that there is a lack of awareness? Do clients and other service providers know about the services currently available?

4. What might be done to assist organizations providing transportation assistance?

   Prompts: Get other organizations involved/better communication?

   Training?

Job Placement/Benefits Counseling

1. What current assistance is available for job placement/benefits counseling for individuals infected with HIV? AIDS?

   Prompts: What organizations are responsible for this?

   Direct assistance versus referrals?

2. What is the current demand for job placement/benefits counseling assistance?

   Prompts: How many individuals need help?

   What kind of help do they need (reduced rate, etc.)?

2a. How do you see this demand changing in the future?

   Prompts: Will the need increase suddenly (as more individuals get AIDS) or gradually?

3. What might be done to improve job placement/benefits counseling assistance?

   Prompts: Realistically, given time and budget constraints?

3a. Do you think that there is a lack of awareness? Do clients and other service providers know about the services currently available?

4. What might be done to assist organizations providing job placement/benefits counseling assistance?

   Prompts: Get other organizations involved/better communication?

   Training?

Other Needs Such as Food, Clothing, and Childcare

1. What current assistance is available for other needs such as food, clothing, and childcare for individuals infected with HIV? AIDS?

   Prompts: What organizations are responsible for this?

   Direct assistance versus referrals?

2. What is the current demand for other needs such as food, clothing, and childcare assistance?

   Prompts: How many individuals need help?

   What kind of help do they need (reduced rate, etc.)?

2a. How do you see this demand changing in the future?

   Prompts: Will the need increase suddenly (as more individuals get AIDS) or gradually?

3. What might be done to improve other needs such as food, clothing, and childcare assistance?

   Prompts: Realistically, given time and budget constraints?

3a. Do you think that there is a lack of awareness? Do clients and other service providers know about the services currently available?

4. What might be done to assist organizations providing other needs such as food, clothing, and childcare assistance?

   Prompts: Get other organizations involved/better communication?

   Training?

MEDICAL

Medical Care Specifically Addressing HIV/AIDS-Related Concerns

1. What current assistance is available for medical care for individuals infected with HIV? AIDS?

   Prompts: What organizations are responsible for this?

   Direct assistance versus referrals?

2. What is the current demand for medical care assistance?

   Prompts: How many individuals need help?

   What kind of help do they need (reduced rate, etc.)?

2a. How do you see this demand changing in the future?

   Prompts: Will the need increase suddenly (as more individuals get AIDS) or gradually?

3. What might be done to improve medical care assistance?

   Prompts: Realistically, given time and budget constraints?

3a. Do you think that there is a lack of awareness? Do clients and other service providers know about the services currently available?

4. What might be done to assist organizations providing medical care assistance?

Prompts: Get other organizations involved/better communication?

Training?

EMERGENCY TREATMENT

NURSING HOME/HOSPICE

MEDICINE/PRESCRIPTION

General Medical Care (Dental, Optical, etc.)

1. What current assistance is available for general medical care (dental, optical, etc.) for individuals infected with HIV? AIDS?

Prompts: What organizations are responsible for this?

Direct assistance versus referrals?

2. What is the current demand for general medical care (dental, optical, etc.) assistance?

Prompts: How many individuals need help?

What kind of help do they need (reduced rate, etc.)?

2a. How do you see this demand changing in the future?

Prompts: Will the need increase suddenly (as more individuals get AIDS) or gradually?

3. What might be done to improve for general medical care (dental, optical, etc.) assistance?

Prompts: Realistically, given time and budget constraints?

3a. Do you think that there is a lack of awareness? Do clients and other service providers know about the services currently available?

4. What might be done to assist organizations providing for general medical care (dental, optical, etc.) assistance?

Prompts: Get other organizations involved/better communication?

Training?

COUNSELING/SUPPORT SERVICES

Psychological Counseling/Support

1. What current assistance is available for psychological counseling/support for individuals infected with HIV? AIDS?

Prompts: What organizations are responsible for this?

Direct assistance versus referrals?

2. What is the current demand for psychological counseling/support assistance?

Prompts: How many individuals need help?

What kind of help do they need (reduced rate, etc.)?

2a. How do you see this demand changing in the future?

Prompts: Will the need increase suddenly (as more individuals get AIDS) or gradually?

3. What might be done to improve for psychological counseling/support assistance?

Prompts: Realistically, given time and budget constraints?

3a. Do you think that there is a lack of awareness? Do clients and other service providers know about the services currently available?

4. What might be done to assist organizations providing for psychological counseling/support assistance?

Prompts: Get other organizations involved/better communication?

Training?

FAMILY

SPIRITUAL

SUBSTANCE ABUSE

BIG PICTURE

Are There Other Specific Services that We Should Discuss?

1. Probe theme. For example, it seems that awareness may be a general problem. What are your feelings about this? What might be done?

2. If you were to prioritize the top three needs of those infected with HIV, what would they be?

   Prompts: So there seems to a consensus that _____ is a problem. Does this sound right? Or both _____ and _____ have been mentioned quite a bit; which of these do you think is a more urgent need?

3. If you were to prioritize the top three needs of service providers, what would they be?

   Prompts: So there seems to a consensus that _____ is a problem. Does this sound right? Or both _____ and _____ have been mentioned quite a bit; which of these do you think is a more urgent need?

It is about time for us to wrap it up. Is there anything else that we have missed? (Try to keep it short).

Well, on behalf of the Needs Assessment Committee, I would like to thank you for participating. Your input is greatly appreciated. We have prepared a brief survey sheet on your perceptions of the three most important needs among those we have discussed. It you could take a few minutes before you leave to fill it out, we would greatly appreciate it. Thank you.

Table B

POST-FOCUS GROUP QUESTIONNAIRE

What do you think are the three most important needs among those we have discussed?

1.

2.

3.

In your opinion, what is the best way to meet those needs?

1.

2.

3.

Affiliation/Occupation: _____

Thank you for your participation!

REFERENCES

Alabama Department of Public Health. (1992). *HIV/AIDS Directory of Alabama Education and Services Programs*. Montgomery, AL: Alabama Department of Public Health.

Alabama Department of Public Health. (1994a). *HIV/AIDS Surveillance: AIDS Cases Reported Through June 1994*. Montgomery, AL: Alabama Department of Public Health.

Aronson, J. (1992). Women's sense of responsibility for the care of old people: "But who else is going to do it?" *Gender and Society, 6*, 8-29.

Blumfield, M., Smith, P. J., Milazzo, J., Seropion, S., and Wormser, G. P. (1987). Survey of nurses working with AIDS patients. *General Hospital Psychiatry, 9*, 58-63.

Bohan, J. S. (1993). Women at center stage: A course about the women of psychology. *Teaching of Psychology, 20*, 74-79.

Brabant, S. (1994). An overlooked AIDS affected population: The elderly parent as caregiver. *Journal of Gerontological Social Work, 22*, 131-145.

Brackley, M. H. (1994). The plight of American family caregivers: Implications for nursing. *Perspectives in Psychiatric Care, 30*, 14-20.

Chafetz, J. S. (1988). The gender division of labor and the reproduction of female disadvantage. *Journal of Family Issues, 9*, 108-131.

Committee on Substance Abuse and Mental Health. (1994). Disease progression and intervention. In J. D. Auerbach, C. Wypijewska, and H. K. H. Brodie (Eds.), *AIDS and Behavior: An Integrated Approach,* 124-156. Washington DC: National Academy.

Dhooper, S. S., Royse, D. D., and Tron, T. V. (1987). Social work practitioners' attitudes towards AIDS victims. *Journal of Applied Social Sciences, 196*, 108-123.

Folkman, S., Chesney, M. A., Cooke, M., and Boccellari, A. (1994). Caregiver burden in HIV-positive and HIV-negative partners of men with AIDS. *Journal of Consulting and Clinical Psychology, 62*, 746-756.

Gergen, K. J. (1985). The social constructionist movement in modern psychology. *American Psychologist, 40*, 266-275.

Hall, S. (1988). The toad in the garden: Thatcherism among the theorists. In C. Nelson and L. Grossber (Eds.), *Marxism and the Interpretation of Culture,* 35-57. Urbana, IL: University of Illinois.

Harre, R. (1979). *Social Being: A Theory for Social Behavior.* Totowa, NJ: Littlefield, Adams.

Harre, R (1984). *Personal Being: A Theory for Individual Psychology.* Cambridge, MA: Harvard University.

Harre, R (Ed.). (1986). *The Social Construction of Emotions.* New York: Basil Blackwell.

Koch, P. B., Preston, D. G., Young, E. W., and Wang, M. (1991). Factors associated with AIDS-related attitudes among rural nurses. *Health Values: The Journal of Health Behavior, Education, and Promotion, 15*, 32-40.

McCann, K. and Wadsworth, E. (1992). The role of informal carers in supporting gay men who have HIV-related illness: What do they do and what are their needs? *AIDS Care, 4*, 25-34.

Miller, B. (1992). Gender differences in caregiving: Fact or artifact? *Gerontologist, 32*, 498-507.

Miller, D. (1991). Occupational morbidity and burnout: Lessons and warnings for HIV/AIDS carers. *Internal Review of Psychiatry, 3*, 439-449.

Morse, J. M. (1994). Designing funded qualitative research. In N. K. Denzin and Y. S. Lincoln (Eds.), *Handbook of Qualitative Research,* 220-235. Thousand Oaks, CA: Sage.

Patton, M. Q. (1990). *Qualitative Evaluation and Research Methods.* Newbury Park, CA: Sage.

Rizzo, J. A., Marder, W. D., and Wilkie, R. J. (1990). Physician contact with and attitudes toward HIV-seropositive patients. *Medical Care, 28*, 251-260.

Schaffer, D. (1988). The feminization of poverty: Prospects for an international feminist agenda. In E. Bonepart and E. Stopper (Eds.), *Women, Power and Policy: Toward the Year 2000,* 223-246. New York: Pergamon.

Schiller, N. G. (1993). The invisible woman: Caregiving and the construction of AIDS health services. *Culture, Medicine, and Psychiatry,* Special issue: *Women, poverty, and AIDS, 17*, 487-512.

Shotter, J. and Gergen, K. J. (1994). Social construction: Knowledge, self, others, and continuing the conversation. In S. A. Deetz (Ed.), *Communication Yearbook, 17,* 3-33. Thousand Oaks, CA: Sage.

Silverman, D. (1993). Psychosocial impact of HIV-related caregiving on health providers: A review and recommendation for the role of psychiatry. *American Journal of Psychiatry, 150*, 705-712.

Turner, H. A., Catania, J. A., and Gagnon, J. (1994). The prevalence of informal caregiving to person with AIDS in the United States: Caregiver characteristics and their implications. *Social Science and Medicine, 38*, 1543-1552.

Viney, L. L., Crooks, L., and Walker, B. M. (1995). Anxiety in community-based AIDS caregivers before and after personal construct counseling. *Journal of Clinical Psychology, 51*, 274-280.

Wardlaw, L. A. (1994). Sustaining informal caregivers for persons with AIDS. Special issue: *HIV/AIDS. Families in Society, 75*, 373-384.

Wilson, J. (1992). Women as carers. In J. Bury, V. Morrison, and S. McLachlan (Eds.), *Working with Women and AIDS,* 117-124. London: Tavistock/Routledge.

Chapter 8

Enacting Care: Successful Recruitment, Retention, and Compliance of Women in HIV/AIDS Medical Research

Nancy L. Roth
Myra Shoub Nelson
Carol Collins
Pamela Emmons
Mary Alderson
Frank Hatcher
Barbara Nabrit-Stephens
Mary Ann South

The NIH Revitalization Act of 1993, implemented in June 1994, mandated the recruitment of diverse populations, especially minorities and women, into federally funded research studies.[1] The policy of the NIH is designed to remedy past inequities concerning under-representation and exclusion from clinical trials and medical research studies. Past research has been conducted largely on white males, in such mass trials as the major Coronary drug project, under the implicit belief that conclusions concerning risks of coronary disease and efficacy of drug treatment would be generalizable to

The authors wish to acknowledge the original staff of Project SHARE and other individuals who have been instrumental in its success over the years: Deborah Coffee; Ayesha Curry; John Estrada, MD; Richard Frankel; Rena Harris, CNM; Joyce Perkins; Larry Smith; and Cynthia Wilder. Project SHARE was supported by grant #RR003032 from the Research Centers in Minority Institutions Program Grant, NIGMS. The research reported in this chapter was supported by the AMPHS AIDS Research Consortium, NIH Grant 3 P20 AI20360-03S2.

females and minority populations (Merkatz and Junod, 1994; McCarthy, 1994).

Prior regulations protecting women and minorities from inclusion in studies arose as a reaction to studies from the mid-nineteenth to mid-twentieth century. Many studies were performed upon dependent populations unable to give consent to research in which they were unwilling participants: slave women,[2] the incarcerated, the mentally ill,[3] concentration camp victims. Perhaps the most infamous example was the Tuskegee experiment. This study, conducted by the United States Public Health Service from 1932–1947, enrolled 400 black men in a "natural history study of untreated syphilis." It continued even after research findings clearly indicated a mortality rate twice as high in untreated cases, and even after penicillin was readily available to treat the infection (Allen, 1994; Washington, 1994). Studies such as Tuskegee are often cited as contributing factors in the mythologies about the reluctance of African Americans to volunteer as medical research subjects (Washington, 1994; Allen, 1994; El-Sadr and Capps, 1992; McCarthy, 1994).

In this chapter, we examine a project at Meharry Medical College, Nashville, Tennessee that was highly successful in attracting and gaining compliance from women, and in particular, African-American women as medical research subjects. Project SHARE was developed to provide support to HIV-positive pregnant women and their (subsequent) children who were subjects in medical research about the children's immunological development. SHARE is an acronym for: Specialized Health Care Aimed at Research and Education.

The literature concerning underrepresented populations in medical research or medical trials in general, and HIV/AIDS in particular, is scant. Research on African-American participation has either been more general in nature (Haywood et al., 1992; Johnson and Arfken, 1992; Scott-Jones, 1993; Washington, 1994), has focused on cancer trials (Hunter et al., 1987; Millon-Underwood, Sanders, and Davis, 1993; Thomas et al., 1994), or has focused on hypertensive disorder trials (Moser and Lunn, 1982).

Research on women in clinical trials has been hampered by federal policies barring women of childbearing age from participation in research, what is referred to as "the exclusion of pregnant, pregnable, and once-pregnable people in biomedical research" (Merton, 1993). Two major arguments are cited by ethicists and researchers for prior lack of incorporation of women into studies: the legal and the sociocultural.

> Important practical barriers are often cited to explain the much lower rate of participation of women even in trials that do not formally exclude them. Women are far more often the principal caregivers for babies, children, disabled and elderly family members or neighbors, and have much less mobility and ability to 'take time off' to attend to their own medical needs. (Merton, 1993, p. 374)

Within the last 20 years, the participation of women in trials has been further eroded—a larger percentage of recent trials enroll men only than in the early seventies (Schmucker and Vessel, 1993).

In order to begin to examine current and future participation in HIV-related medical research pursuant to the new guidelines, we must integrate what has been previously found about women who are HIV/AIDS-positive (Merkatz and Junod, 1994) with the literature about African Americans. This can be accomplished by examining the factors involved in recruitment, retention, and compliance (RRC) in clinical trials and other medical research through the overlapping lenses of gender, HIV/AIDS, and race.

RECRUITMENT

Recruitment entails the persuasion of a potentially eligible person to be screened for inclusion in a medical or clinical trial, presentation of informed consent and other explanatory materials, and procurement of informed consent to participate (usually in the form of a signature). The literature generally suggests that participants offer two types of explanations for deciding to enter a trial: perceptions of benefits to self—extend life, delay disease progression, continue working, gain control over disease—and perceptions of benefits to society—help community affected by disease and contribute to medical science (Millon-Underwood, Sanders, and Davis, 1993; Ross, Jeffords, and Gold, 1994). Specific psychological factors may mediate against recruitment, such as the demands of time required for participation, travel difficulties, and perception of lack of quality of life inherent in participation in clinical research (Schain, 1994; McCabe, Varricchio, and Padberg, 1994). Ryan (1994) argues that such research confuses two variables which should be considered separately: (1) what prompts a potentially eligible person to seek participation in a study; and (2) what they expect the benefits and costs of such participation to be. Ryan found that reasons for entry included: having an identifiable symptom, inability to obtain experimental drug without participating in clinical trial, inability to pay for drugs without participating in clinical trial, "pressure" from physician, and hope in addition to balancing self-interest and altruism, as identified by previous research (Schain, 1994).

An intertwined issue that might influence decisions to participate in clinical trials is relational. "As the traditional physician-patient relationship continues to evolve, patients are taking a more active role in assessing potential risks and benefits and have become more aware health care consumers" (Wermeling and Selwitz, 1993). All of the studies examined identified the individual's physician as having greater influence on decisions to enter a protocol than the media, friends, families, lovers, or other sources of such information (Ross, Jeffords, and Gold, 1994; Thomas et al., 1994). Thus, not having an established relationship with a physician may be a powerful barrier to participation in medical research for members of lower socioeconomic groups who lack access to an ongoing relationship with a specific medical provider. Research on women as medical patients suggests that perceptions of power differences in the physician/patient relationship might also affect decisions to participate (Weijts, 1994).

Recruitment to HIV Trials

Research specific to HIV/AIDS trials highlights the experience of gay men—race is generally not specified (Ross, Jeffords, and Gold, 1994; Ryan, 1994; 1995). The specific nature of HIV/AIDS may influence people's decisions to enter trials. People infected with HIV live an average of ten years without becoming symptomatic (Marlink et al., 1994). Asymptomatic people may be more likely to want to join trials because they wish to extend their period of symptom-free life. On the other hand, they may wish to avoid such trials to prolong their period of life free from regular interactions with the health care system. Such decisions may be based on different ways that individuals weigh quality of life issues (Ryan, 1994; Wachtel et al., 1992).

Because of the stigmas that many people associate with HIV/AIDS, as well as concerns about loss of employment or medical coverage (in the United States), many people who have HIV infection prefer to keep their antibody status confidential—even when they are among others who are similarly infected. Within the gay male communities, some prefer to maintain confidentiality about their status for fear of affecting their social status. For this reason, some eligible candidates may decline to participate if being seen in the places where trials are conducted might label them as having HIV infection (Ryan, 1995).

Recruitment of African Americans to HIV Trials

African Americans and Latinos are affected disproportionately in the AIDS epidemic. While representing only 12 percent of the United States population, African Americans account for 34 percent of AIDS patients cumulatively and 38 percent of new AIDS cases between 1993 and 1995 (CDC, 1995). Racial and ethnic minorities have been clearly underrepresented in HIV trials (El-Sadr and Capps, 1992). Associations of HIV with homosexuality may make participation in clinical trials unappealing to nongay African Americans who might fear that participation in clinical trials would label them as gay (Ryan, 1994).

Another possible reason for low rates of recruitment among African Americans in HIV trials is the high rate of AIDS transmission associated with intravenous drug use in the African-American community. Rates of HIV in the African-American community are linked to systemic racism that contributes to a tangled web of poor socioeconomic conditions, intravenous drug use, and heterosexual transmission of the virus to sexual partners of IDUs (Brown, 1993). All of these factors may inhibit access to medical practitioners who might refer members of the community to trials and may influence providers to assume that such patients would not be compliant if they were recruited to a trial.

Intravenous Drug Use and Recruitment to HIV Trials

As of 1995, 27.3 percent of AIDS cases were among intravenous drug users (IDUs) (CDC, 1995). A perception exists (among directors of clinical trials units) that drug use is directly associated with poor recruitment and compliance. However, recent research has found that accrual and compliance of IDUs to HIV trials is associated with many factors. This research concludes that issues such as access to care (both medical and psychosocial) are particularly important in the recruitment of this especially disadvantaged subpopulation. Individual behavioral issues (such as drug use) were not predictive of recruitment and compliance rates, but access to care was predictive of recruitment and compliance among IDUs (Brown, 1993, p. 49).

Women and HIV Trials

The proportion of AIDS cases among women increased from 8 percent of cases reported in 1981 to 1987 to 18 percent in 1993 to 1995 (CDC, 1995). AIDS disproportionately affects women of color: fully 53.3 percent of women diagnosed with AIDS are African American, 20.3 percent Latina, and 25.2 percent white (Allen, 1994). Women have not been recruited to clinical trials at the same rates as men in the African-American community (Cotton et al., 1993). Many barriers to recruitment may be common to both African American males and females such as a widespread mistrust of clinical trials after Tuskegee (Scott-Jones, 1993; Thomas et al., 1994; Washington, 1994). Some barriers such as noncompliance due to incarceration affect African-American male populations, while other barriers to recruitment tend to be more salient for women:

- *Location*—Women may face more geographic barriers and be more constrained to particular locations—the seven New York City for sites for the ACTG trials enrolled variable percentages of women (Cotton et al., 1993, p. 1326).

- *Gender of primary investigator*—Sites with a female primary investigator enrolled a larger percentage of women (Cotton et al., 1993, p. 1326).
- *Child and family care*—Women are more often the primary family caretakers and are thus constrained from participation by lack of assistance in family care (Merton, 1993).
- *Transportation*—Community-based studies such as CPCRA have found that nontraditional services such as childcare and transportation have an impact on recruitment of women (Morse et al., 1995).

RETENTION AND COMPLIANCE

Retention refers to the continued participation in a clinical trial once an eligible candidate has given informed consent. Little research has addressed the issue of retention in trials. It is suggested that "retention of study participants is enhanced if the initial recruitment is handled properly" (Haywood et al., 1992). In addition, attention by study staff to patients' problems and needs as well as the study staff's empathy, acceptance, and courtesy are important. Meeting participants' needs is often the key to effective retention. Such needs have been previously defined as transportation, financial recompense, or provision of medical care (Haywood et al., 1992). Similarly, negative attitudes of staff can interfere with retention in a project (Morse et al., 1995).

In addition, there is some (anecdotal) evidence that individuals' perceptions of their own needs are often quite different from those of their caregivers. Kroger (1994) notes a case where caregivers identified the primary needs of participants to be transportation and more education in order to ensure retention and compliance. Participants noted that they had missed appointments because they were sick, and disliked the waiting, crowding, and lack of privacy encountered at the site. Retention in community-based trials occurs when attempts to balance the "seemingly antithetical demands of research and service delivery," are successful (Morse et al., 1995, p. 14).

Compliance refers to the extent to which participants in clinical trials appear for scheduled appointments, take the appropriate quantity of the drug on trial, at the appropriate times and for the prescribed period of time, and otherwise engage in the behaviors required by the study protocol. It is generally suggested that there is a relationship between the communication of caregivers and study participants and the outcomes of a clinical trial—including participant compliance (Kreps, O'Hair, and Clowers, 1994; Kroger, 1994). However, work by Burgoon et al. (1987) suggests that while there is a strong association between communication factors and patient satisfaction, the relationship between communication and compliance gaining strategies employed is weak. They note that while research consistently shows that patients' understanding of their situation is positively related to compliance, "how the medical practitioner communicates with the patient may be more important than the content itself" (Burgoon et al., 1987). They note that the extent to which a provider engages in relational communication—that which demonstrates how s/he feels about his/her relationship with a patient—may have a stronger influence on compliance than what the provider says.

In medical research in general, where new drugs are not being tried, it is not necessary to divorce the issues of compliance and retention. As the participants are not responsible for taking medication, compliance can be seen as equal to retention. What is required of the patient is the same: return visits to monitor status and participation in study activities. Poor compliance and retention are associated with lower levels of education, poverty, and language barriers,[4] as well as lack of relationship with a specific medical care provider or providers and use of private practice (Blackwell, 1975).

HIV Trials

Many different strategies have been used to increase compliance and retention in HIV trials. They tend to focus on overcoming instrumental barriers:

- *Appointment tracking*—Reliance on databases to ensure return of patients. For example, the staff can send appointment cards and letters one and two months in advance, call patients before appointments as a reminder, or after missed appointments, to reschedule (Woody, Metzger, and Mulvaney, 1994).

- *Transportation*—Provision of transportation to the site, either taxis, bus tokens, or vouchers for gas.
- *Nutrition*—Meals served at the site for patients on-site at a mealtime (Woody, Metzger, and Mulvaney, 1994).
- *Home visits*—Visits to hospitals, homes, and prisons to see patients (Woody, Metzger, and Mulvaney, 1994).
- *Clinical flexibility*—Provide privacy or anonymity, short waiting time, flexible clinic hours, and availability of staff at times other than clinic hours (Besch, 1995; Morse et al., 1995; Woody, Metzger, and Mulvaney, 1994).

In addition, other noninstrumental factors have also been shown to have been very important in the provision of care to persons in clinical trials. These issues can be considered "quality of life issues." The clinical environment can be considered very important in the construction of a new identity for the person with AIDS (PWA). Just participating in a trial alters the life of the person who has decided to enroll. A PWA who chooses to be in a trial puts himself or herself in a position of having medical care become a larger and more explicit piece of his or her existence. Attendance at a clinic with persons showing signs of the terminal stage of AIDS can force a person to come to terms with his or her own mortality (Ryan, 1995). The participation in a trial might also offer a person access to medical care and social services they might otherwise not know about or be able to afford. A key issue in the retention of patients in HIV trials is linking them to systems of care, both medical and psychosocial, through the intervention of project staff (Besch, 1995; El-Sadr and Capps, 1992), thus serving the needs of the person in the context of his or her life experience as well as in the context of his or her illness.

African-American Women

African-American women are more likely to be single parents and live in poverty than other women in American society. These factors are often associated with lack of access to medical care on a continuing basis. The provision of links to social and medical services becomes an important motivation for the women to continue to participate in HIV trials. This higher retention rate for females, though, has been shown to not differ by employment or marital status (Woody, Metzger, and Mulvaney, 1994).

In this chapter, we explore the experience of Project SHARE (Specialized Health Care Aimed at Research and Education), a program in middle Tennessee specifically designed to recruit HIV-positive pregnant females and their babies as subjects for a series of HIV medical research projects. Project SHARE coordinated subjects' research visits, provided transportation and childcare, and offered a range of social support services for the subjects and their families including prenatal care, baby care education and counseling for new mothers, HIV education, and baby care necessities such as diapers, baby food, and baby blankets. The project was highly successful in recruiting and retaining HIV-positive women, particularly African-American women and their at-risk babies. It is our belief that understanding the experience of Project SHARE may help us to understand why minority women would choose to participate in a community trial and stay with the trial from start to finish. This chapter presents data collected from both the study nurse and her assistant, who coordinated Project SHARE during its last two years of operation, as well as data from 10 of the 38 women who participated in the project.

METHODS

Sample

This chapter reports on a case study of the recruitment, retention, and compliance efforts of one middle Tennessee project designed to enhance the lives of women and their children who were subjects for AIDS medical research studies. This site is one of five included in a larger study of middle Tennessee medical research and support programs that have been successful in the recruitment, retention, and compliance of underrepresented populations in AIDS clinical trials. Project SHARE was chosen as a study site because of its success in the recruitment, retention, and compliance of women, particularly African-American women, with babies. Middle Tennessee was chosen as a study site because it was the location for an

AIDS clinical trials unit specifically designated to focus on the recruitment of populations that are underrepresented in clinical trials.

Three visits were made to Project SHARE during the course of a year to learn about its mission and how it functioned, to become familiar with project staff, to interview project staff, and to train staff to interview project patients. Project SHARE served a total of 35 women during its five years of operation—26 were HIV infected and nine were healthy controls. Seventy percent were African American and their ages ranged from 17 to 40. Ten of the 35 SHARE patients were randomly selected to be interviewed for this study: two were healthy controls, two were white, one was married, and their ages ranged from 20 to 30. Eight of the ten were unemployed at the time of the interview, and all and were either covered by Medicaid or TennCare (Tennessee's program of universal medical coverage).

Data Collection

Project staff were formally interviewed during the third visit to the project. Ethnographic interviewing techniques were employed (McCracken, 1988; Spradley, 1979). A brief question guide was used to ensure that all major desired topics were covered, but the interview was jointly structured by the interviewers and the interviewees. After project staff were interviewed, the clinical nurse coordinator was trained to interview clients using the same procedures. The research team for the larger study did not conduct the interviews, as that might have compromised patient desires for anonymity. All interviews were audio recorded and transcribed verbatim.

Data Analysis

Interview transcripts, archival data, and researchers' notes from the preliminary site visits were analyzed using grounded theory techniques (Glaser and Strauss, 1967; Strauss et al., 1990). Analysts reviewed transcripts and notes for categories and patterns, then amended categories as additional data were reviewed. This analysis resulted in a preliminary theory about the factors associated with successful recruitment, retention, and compliance of women in AIDS-related medical research.

DIMENSIONS OF SUCCESS

Two primary categories emerged that explained project SHARE's success in recruitment: (1) it offered needed services and support; and (2) it provided an opportunity for altruistic behavior. Several categories ·emerged to explain the project's success in retention/ compliance (the two issues are collapsed in the analysis because SHARE was a medical research project, therefore retention and compliance cannot be differentiated as they are in clinical trials): (1) mutual connectedness between the patients and caregivers described as friendship and family-like connections; (2) a sense of caring for the patient that went beyond the usual bounds of caregiver/patient relationships; (3) an enormous sense of patient trust in their caregivers; and (4) patient comfort with the staff.

Recruitment: Getting Needs Met and Giving to Others

The project maintained quantitative data concerning recruitment which do not begin to do justice to the myriad reasons women had for being recruited into the study. The numbers indicate that HIV-positive women of all races reported the availability of counseling as the most frequent motivation for participation. HIV-negative African-American women were motivated most frequently by the promise of free well-baby care, while the one Caucasian HIV-negative control indicated that her primary reason for participation was free HIV testing (Nabrit-Stephens et al., 1995). The qualitative data depict a much richer picture of motivations for participation.

Often women joined for multiple reasons. The need for counseling was often mentioned, and certainly functioned as an important reason for recruitment, as part of a constellation of expressed needs for personal help:

> When I first found out about my situation, I knew I needed more information about it, so I decided to attend the project.

I knew I needed to be in somebody's program, so . . .

I didn't have anything to lose and had a lot to gain, any help that I can get is welcomed.

Education concerning HIV was seen as a dimension of counseling/help for the participants. One of the controls in the study signed up for the study specifically because a member of her family is HIV positive. She indicated, "I was directly affected by the AIDS virus, and I wanted to do and learn as much as I could about the disease." She looked at her participation in terms of providing her son with vaccinations and well-baby care as well as keeping her "up to date as far as my AIDS awareness or AIDS checkup."

Both the staff and the participants saw altruism as a reason for participation in the study. The clinical nurse coordinator indicated that the participants "wanted to help somebody else." Taking an active role in helping others coexisted with self-interested reasons. For women in the community without resources, a possibility existed for a positive outcome, as echoed by one mother, "I wanted to help other people, and I figured that this was the best way that I could do that." Another mother noted:

I feel like I'm doing my part to help understand the disease better and form new procedures on how to deal with HIV in children and adults, and anything that we can do to help each other get through is a benefit that people ought to consider.

While much of the prevailing literature about motivation for participation in clinical trials and medical studies suggests an "economic exchange" model of motivation for participation, our research suggests that while many patients agree that they participated to receive needed services, many also did so for altruistic reasons. Under the "economic exchange" model, researchers gain subjects for their studies in return for free testing and medical care, monetary or material incentives, and information provision (McCabe, Varricchio, and Padberg, 1994). Eligible patients weigh the risks and benefits of expenditures of resources (Schain, 1994: Morrow, Hickok, and Burish, 1994), as well as the perceived efficacy of treatment.

The SHARE project provided women with many benefits in addition to those explained at the time informed consent forms were signed. Data from our study suggest that the desire for services was for many women intertwined with a desire to give something back to the community. Thus, the "economic exchange" framework does not appear to adequately describe Project SHARE's recruitment success.

Retention/Compliance: Interaction and Mutual Connectedness

Interpersonal interactions between medical care providers and patients are often seen as role based—taking place within a formal, circumscribed setting (Capella, 1987). Research tends to look only within rigid role boundaries at communication activities and relationship building between the interactants. Communication and interdisciplinary theorists interested in health care such as Schegloff (1988) have questioned the appropriateness of this assumption. Should one assume, barring evidence to the contrary, that women in medical studies who interact with a set of medical care providers continually over a period of years have the same type of relationship with their care providers as persons involved in a singular clinical encounter lasting ten to fifteen minutes (or less)? Qualitative evidence suggests that the relational component of the ongoing process of interaction between the patients and the staff is the key to retention in the study. This relationship is based on caring about the patient, and a mutual connectedness between the patient and the staff person.

Everyone Seemed to Care Who You Were; You Weren't Just Some Number

The above phrases echoed throughout the interviews with the participants, focusing on caring and individual attention. This type of relationship in a medical setting reflects a holistic approach (Schubert and Lionberger, 1995), and the growth of a recognition of the need for medical care providers to be "sharers" of care (Shillitoe and Christie, 1990) rather than providers. This feeling of caring was expressed by Project SHARE's clinical nurse coordinator: "We treat her like she was a friend instead of like a patient." Another SHARE staff member stated in a conversation with the first author of this chapter that she wanted the women to know she was more concerned with *them* than their *blood*, and that the patients were valued members of the team. Clearly, the patients were cognizant of provider attitudes. The patients felt that they "always have somebody to talk to," and that "they've always been there for me." When asked to evaluate the study, the patients indicated a high level of satisfaction tied to their level of comfort:

> I liked the way things were done and the people. Everyone seemed to care about who you were; you just weren't some number.

> I like it the way it is. You get to know the people and they know who you are. The people in the clinic are nice; they care about you. They give . . .

> The genuine concern I felt from the people that work here. The attention that's been given to not just our health, but our emotional stability, and even at times, financial stability. The fact that people genuinely care.

> I felt comfortable. I don't know—something made me come back, I just felt comfortable. I felt like they were going to take care of me.

Other patients indicated a perception of an emotional response going beyond any provider-client service relationship. The metaphors they chose to express themselves are a powerful glimpse into the depths of feelings engendered by the project staff in conjunction with the SHARE subjects. One women said that, "for the past three years, I've made a lot of *friends*, and I agreed to help, so I always keep my word." This is indicative of a very strong intrinsic motivation for adherence to protocol. Others expressed continuing involvement "'cause this is part of my *family*." One HIV-positive mother was involved in the project for the second time—with a second child born during the duration of the study. She said, "Yes, I like it. And they are good here. They are very good here. I *loved* them and I'm sure they *love me* . . . they're good people."

Connectedness: Using Feminist Theory to Understand the Data

By looking at the data through the lens of feminist psychology first articulated by the psychoanalyst Nancy Chodorow, many of factors that motivated women to participate in SHARE and to stay with the project can be seen. Feminist psychoanalytic theory broke new ground with a theory that denied Freud's androcentric ideas of individuation and the growth of the self in opposition to the all powerful mother figure. Rather, these theories suggested that women grow up "with a sense of continuity and similarity to their mother, a relational connection to the world" (Chodorow, 1990, p. 260). The term "self-in-relation" is used to describe female development rather than the "individuation" that is stressed in Freudian theories. In these feminist theories, a continuous psychological connection is posited that links females during normal development of the self. Further, the growth of identity in women and the fostering of relationships happen simultaneously. Instead of psychological growth being measured by the (male) criterion of "degree of separation," it is measured by the "female" criterion "degree of connectedness" (Surrey, 1991).

In medical settings, these theories have been used to help explain the conflict experienced by chronically ill mothers who seek treatment and feel that getting treatment for themselves interferes with their ability to parent (Thorne, 1990). Project SHARE helped mothers integrate their needs for well-baby care, HIV associated care, and the mothers' own needs to connect with other women for support, friendship, and medical care.

The relationships between the staff and clients were developed by the creation of intimacy. Intimacy in health care relationships can be seen as "the process of getting to know one another by sharing personal and private worlds in [the health care] environment" (Schubert and Lionberger, 1995, p. 109). Intimacy in this case was built by staff home visits, availability of staff beeper numbers (and in many cases, home phone numbers), and the availability of staff above and beyond medical necessity. One experience which both the staff and the clients saw as a "bonding experience" was the availability of the staff to be at the births of the babies. Staff were required to be at the births to obtain blood samples, but again, they offered support above and beyond that which was required by the study protocol by volunteering to be birthing coaches and to serve as support persons during the births in addition to their formal duties. According to the clinical nurse coordinator, "One of the things we said [in recruiting mothers-to-be] was, 'You know, you don't have to be by yourself.'" A participant who went through the birth process with a staff person mentioned that it was the support during labor that made her come back time and again to the project, because she "felt like she [the staff person] was here."

Through their relationships with staff, women gained the freedom to talk about their fears about mothering, coping with seropositivity, the uncertainty of the health of their babies, and living with partners and others with HIV. "I feel that I can have somebody to talk to about my situation. Like [the clinical nurse coordinator and her assistant]. I feel that I can have them two that I can talk to." Tied into disclosures in the reach toward intimacy with providers was the confidentiality of the program. Initially, many women were frightened of disclosure and felt they had to build up trust.

Trusting Providers Not to Broadcast Patient Business on the Street

The growth of trust between patients and providers can be seen as a function of the relational self of women. This relational self, the self engaged in caring with and for others, is mutually constructed through intimate disclosure, active participation with others, and empathy (Chodorow, 1990). In this model, the growth of intimacy between patient and provider can be defined as the "process of getting to know one another by sharing personal and private worlds in this environment" (Schubert and Lionberger, 1995, p. 109). The following exchange indicates how this trust was a mutual construction of the patient and provider relationship. The interviewer questions the patient's perceived need for other services.

> **Patient:** You'd probably have people open up more . . . if they could reach you or knew somebody else they could trust. I had to build my trust up.
> **Interviewer:** Building trust was important to you?
> **Patient:** Yeah. 'Cause it's not something you just want to blurt

out to the world, and ya'll are very good at keeping . . .
[confidentiality] . . .

Another patient noted: "I was afraid at first because I didn't know if
my business was going to be in the street," yet she returned because
she felt "everybody seemed to be really nice—that's the main reason. So that's the main reason to go ahead."

The clinical nurse coordinator indicated in her interview that
whenever the project needed to contact a patient at home, they
maintained the confidentiality of the project. Many of the patients
had not told their families or partners of their HIV status.

> When I place a call to their home, I say my first name,[ ].
> Family members may ask what group is this; what organization,
> what hospital, what clinic or that kind of thing. So, we were
> always cautious regarding confidentiality. When asked what
> Project SHARE is, we never tell them that we're an HIV/AIDS
> project. We say that we're a mother-baby research project.

This use of first names in calls to the house, the maintenance of
informality in phone conversation, and the sharing of the home
phone numbers by staff, illustrate how relationships between SHARE
mothers and staff are not necessarily built upon role-based encounters. From the initiation of the project, the women were not treated
as typical research subjects. The patient care liaison for the project
stressed that she treated the first meeting with a potential participant
as a social contact, and used the initial contact to start up a conversation. Often, whoever did the intake interview would become
the special contact for the mother throughout the project. A feeling
of responsibility and connection was fostered between the recruiter
and the mother. According to the clinical nurse coordinator:

> . . . whoever did the initial intake on the patient, was that
> patient's "person" throughout the whole project—day or night.
> One lady called during the day, to say that she that she needed
> somebody to come see her in the hospital because she thought
> she was dying. I was the person who interviewed her and brought
> her into the study and did the referral and intake—she would
> always call me. Then, the people who [the patient care liaison]
> had interviewed and brought into the project, would call her.

We Treated Her Like She Was a Friend Instead of Like a Patient

The developing relationships between the staff and the mothers were built upon more than confidential and intimate discourse. Program staff provided the mothers with material goods as well as pleasant experiences, indicating that the patients were treated in a model of a caring relationship not circumscribed by provider-patient roles. Yet, as in other research studies, access to material goods such as baby formula were used very self-consciously as incentives. Women had to be compliant, to come to their appointments with their babies, in order to obtain the goods and services:

> That's how the moms got the baby's milk—if they came and got the immunizations. If they haven't done the immunizations, they can't go to the WIC office and get milk. So one of the reasons that they are going to be compliant is that, if they get the vaccinations done, they'll get the milk.

Yet even the success of the milk program was not necessarily seen in relation to compliance with the study, rather in terms of the well-being of the children:

> The milk program has been a successful program because the babies got to have what they needed and got immunizations. They would be on the correct immunization schedule. This would help them not to come down with other kinds of diseases. That was one of the good things about having a program set up like that.

The staff also gave the mothers "little things" such as a few diapers or Tylenol—that they had obtained by actively seeking donations within the hospital and the community, so that the mothers did not have to utilize their limited resources:

> . . . little things, from a little medication to everything from thermometers to bulb syringes to clean out the mucus in the nose. Some babies didn't have many things. Moms didn't have clothes for them. We had little socks, diapers, and T-shirts.

The distribution of Tylenol was seen by the staff as a way of not straining the mother's personal budgets to include an avoidable visit to a physician, and so the babies would not be "sick and irritable."

When the HIV-positive mothers were in the hospital for births, the staff brought the participants both bottles and a handmade baby quilt made by the Quilt Project—a national volunteer group that provides homemade baby quilts to indigent, HIV-positive new mothers. The provision of baby presents and baby paraphernalia that in other socioeconomic groups would most likely be given by friends and relatives, seemed to create a bond between the mothers and staff. It led to the participants and staff alike feeling as if they were friends who participated in material and verbal exchanges that more closely characterized a relationship between social intimates than a provider-patient relationship.

The growing relational network between staff and participants was fostered by special events that took place within the confines of the clinic. The genesis of the project was a feeling shared by the clinical nurse coordinator that, "We just realized, I guess, how short life may be for a patient and her child who may be infected, because you really don't know." The project staff and volunteers decided to have parties for the children during clinic time for their first and second birthdays. With no budget for such activities, the staff and volunteers needed to band together to obtain the supplies:

> We had people who'd give us stuff. We'd go out and buy out of our own pockets—balloons and other party items. We'd have $2 left from the coffee fund and we'd buy a birthday cake and we'd buy some streamers. We had a volunteer who gave us some things.We'd use our own cups and other things from home. We'd just [have] cake and ice cream pretty much, at the end of a clinic visit.

The staff and mothers even took photographs at the parties, while taking precautions to preserve anonymity. Sharing pictures with the other staff members who knew the patients, as well as visitors from out of town who could not identify any of the participants, seems to be a social activity in which women in social and workplace situations commonly participate.

Most of the participants in the project seemed to feel positive about the parties, indicating that "we enjoyed it." One HIV-positive participant often sent her husband and child to parties when she had to work—feeling that "this is part of our extended family." She saw the parties in the following way:

> When we've come to social events here, it's been strictly social events. "How are you?" "It's a nice day." "This is a cute idea." Whatever, but the social atmosphere here is not revolving around illness and it's uplifting, not depressing. Everybody needs that. They don't always need to talk about how sick you are that particular day.

Only one of the interviewees indicated a discomfort with the party idea, and felt stigmatized at social events. "It might just be me; I'm looking at people and they're probably looking at me, and we're thinking, 'I wonder what's wrong with her,' so, you'd never say it, but . . ." This feeling of being stigmatized does not appear to be true of the healthy controls. One of the controls didn't mention the parties in her interview at all, and the other indicated that they participated in two Christmas parties, and her son was given "nice gifts."

These experiences are consistent with the work of Burgoon et al. (1987) who consider the affective factors in communication between providers and their patients to be more important than the exchange of information. Their findings indicate that:

> . . . affective satisfaction—trusting the physician, feeling the physician is concerned, feeling accepted and liked and feeling free to self-disclose—increases as a physician is perceived to express less dominance, more similarity, and more immediacy, as well as more receptivity. (p. 320)

The model of mutual sharing and connectedness exemplified by the Project SHARE experience is also consistent with the work of Jordan (1991), who suggests that:

> A model that acknowledges that therapy is a dialogue also recognizes that therapy is characterized by a process of mutual change and impact. Both the therapist and patient are touched

emotionally by each other, grow in relationship, gain something from one another, risk something of themselves in the process—both are affected, changed—part of an open system of feeling and learning. There is significant mutuality. . . . The therapist offers herself to be used for the healing. But within this context there is real caring in both directions, and is an important feeling of mutuality, with mutual respect, emotional availability, and openness to change on both sides. (p. 288)

CONCLUSION

Our study of Project SHARE is part of a larger study of the factors that are associated with successful recruitment, retention, and compliance of underrepresented populations in medical research. The success of Project SHARE with women—particularly with African-American women—suggests that it might serve as a model for future medical research projects and clinical trials that are interested in attracting similar patients. Our study suggests that women are attracted to such projects both to fulfill their own medical and psychosocial needs and in order to help others. These findings are consistent with the literature which posits the desire for services and altruism as factors in successful recruitment. However, the literature does not address the importance of the nature of the relationship created between the staff who recruit the patients and the patients themselves. Our research suggests that the bonds between study staff and patients are formed at the time of recruitment and that those bonds are so strong that patients continue to seek out the staff member who recruited them for assistance throughout their association with the project.

The caring relationships begun at the time of recruitment are the key to successful retention, according to our data. Previous research has suggested that retention and compliance are associated with meeting patients' physical needs for transportation, childcare, or financial recompense and meeting patients' social needs for empathy, acceptance and courtesy. Our research suggests that Project SHARE was successful because it not only met patients' physical and social needs, but it also met patients' needs for reciprocal caring relationships with other women. While the physical gifts and assistance with transportation were necessary and appreciated, the medical care and monitoring were very important, and the counselling and education were seen as useful, patient and provider interviews consistently emphasized the importance of the relationships that developed between patients and providers during the course of the project. Previous research has neglected this key component in successful retention and compliance.

These conclusions have several implications. For those interested in theory, they suggest that "exchange" models of patient motivation for involvement in research ought to be revisited. Theorists might create models that emphasize the relational dimensions as well as the physical and psychosocial dimensions of patient motivation.

For those interested in future research, our work suggests that close examination of medical research projects that have been successful in the recruitment, retention, and compliance of underrepresented populations provides insights not available in the literature. Future work should examine projects that were successful with other underrepresented populations including IDUs and African-American men. In addition, future work should examine the communication dimensions of development of the types of mutual caring relationships found in this study.

For those interested in practical applications, our research suggests that while the provision of necessary services such as transportation and child care are necessary for the successful recruitment, retention and compliance of women as medical research subjects, they are not sufficient. In addition, women seek opportunities for developing close relationships with providers with whom they can share their fears and their joys. Practitioners might consider how clinic visits can be structured to facilitate the development of such mutually caring relationships.

Project SHARE's success can serve as a model for other medical research projects. It suggests that the development of a unit that provides physical, psychosocial, and relational care as an integral component of medical research projects designed for women can enhance both the success of the research and the lives of the women (and their families) who participate. The ability to attract and maintain subjects while providing ethical service and care should be the goal of all medical research.

NOTES

1. U.S. Congress Public Law 103-43. National Institutes of Health revitalization Amendment. Washington, DC, June 10, 1993.
2. Dr. Marion Sims, the "Father of American Gynecology" in his experiments on vaginal fistulas.
3. "Mentally ill retarded infants at Willowbrook State School were deliberately infected with hepatitis" (Levine, 1986, quoted in Allen, 1994, p. 106).
4. There is some disagreement concerning these factors. See Besch.

REFERENCES

Allen, M. (1994). The dilemma for women of color in clinical trials. *JAMWA*, *49*(4), 105-109.
Besch, C. (1995). Compliance in clinical trials. *AIDS*, 9(1), 1-10.
Bishop, G.D., Alva, A.L., Contu, L., and Rittiman, T.K. (1991). Responses to persons with AIDS: Fear of contagion or stigma. *Journal of Applied Social Psychology, 21*, 1877-1888.
Blackwell, B. (1975). Drug therapy: Patient compliance. *New England Journal of Medicine, 289* (5), 249-252.
Brown, L. (1993). Enrollment of drug abusers in HIV clinical trials: A public health imperative for communities of color. *Journal of Psychoactive Drugs, 25*(1), 45-52.
Burgoon, J.K., Pfau, M., Parrott, R., Birk, T., Coker, R., and Burgoon, M. (1987). Relational communication, satisfaction, compliance-gaining strategies, and compliance in communication between physicians and patients. *Communication Monographs, 54*, 307-324.
Capella, J. (1987). Interpersonal communication: Definitions and fundamental questions. In Berger, C. and Chaffee, S. (Eds.), *Handbook of Communication Science,* 184-238. Newbury Park, CA: Sage.
CDC. (1995). First 500,000 AIDS Cases—United States, 1995. *Morbidity and Mortality Weekly Report, 44* (46), 849-853.
Chodorow, N. (1990). What is the relationship between psychoanalytic feminism and the psychoanalytic psychology of women? In D.L. Rhode (Ed.), *Theoretical Perspectives on Sexual Difference,* 114-130. New Haven, CT: Yale University Press.
Cotton, D., Finkelstein, D., Weili, H., Feinberg, J. (1993). Determinants of accrual of women to a large multicenter clinical trials program of human immunodeficiency virus infection. *Journal of Acquired Immune Deficiency Syndromes, 6*(12), 1323-1328.
El-Sadr, W. and Capps, L. (1992). The challenge of minority recruitment in clinical trials for AIDS. *JAMA, 267*(7), 954-957.
Glaser, B. and Strauss, A. (1967). *The Discovery of Grounded Theory: Strategies for Qualitative Research.* Chicago: Aldine.

Haywood, L.J., deGuzman, M., Jackson, L., Venegas, J., and Blumfield, D. (1992). Patient recruitment for hospital- and clinic-based studies in the inner city. In Becker, D.M., Hill, D.R., Jackson, J.S., Levine, D.M., Stillman, F.A., and Weiss, S.M. (Eds.), *Health Behavior Research in Minority Populations: Access, Design, and Implementation,* 47-52. Bethesda, MD: NIH.

Hunter, C., Frelick, R., Feldman, A., Bavier, A., Dunlap, W., Ford, L. et al. (1987). Selection factors in clinical trials: Results from the community clinical oncology program patient log. *Cancer Treatment Reports, 71*(6), 559-565.

Johnson, K.M. and Arfken, C.L. (1992). Individual recruitment strategies in minority-focused research. In D.M. Becker, D.R. Hill, J.S. Jackson, D.M. Levine, F.A. Stillman, and S.M. Weiss (Eds.), *Health Behavior Research in Minority Populations: Access, Design, and Implementation,* 24-29. Bethesda, MD: NIH.

Jordan, J. (1991). Empathy, mutuality, and therapeutic change: Clinical implications of a relational model. In J. Jordan, A. Kaplan, J.B. Miller, I. Stiver, and J. Surrey (Eds.), *Women's Growth in Connection: Writings from the Stone Center,* 283-290. New York: The Guilford Press.

Kreps, G.L., O'Hair, D., and Clowers, M. (1994). The influences of human communication on health outcomes. *American Behavioral Scientist, 38,* 215-223.

Kroger, F. (1994). Toward a healthy public: Models, messages, and meaning. *American Behavioral Scientist, 38*(2), 215-233.

Marlink, R., Kanki, P., Thior, I., Travers, K., Eisen, G., Silby, T., Traore, I., Hsieh, C.C., Dia, M.C., and Gueye, E.H. (1994). Reduced rate of disease development after HIV-2 infection as compared to HIV-1. *Science, 265,* 1587-1590.

McCabe, M., Varricchio, C., and Padberg, R. (1994). Efforts to recruit the economically disadvantaged to national clinical trials. *Seminars in Oncology Nursing, 10*(2), 123-129.

McCarthy, C. (1994). Historical background and clinical trials involving women and minorities. *Academic Medicine, 69*(9), 695-698.

McCracken, G. (1988). *The Long Interview.* Newbury Park, CA: Sage.

Merkatz, R. and Junod, S. (1994). Historical background of changes in FDA policy on the study and evaluation of drugs in women. *Academic Medicine, 69*(9),703-707.

Merton, V. (1993). The exclusion of pregnant, pregnable, and once-pregnable people (a.k.a. women) from biomedical research. *American Journal of Law & Medicine, 19*(4), 369-451.

Millon-Underwood, S., Sanders, E., and Davis, M. (1993). Determinants of participation in state-of-the-art cancer prevention, early detection/screening, and treatment trials among African Americans. *Cancer Nursing, 16,* 25-33.

Morrow, G., Hickok, J., and Burish, T. (1994). Behavioral Aspects of Clinical Trials: An Integrated Framework from Behavior Theory. Paper presented at the National Conference on Clinical Trials, Atlanta, 2676-2682.

Morse, E., Simon, P., Besch, C., and Walker, J. (1995). Issues of recruitment, retention, and compliance in community-based clinical trials with traditionally underserved populations. *Applied Nursing Research, 8*(1), 8-14.

Moser, M. and Lunn, J. (1982). Responses to captopril and hydrochlorothiazide in black patients with hypertension. *Clinical Pharmacology Therapy, 32,* 307-312.

Nabrit-Stephens, B., Emmons, P., South, M., Estrada, J., Harris, R., Curry, A., and Hatcher, F. (1985). *Challenges in Clinical Research Activities Among Minorities Infected with Human Immunodeficiency Virus (HIV).* Paper presented at the National Medical Association Scientific Assembly, Atlanta, GA.

Pollack, P.H., Lilie, S., and Vittes, M.E. (1993). On the nature and dynamics of social construction: The case of AIDS. *Social Science Quarterly, 74,* 123-33.

Ross, M.W., Jeffords, K., and Gold, J. (1994). Reasons for entry into and understanding of HIV/AIDS clinical trials: A preliminary study. *AIDS Care, 6,* 77-82.

Ryan, L. (1994). *Reasons for Entry into Anti-V Trials.* Manuscript submitted for publication.

Ryan, L. (1995). "Going Public" and "Watching Sick People"—the Clinic Setting as a Factor in the Experiences of Gay Men Participating in AIDS Clinical Trials. *AIDS Care, 7* (2), 147-158.

Schain, W. (1994). Barriers to clinical trials—Part II: Knowledge and attitudes of potential participants. Paper presented at the National Conference on Clinical Trials, Atlanta, 2666-2671.

Schegloff, E. (1988). Between micro and macro: Contexts and other connections. In J. Alexander, B. Geissen, R. Munch, and N. Smelser (Eds.), *The Macro-Micro Link,* 207-234. Berkeley: University of California Press.

Schmucker, D. and Vessel, E. (1993). Underrepresentation of women in clinical drug trials. *Clinical Pharmacology & Therapeutics, 54,* 11-15.

Schubert, P. and Lionberger, L. (1995). Mutual connectedness: A study of nurse-client interaction. *Journal of Holistic Nursing, 13*(2), 102-116.

Scott-Jones, D. (1993). *Ethical Issues in Reporting and Referring in Research with Minority and Low-Income Populations.* Paper presented at the biennial meeting of the Society for Research in Child Development, New Orleans, LA.

Shillitoe, R. and Christie, M. (1990). Psychological approaches to the management of chronic illness: The example of diabetes mellitus. In P. Bennett, J. Weinman, and P. Spurgeon (Eds.), *Current Developments in Health Psychology,* 177-208. Chur, Switzerland: Harwood Academic Publishers.

Spradley, J.P. (1979). *The Ethnographic Interview.* Orlando, FL: Holt, Rinehart & Winston.

Strauss, A.L., Corbin, J., Fagerhaugh, S., Glaser, B., Maines, D., Suczek, B., and Wiener, C.L. (1984). *Chronic Illness and the Quality of Life.* (second edition). St. Louis, MO: Mosby Company.

Surrey, J.L. (1991). Relationship and empowerment. In J. Jordan (Ed.), *Women's Growth in Connection: Writings from the Stone Center,* 162-180. New York: The Guilford Press.

Thomas, C., Pinto, H., Roach, M., and Vaughn, C. (1994). Participation in clinical trials: Is it state-of-the-art treatment for African Americans and other people of color? *Journal of the National Medical Association, 86*(3), 177-182.

Thorne, S. (1990). Mothers with chronic illness: A predicament of social construction. *Health Care for Women International, 11,* 209-221.

Wachtel, T., Piette, J., Mor, V., Stein, M., Fleishman, J., and Carpenter, C. (1992). Quality of life in persons with human immunodeficiency virus infection: Measurement by the medical outcomes study instrument. *Annals of Internal Medicine, 116* (2), 129-137.

Washington, H. (1994). Human guinea pigs. *Emerge*, October, 24-35.

Weijts, W. (1994). Responsible health communication: Taking control of our lives. *American Behavioral Scientist, 38*(2), 257-270.

Wermeling, D. and Selwitz, A. (1993). Current issues surrounding women and minorities in drug trials. *The Annals of Pharmacotherapy, 27,* 904-910.

Woody, G., Metzger, D., and Mulvaney, F. (1994). Preparations for AIDS vaccine trials: Recruitment and retention of in- and out-of-treatment injection drug users. *AIDS Research and Human Retroviruses, 10,* (supplement 2), 197-199.

PART III:
NEGOTIATING REPRESENTATION

Chapter 9

Women and the AIDS Memorial Quilt

David F. Shaw

Francine say she gonna send this quilt to Washington
like folks doing from all 'cross the country,
so many good people gone. Babies, mothers, fathers
and boys like our Junie.

—Melvin Dixon
(extracted from "Aunt Ida Pieces a Quilt," 1993)

Since its October 1987 inaugural display in Washington, DC, The NAMES Project AIDS Memorial Quilt (the Quilt) has grown from 1900 memorial panels to more than 40,000 panels for the display on the Capitol Mall in October 1996. The small storefront on San Francisco's Market Street where neighborhood residents gathered to "take all of our individual experiences, and stitch them together to make something that had strength and beauty" (NAMES Project, 1995, p. 1) has spawned 39 NAMES Project chapters across the country, and 28 international chapters.

In addition to conveying the enormity of the AIDS pandemic, an integral goal of the AIDS Memorial Quilt is to offer a creative form of expression for all whose lives have been affected by HIV and AIDS and to preserve the memory of those who have died as a result of the disease. In this light, the Quilt honors those who have lost a loved one to AIDS as much as it honors those who died as a result of AIDS.

Cleve Jones, a San Francisco gay rights activist, conceived the NAMES Project AIDS Memorial Quilt during a 1985 candlelight march memorializing the 1978 assassination of San Francisco Supervisor Harvey Milk. By the time of the 1985 march, the number of San Franciscans lost to AIDS had passed 1,000. Jones asked the marchers to write the names of friends and loved ones who had died of AIDS on placards which they could carry in the march. When the march ended, marchers taped the placards on the side of the Federal Building. The assembly of placards, each unique in script and style, reminded Jones of a patchwork quilt. He later commented:

> . . . and that idea evoked such warm old memories of comfort. I had been consumed with rage and fear. Most of my old friends were dead. I felt that we lived in this little ghetto on the West Coast which would be destroyed without anyone in the rest of the world even noticing. I knew we needed a memorial. (Bellm, 1989, p. 35)

The idea came to life in 1987 when Jones created the first panel, a memorial made from stencils, spray paint, and a white sheet, for his best friend Marvin Feldman to whom the NAMES Project AIDS Memorial Quilt is dedicated:

> I spent the whole afternoon thinking about Marvin. I thought about why we were best friends and why I loved him so much. By the time I finished the piece, my grief had been replaced by a sense of resolution and completion. (Ruskin, 1988, p. 18)

Several months later, The NAMES Project displayed the Quilt for the first time in Washington, DC as part of the National March on Washington for Lesbian and Gay Rights. There were 1,920 memorial panels, 2,000 yards of white walkway, nearly 7,000 pounds of materials, and half a million visitors. Since the first display, the Quilt has grown steadily to its current mark of more than 40,000 panels. Portions of it have been displayed at fundraising events across the country raising more than $1,700,000 for AIDS service organizations throughout North America. The October 1996 display in Washington, DC, marked the fifth time the Quilt had been displayed in its entirety.

Images of the Quilt permeate American popular culture. The Quilt was featured on a daytime soap opera and in the Academy

Award-winning documentary, *Common Threads: Stories from the Quilt*. Its panels decorated the windows of a Neiman-Marcus department store and an image of its display is pictured in a series of images of American life in a Boeing commercial. It has inspired literature and poetry and, most notably, the Quilt was nominated for a Nobel Peace Prize in 1989.

The vast media promotion and iconic status of the Quilt is, however, only part of its complex effect. Sturken (1992) argues that the major part of the Quilt's effect exists in the tension between the two levels Jones conceived: the Quilt as a national memorial versus the Quilt as a product of intimate and local communities. In short, while the Quilt as memorial memorializes a largely gay male population, the Quilt as a grassroots effort rising from within intimate communities necessarily includes women who through their work, friendships, filial, and other familial relationships have been affected by AIDS.

This chapter investigates the ways in which a number of Denver-area women have come to volunteer their time, energy, and skill in constructing panels for the Quilt. Collectively, the panels created by these women memorialize the lives of two sons, two friends, a sister, a brother, and a niece. Further, it asks how women's subjective experiences with AIDS and loss have been made meaningful through their experiences with and responses to the Quilt. It also queries the function of the Quilt in the creation of new kinship communities and the maintenance of other AIDS-related communities.

QUILTING AND WOMEN'S COMMUNICATION

Quilting has traditionally been viewed as domestic, and therefore female, work. Made with spare time and spare fabric, quilts were regarded with little import other than that of their utility. John Howat, Chair of the Departments of American Art for the Metropolitan Museum of Art, (Peck, 1990, p. 10) chronicles the shifting emphasis in the collecting and artistic study of quilts. Initially, quilts were collected primarily as testaments to the historical figures who owned them, rather than for the beauty or significance of the objects themselves. This collecting pervaded much of the antique craze that began with the nation's centennial. The first quilts to

enter the museum's collection were donated as part of family trea-
sures.

By the late 1960s, the collecting of quilts based on historical
ownership was subsumed by collections based on graphic sensibilities. Off the bed and onto the wall, the quilt became a validated
object of scholarly study. By the 1980s, the new questions revolved
around the place of quilting in women's lives, regionalism, technique, and technology. Because many quilts were of anonymous
origin, not only was the quilt itself a worthy object of interpretive
theories, but so were the diaries, journals, and letters by and
between quilters of the era (Peck, 1990).

Quilts, however, are more than records of family histories and
indexes of North American textiles and design. They are an art that
comes from the home and the relationships formed within it. The
bulk of communication research surrounding quilts focuses on the
rhetorical power of the quilt as women's speech—essentially positing the quilt as an artifact that communicates (e.g., Williams, 1994).
This, however valid, ignores the act of quilting itself as communication which fosters strength and community.

In "Fragile Families: Quilts as Kinship Bonds," Clark (1987)
discusses the dissolution of the family into gender-based spheres
during the period of increasing industrialization in the nineteenth
century. The worlds of commerce and industry were deemed the
domain of men. In search of employment, men were often separated
from their families for extended periods of time. Women were often
separated from their mothers, sisters, and grandmothers as they
followed their husbands' searches for work. The toll of physical
labor on men also left many young women and children widowed
and fatherless. Women found security in a family-based female
world and an extensive network of female relatives and friends. In
addition to being part of the domestic economy of women, the quilt
was also a vital part of this extended family bond. Women gathered
in support of one another sharing advice, happiness, and grief over a
large wooden quilting frame. When a man died before his wife, the
community of women gave quilts to the widow to show their continued support. As Clark writes, quilts were not only the "symbols
of the strong and loving ties that underlay women's family relationships. They were truly comforters" (Clark, 1987, p. 7).

Williams (1994) writes that in addition to their utility in providing warmth and the social bonding inherent in the production of a
quilt, quilts must be seen as historic vehicles for women's speech:

> Even in a culture that largely denies women a public voice,
> women have discovered that through their private work, they
> can speak about private and public concerns. Women have
> used their quilts to record historical events; pass family values,
> stories, and histories from one generation to the next; cast
> ballots; register their support for or opposition to various polit-
> ical policies; and draw road maps to freedom. (p. 21)

In this light, the panels women make for the AIDS Memorial Quilt
can also be seen as potent vehicles of women's speech in support of
AIDS communities and, in some instances, in opposition to political
and governmental inaction around AIDS.

Jones was acutely aware of the strong tradition of the feminized
art form when he conceived the Quilt:

> I think of (the quilt) as a strong durable fabric that is made by
> collaborations of prairie women who have marched with their
> Conestoga wagons across the plains; it is something that is
> given as a gift, passed down through generations, that speaks
> of family loyalty. (Sturken, 1992, p. 77)

Again, while the Quilt represents the handiwork of many women,
it also represents the loss of a largely gay and male population. For
Jones, this is integral to the Quilt's symbolic power: "We picked a
feminine art to try to get people to look beyond this aggressive male
sexuality component." Sturken further argues that "connotations of
the quilt as nurturing, comforting, and protective are thus aligned
with the changing identity of the gay community as taking care of
its sick and responding with compassion to the dying" (Sturken,
1992, p. 82).

The three types of traditional quilts that provide a framework for
discussing the AIDS Memorial Quilt and the individual panels com-
prising it are the Crazy quilt, the Mourning quilt, and the Album
quilt. The first, coined "Crazy" because of its complex pattern and
wide array of materials and shapes, best describes the Quilt in its

entirety—the Quilt is, in effect, the world's largest Crazy quilt. In *How to Make an American Quilt*, Whitney Otto (1991) writes of the Crazy quilt's "lack of order, its randomness, its shrouded personal meanings," and invites her reader to "deplore its lack of skill and finesse" (p. 49).

The Mourning quilt reflects the nineteenth century obsession with death (Clark, 1987, p. 11). When families were broken by death, women used quilts as a way to preserve ties to their deceased loved ones. Fragments from the deceased's clothing decorated the Mourning quilt. The traditional Widow's quilt is similarly a Mourning quilt and was given as a gift from women to woman as a sign of support and love. The AIDS Memorial Quilt is a menagerie of Mourning and Friendship quilts, but in reverse exchange, the panels are gifts from the individual to the community.

Finally, the Album quilt is evident in both the Quilt in its entirety and in the individual panels. In an Album quilt, each block is created and signed by a different contributor. The individual blocks are then sewn together in a larger quilt. While many of the individual panels in the Quilt are styled after traditional Album quilts, all of the Quilt's individual panels combine to create a large Album quilt.

THE LIVING, THE DEAD, AND AIDS

While each panel in the Quilt represents one death, or on rare occasion, two deaths to AIDS, the panels also represent the collaboration of those who have survived the deceased. From this duality comes the narrative power of the Quilt—it provides the bereaved with a vehicle to tell the stories of their loved ones while telling the stories about the effects of AIDS on their own lives.

Kathy's sister Annie had just given birth to her daughter Clarice when Annie learned that her IV-drug-addicted boyfriend had AIDS. She immediately tested herself for the virus and discovered that she too was positive. At three months old, Clarice also tested positive for HIV. As her relationship with her boyfriend deteriorated, the family thought it best that Annie and Clarice move from Nebraska to Colorado.

Less than a year after the triple diagnosis, Kathy, a police officer who was single at the time, had her sister and niece move into her two-bedroom apartment. Annie took care of the home and her daughter while Kathy worked and cared for both. A year later, Annie died. Over the period of that first year, Kathy and Clarice developed a strong bond—so strong that strangers could not tell which of the two sisters was Clarice's biological mother. Kathy's career with the Arvada, Colorado Police was in full swing. She was working undercover in narcotics and had just been invited to work with the Drug Enforcement Agency. Her hours were long and scattered, yet she could not imagine turning care of Clarice over to anyone else. Harriet, Kathy's mother and Clarice's grandmother, took an early retirement in order to move in with the two, care for Clarice, and get the child to the hospital for her many visits. Clarice died four years later. She was six years old.

Pat is a mother and grandmother who is active in various quilting communities in Colorado. She works at the Rocky Mountain Quilt Museum in Golden, Colorado where she provides quilts for the museum shop. When she learned that her son Kim was gay her response was somewhat typical: "Just don't act gay at family events." Kim's coming out was somewhat difficult for Pat to understand; he had been married and had a young son.

When Kim was diagnosed with AIDS in 1992, Pat became active in a practitioner class at a local church. Through her involvement with the group, she came to understand and accept her son's sexuality even more. During one of his many stays in the hospital, Kim told his mother, "I wish I knew how to knit or something to help pass the time." Pat brought him one of the small quilting projects that she assembles for the Quilt Museum—an all-inclusive package for the beginner. Kim enjoyed quilting very much; it was an integral part of his relationship with his mother until he died in February of 1993.

Rebecca is an interior architect in Denver. In 1987, her older brother Jeremy, who was also an interior architect, was diagnosed with AIDS. Rebecca moved to Los Angeles and lived with and cared for her brother. She was readily accepted into his circle of friends—many of whom had tested HIV positive or already had full-blown AIDS. She lived with Jeremy for the last 18 months of his life and moved back to Denver six months after his death.

As a teen lesbian in the early 1980s, Nancy became best friends with Thomas, another gay student from her Thornton, Colorado high school. The two were inseparable: they double-dated, registered for the same classes, and snuck into Denver gay bars with fake IDs. As part of a Home Economics class the two shared, Thomas and Nancy learned to quilt. Nancy recalls thinking how bizarre her friend was when he started sewing his baby toys and pictures of himself onto the queen-size backing he had prepared.

When Thomas, who had been sexually active with men since his early teens, became ill after high school graduation, he asked Nancy and his sister to finish the quilt he began in Home Economics class. He had only completed a two-square-foot section of the queen-size quilt. He died less than a year later. The quilt remained unfinished. There was no AIDS Memorial Quilt yet, but the two young women worked sporadically for more than two and a half years to finish the quilt their friend and brother had started.

Barb was a full-time student and worked as an Early Childhood Specialist for Douglas County, Colorado in the spring of 1991 when she met Raymond, an eighteen-month-old infant who had been born HIV positive and addicted to drugs. She was assigned as a case worker for the hospice foster home which housed Raymond and about ten other children. When she met Ray Ray (as she came to call him), she immediately noticed that he was not functioning at the level a child his age should. His doctors attributed his delayed growth and lack of affect to his medical condition, but Barb was convinced that it had more to do with his environment. She intervened and started taking Ray Ray for one day a week and over the weekends. She noticed an immediate improvement in his development and decided that she would take him as her own foster child. Finally, when he was three and a half years old, Ray Ray moved to his new mother's apartment.

"We were going to have fun" was Barb's attitude. She took Ray Ray camping in the mountains, to Disney World, horseback riding, skiing, swimming, and to her parents' home for Christmas. He even got to meet Garth Brooks. It was, however, a difficult road. In addition to a broken engagement, Barb could not find a daycare center that would accept Ray Ray. Her friends, largely a group of childhood specialists like herself, would take Ray Ray whenever they could. When there was no one to watch him, Kathy took him to work and school with her. She missed both school and work frequently because of necessary trips to Children's Hospital.

Ray Ray blossomed. An integral part of Barb's life, he became part of a large extended family of her friends. After three weeks in his first daycare center, Ray Ray caught strep throat and died at four and a half years old. Barb had only recently begun the process of legally adopting her son.

Maria worked at the I-Beam, a gay bar in San Francisco, for ten years. She was the only female bartender on the staff. The money was great and the I-Beam was the place to be, thus there was little turnover in the staff. Consequently, Maria came to see her co-workers as an extended and constant family.

As a lesbian working in a gay bar in San Francisco during the height of the AIDS epidemic, Maria was well aware of the disease and its devastation. Just as many people, her friend and co-worker Mark had lived a somewhat wild life before becoming aware of AIDS. In the late 1980s, he was still in good health and took good care of himself. Maria recalls that Mark appeared to be fine in October and suddenly died two months later in December 1988. He was the second of many good friends Maria has lost to AIDS.

THE SYMBOLIC REPRESENTATION OF THE DEAD

The NAMES Project has only one requirement for contributing a panel to the AIDS Memorial Quilt: it must measure three feet by six feet, approximately the size of an adult grave site. Creativity abounds in the panels. Some panels are quilted, others painted. Some contain only text, others contain only images. Some are somber in tone, others are whimsical. The list of materials used in the panels reads like a trip to the craft store, hardware store, flea market, toy store, and thrift shop: antique quilts, Barbie dolls, bubble-wrap, cowboy boots, credit cards, leather chaps, photographs, sequins, stuffed animals, and wedding rings.

Once the panels have been submitted, volunteers sew them in 12-foot square blocks of eight. When the Quilt is on display, four of these larger blocks create a larger square of 32 panels. When the Quilt is in storage in San Francisco, visitors can call ahead and schedule a viewing of specific panels. Names from all the panels are stored in a database which tells volunteers where to find each individual panel.

Kathy had numerous mechanisms for coping with the grief of losing Clarice—a process she started while Clarice was still alive. She kept volumes of journals out of which she published a chapter on her life with Clarice in a book for AIDS caregivers. Kathy also went to a local PFLAG group (Parents and Friends of Lesbians and Gays) for support, but found that her issues in dealing with a small child with AIDS were different. She talked to one of Clarice's doctors at Children's Hospital about starting a support group for families with children affected by AIDS. When she founded Angels Unaware in February 1992, there were four families at the first meeting. Nearly four years later, Angels Unaware has 52 member families.

Making a quilt panel was another way Kathy dealt with her grief. She had learned about the Quilt through news features. She had also heard that a panel dedication ceremony was scheduled in Greeley, Colorado, for the fall of 1994:

> After Clarice died, my mom and I knew we wanted to do a panel. We got together with some other women who had lost their sons to AIDS and we did a quilting day. We had a quilting book that had all kinds of different ideas from the panels. We all drew pictures and talked about what we wanted to do. Out of that initial meeting came this panel for Clarice.

Clarice's panel depicts an angel floating with several balloons. Three small balloons contain images of Sesame Street characters. Clarice was cremated with a stuffed Elmo toy, her favorite of the characters. The silver balloon in the upper left corner contains a photo transfer image of Clarice with quilted angel wings sewn to her shoulders. The balloon next to it has a photograph of Clarice and her mother that was taken when they moved in with Kathy; the words "Mother and Daughter" appear underneath it. Another balloon depicts two unicorns in needlepoint that Annie had stitched before she died. Kathy and her mother chose this image because it reminded them of a mother and daughter. When Clarice was sick, it was often difficult to change her clothes. Kathy and Clarice, always involved in crafts, made a Barney T-shirt that tied in the back to facilitate simple clothing changes. The shirt constitutes another balloon. The final balloon has a drawing Clarice made of herself. A stick figure with a feeding tube coming from her stomach, it simply says "ME." The word "LOVE," written three times, appears in the lower left corner of the panel.

Barb, too, was at the initial quilting day with Kathy. Through Ray Ray, she had become involved with Kathy's group, Angels Unaware. She was seeing a therapist to help her through her grief and was still active with Angels Unaware. About making a panel, she recalls:

> At first, I didn't think this was going to be part of my grieving process—I didn't think, "This is something that will help me." Like a journal, I know that I'm doing that as part of my healing process. The key was that the quilt was part of a way of staying his mom. At first, I did it as his mom for him. I needed to make it good to represent him. I really didn't think how it was affecting me.

Barb had seen several images from the Quilt. She knew that many people used clothes and toys in constructing their panels, but she did not want to give those items up. Instead, she searched for fabrics and images that captured the essence of a little boy—specifically, those images that reflected Ray Ray's interests.

Barb went to visit her parents in North Dakota and worked on the panel for about a week. Barb conceived the panel, her mother did most of the sewing, and her sisters helped from time to time. Ray Ray's panel is white with a red border and red crossbars dividing it into four quadrants. Each quadrant is filled with images of cowboys, sports, and cars—the stuff of childhood. In the center is a yellow cloud that says "Ray Ray Age 4." Emerging from the cloud is a yellow beam with the words "our Ray of sunshine" sewn into it. In one corner are several small balloons. Barb left many of these balloons blank so that if she ever saw the panel again, she could write in them. Scattered throughout the panel are stamped handprints cut from a printed sheet. Barb explains that Ray Ray left an indelible print on all who met him and she hoped that somehow, through the panel, he "might touch someone else."

On one of Pat's hospital visits to see her son Kim, he asked her to make him a panel for the Quilt. They talked about it only briefly. Kim's only request was that the panel contain irises:

> He had seen that movie on the Quilt and was very touched by that and he wanted me to make him a panel for the NAMES Project. He was very specific that he wanted to have irises on it. He loved irises. If I hadn't been a quilter, he would probably have asked someone else. Kim wanted a panel on that quilt.

Pat distributed fabric squares at Kim's memorial service. Telling people of Kim's request for irises, she asked them to take the squares home and create a patch for Kim's quilt. She was making a traditional friendship quilt—one in which members of a community would contribute their own squares to a larger commemorative quilt. Pat recalls, "I wanted it to reflect all the lives he had touched."

Several months later, she had collected nine squares and began to lay them out in her sewing room, carefully arranging them on the iris print fabric she had selected for the top of the quilt. Among the squares was one she had made Kim's son sign, and another stitched by her religious and conservative mother-in-law. In the center of the quilt is a square with a red ribbon and the following text: "IN MEMORY OF KIM ALLEN DAVIS JANUARY 24, 1963-FEBRUARY 18, 1983. BELOVED SON BROTHER HUSBAND FATHER FRIEND LOVER." The finished quilt did not meet the NAMES Project's three-by-six-feet requirement for panel submission. Pat laughs, "I knew what they wanted and I knew what I wanted. I was making a quilt!"

Four months after Rebecca's brother Jeremy died, four of his friends approached her with the idea of making a panel in his memory. Of the men who had approached her, all were HIV positive and two had developed AIDS. Because Rebecca was a designer and had lived closely with Jeremy for the last 18 months of his life, the men thought that she would be a valuable asset in designing the panel in a way true to Jeremy's own design sensibilities.

At the time, Rebecca thought that the panel was nothing Jeremy would have instigated for himself or anyone else. The Quilt, to Rebecca, was a way for the living to deal with AIDS. Opting for more proactive work, Rebecca knew that this was probably the only panel she would ever work on. The panel that she helped design was completed by the four men two months after she left Los Angeles. It is a noniconic ivory and black grid pattern made of woven fabric. The weaves generate from the middle of the panel, reaching out to the larger Quilt. In the corner is a small red patch which read: "In Loving Memory of Jeremy Kenny, from Friends and Family." Rebecca stated:

> Jeremy had a really fine sensibility and a really classical and truthful nature. There was a real simplicity to what we did and as much as it reflected his own character it was universal. We dealt more with the issue—obviously, because it was created by four guys who had AIDS and me who knows so many people with it.

Nancy first read of the Quilt in *Outfront*, a Denver-area gay and lesbian weekly newspaper. She was struck by the fact that Thomas had started his own memorial quilt before he died, moreover, that she and his sister had finished it for him nearly three years later. Rather than creating a new panel for the Quilt, the two women decided to contribute a section of the memory quilt that Thomas had begun himself. They cut a three-by-six section out of the middle of the queen-size quilt, covered the photographs and trinkets with plastic and submitted it to the NAMES Project.

Thomas's sister sewed the words "this was my brother" into the panel. Nancy moved a photograph from their senior prom to the center of the Quilt to make sure it would be included with the section that Thomas had started. Among the menagerie of objects on the panel are a section of baby blanket, a baby tooth, a beer cap, and an empty one-shot vodka bottle. They cut the remaining part of Thomas's quilt into several small blocks. They each still have pieces. Several years later, when Thomas's father died, his mother was finally able to ask what became of Thomas's memory quilt. The two women told her and she accepted one of the remaining blocks.

Shortly after Mark died, Maria was having dinner with her partner and two of Mark's friends. One of the friends, Ralph, suggested they all make a panel for Mark. The idea stuck and the four talked about who else they would ask to help. Soon after that, Maria, the others from that dinner, two neighbors, and a friend Mark had grown up with in New York met to talk about Mark and a panel. The theme that kept coming up was music; Mark had worked in record stores when he was younger, DJ'd at the Stud in San Francisco, and tended bar with Maria at the I-Beam.

The panel they made for Mark brings new meaning to the term Album quilt. In the center of the panel is a large black record. The label reads "Mark Cheroff." A diagonal rainbow strip runs from the lower left corner to the upper right corner. Several smaller record discs cut from iridescent fabric fill the rest of the panel. The label on each of these discs tells of a period or place in Mark's life. The group worked steadily for weeks, laying the pieces out on paper, cutting discs, telling stories, and finally sewing the panel together at the NAMES Project's workshop. In the fashion of traditional Album quilts, the quilters all signed the underside of the panel.

HEALING THROUGH THE QUILT: TURNING PAIN INTO ACTION

Raphael (1983) writes that the rituals and ceremonies such as funerals and memorials surrounding the dead "make the death public" (p. 37). Hawkins (1993) similarly argues that the Quilt has "enabled quite private reality to come out in public" (p. 770). These rites of passage enable the bereaved to accept the death of the loved one. Symbolically, the rites serve as an opportunity for the living to experience the presence of the dead person one last time before bidding a final farewell. More important, the rites "provide an opportunity for reestablishment of the social group, for a reinforcement of its life and unity" (p. 37). When the pain of separation is too awesome to deal with, the bereaved may take active measures to cultivate a sense of presence of the deceased (p. 41).

For each woman who worked on a panel, the part the Quilt serves in healing their loss varies. Sometimes the panel presented the decisive moment when they became aware of the enormity of the AIDS epidemic. The mother of a gay man likened working on the Quilt to coming out of the closet. For others, as Raphael (1983) suggests, it was an experience that bonded them with friends and family. All agree, however, that the Quilt was one of the many mechanisms used in healing the grief of loss. The different reactions to the Quilt are an integral part of its effect, and the ways in which each woman has taken her individual experience with the Quilt and turned it into other AIDS-related work vary as widely as the panels they designed. In short, for those not already actively working in AIDS communities, the Quilt represented a viable segue to political and social action. For those already working through and with AIDS, the Quilt offered an opportunity to refocus and reexamine the work they had already undertaken.

Butler (1993) writes that, "Insofar as grief remains unspeakable, the rage over the loss can redouble by virtue of remaining unavowed." She also cites the importance of collective institutions for grieving inasmuch as they allow for the "reassembling of community, the reworking of kinship, and the reweaving of sustaining relationships" (p. 236). The panels made by the women I interviewed were only part of their responses to AIDS and, in many ways, fulfill those virtues of collective institutions Butler cites. Many of the women remain active in AIDS communities. Young (1990) critiques the notion of community, arguing that the leveling over of difference in favor of unity exists in tension with the goal of feminist research, further that "such an ideal of shared subjectivity, or the transparency of subjects to one another, denies difference in the sense of the basic asymmetry of subjects" (p. 307). However, the Quilt, by it's very design, promotes unity while acknowledging difference.

Barb, unaware how the Quilt would affect her, had made Ray Ray's panel out of a sense of motherly duty. It was not until she presented the panel at a ceremony with hundreds of panels that she realized how the Quilt affected her:

> The ceremony was probably the most overwhelming and emotional experience I had had since he died. When I walked in and saw all the panels and I walked around looking at them, I felt like I was in a huge warehouse with all these unwrapped gifts that were never going to get to be opened. They were sitting there wasted and when I'd look at the panel I'd think, "God, I know what's in this present and no one's going to get to experience it again." It just hit me how horrible AIDS was. I mean I knew how horrible it was watching it take Ray Ray's life away, but to see how much it affected other people and to

know that this was only a very small section of the Quilt—it just hit me. It motivated me to stop thinking about me and my hurt and to do something for other people.

Barb kept working with Angels Unaware, but it became increasingly difficult for her to watch families living with AIDS while she was mourning Ray Ray's death. She decided that she had to do something to make families enjoy the time they still had together. Remembering the wonderful times she and Ray Ray had together in the mountains, she solicited volunteers and donors and started Camp Ray Ray, a camp for families and children affected by AIDS, on Memorial Day Weekend in 1995. At least, Barb hopes to make it a once-per-year event.

Kathy waited for four months after Clarice's death before beginning her memorial panel. Burdened with grief, she didn't feel like she could start any earlier:

> It was really difficult because nobody wants to talk about this stuff. It helped because my mom and I put it together and we spent time together and we were talking a lot about our feelings. It was good for both of us because it made us talk. Usually it's out of your mind—you keep yourself busy so you don't have to think about it. Sometimes you want to think of them not being here anymore and sometimes you need to talk about it.

The panel was on the livingroom floor for months while Kathy and her mother decorated it. It seemed the appropriate place because Clarice had loved being in the livingroom with everyone else. When she was sick, Kathy would bring her into the livingroom and make a bed in the middle of the floor. Clarice died at home, on the livingroom floor. Kathy continues her work with Angels Unaware, the organization she founded.

Pat took the panel she made for Kim to a Colorado Quilt Council (CQC) meeting. She hadn't heard any talk about the Quilt among her quilting contemporaries, so she had some concerns about whether or not she wanted to show the quilt at the CQC meeting. She talked to one of her friends who is an officer and she said she thought Pat should show it to the group:

In my process of coming out as the mother of a gay person, part of that process has been this quilt. I didn't want to show it to get sympathy from people. I wanted to do it to say this is in your backyard, your neighborhood, and with the people you deal with. I wanted to stand up for that. To come out. So I did.

After presenting and talking about the quilt, Pat received overwhelming support from her quilting friends. As part of her process of coming out as the mother of a gay person, she got involved in a local support group for gays and lesbians. She has mailed the quilt she made to all of Kim's friends who made squares so that they can see the final project. Because of the panel's odd size, hectic travel schedule, and personal meaning, Pat eventually made a different memorial panel for Kim. She submitted it to the NAMES Project in time for the October 1996 display, where she worked as a volunteer.

Nancy recalls being angry when Thomas died, but finding solace in working on the quilt he had started:

It was kind of funny. It started out as something he had to do for Home Ec, and then it ended up helping us grieve. Then it ends up in the Quilt that we didn't even know about when we were finishing it.

She has worked on several other panels, but has never instigated another:

If I made a panel for everyone I knew I'd be sewing all day, every day. I've helped with some panels, but just sewing. There's nothing of me on any of those except for my care of sewing.

For Rebecca, helping Jeremy's friends make his panel was more about accepting their grief than dealing with her own. When Rebecca visited her brother in the hospital, she saw several young men left alone to die. After Jeremy died, she volunteered at a Santa Monica hospital for six months before coming back to Denver:

The way I actually dealt with it was going and volunteering in the AIDS ward. I think the Quilt is an incredibly symbolic gesture, but there are also plenty of proactive things you can do instead of that. Like donating your time and money to local AIDS services. I get a lot of solace from being proactive. I already knew AIDS well, and was part of a support community before this idea for Jeremy's panel came up.

Maria was struck by how making the panel with a group brought her closer to both the people in the group and Mark, for whom the panel was made. Making the panel was very therapeutic:

It was a really great way of putting Mark to rest in an upbeat way. As we sewed each of these little discs to the panel, we shared with each other what they meant. I learned a lot about Mark that I never knew. We just told stories and had fun. Remember, I didn't even meet some of these people until our first meeting to talk about the panel.

The group had started working on the panel nearly immediately after Mark's funeral. When she relates losing Mark to the other losses she has experienced, Maria looks to the panel for answers:

It was an uplifting experience—a retelling of funny stories. I think of my father. He died suddenly and unexpectedly—the memory of my his death is sad and heavy, whereas when I think of Mark, I remember happier things—all the stories we told when we made the panel. It was a good way to say good-bye to him. This was a sort of follow-up to all that heavy stuff you're left with after someone dies . . . the death, the funeral, the service, the sadness.

CONCLUSION

For all the women I spoke with, the Quilt was one of many ways of dealing with loss to AIDS. But as Kathy observed, with AIDS the grieving process begins well before the loss. Because the symbolic representation of the dead is an active and social process, the Quilt functions to resurrect the memory of the dead in an emotionally consoling way through its blend of artifact and sentiment. In short, like a Mourning quilt or tombstone, it summons the body of the dead.

The transformative nature of the Quilt is evident in the sense of community it spawns among the living. In the construction of a panel, friends and families become conjoined, new friendships are made, and family relationships are nurtured. While many criticize the Quilt for its apolitical stance, the Quilt's import in the maintenance of other AIDS-related communities is twofold: first, the funds raised through its exhibition support local AIDS service organizations, and second, it eradicates disavowal and promulgates action. Jones once commented:

> We want the grandmother from Iowa who handstitched her boy's flannel shirts together to be comfortable enough with us to come and see the panel. (Bellm, 1989, p. 35)

Most significant, in a day where the quilt has become a commodity and quilting has become a largely solo and artistic endeavor, the Quilt resurrects the rich tradition of women supporting both one another and their community through the bonds fostered in this contemporary quilting bee.

REFERENCES

Bellm, D. (1989). And sew it goes. *Mother Jones, 14* (1), 34-35.

Butler, J. (1993). *Bodies That Matter.* New York: Routledge.

Clark, R. (1987). Fragile Families: Quilts as Kinship Bonds. In M. M. Kile (Ed.), *The Quilt Digest,* 4-19. San Francisco: The Quilt Digest Press.

Dixon, M. (1993). Aunt Ida Pieces a Quilt. In J. L. Pastore (Ed.), *Confronting AIDS Through Literature,* 149. Urbana, IL: University of Illinois Press.

Hawkins, P. S. (1993). Naming names: The art of memory and the Names Project AIDS Quilt. *Critical Inquiry, 19*(4), 752-79.

NAMES Project. (1995). The AIDS Memorial Quilt. Introduction to public relations kit.

Otto, W. (1991). *How to Make an American Quilt.* New York: Ballantine Books.

Peck, A. (1990). *American Quilts and Coverlets.* New York: The Metropolitan Museum of Art and Dutton Studio Books.

Raphael, B. (1983). *The Anatomy of Bereavement.* New York: Basic Books.

Ruskin, C. (1988). *The Quilt: Stories from The NAMES Project.* New York: Pocket Books.

Sturken, M. (1992). Conversations with the dead. *Socialist Review, 22*(2), 65-95.

Williams, M. R. (1994). A Reconceptualization of Protest Rhetoric: Women's Quilts as Rhetorical Forms. *Women's Studies in Communication, 17*(2), 20-44.

Young, I. M. (1990). The ideal of community and the politics of difference. In L. J. Nicholson (Ed.), *Feminism/Postmodernism,* 300-323. New York: Routledge.

Chapter 10

Redressing *Sanuk* : "Asian AIDS" and the Practices of Women's Resistance

John Nguyet Erni

The emergence of the HIV/AIDS pandemic in South and Southeast Asia in the mid-1980s has painfully confirmed many Third World women's global dispositions. In order to understand more fully the contour of women's lives in "Asian AIDS" and how they cope with the epidemic, I suggest three vectors in this chapter that are particularly prevalent in our attempt to frame this discussion. First, we need to look at the mediascape that produces the First World's cultural chronicle of "Asian AIDS." We need to compare the specificity of the First World's narrative of the crisis of AIDS in South and Southeast Asia with the existing narratives about AIDS in other regions of the world, especially AIDS in other Third World regions. Second, we need to trace women's response to the crisis. We need to compile their history of resistance, not only to the spreading virus, but also to the structural conditions of society, economics, nationalism, and cultural and political patriarchy that accompany and *precede* the epidemic. Third, we need to struggle with the kind of language we use to talk about "Third World women" and "Asian AIDS," particularly for those us writing from a non–Third World location and with a non-Third World voice. If the language we use, even as we attempt to craft it in feminist terms, is invariably a political act, then we need to be critically aware of what and whose story we are attempting to tell, and what political and discursive consequences our story brings.

I am convinced that the story of women with HIV/AIDS in Asia is realistically a fragmented narrative, punctuated by orientalist, anti-orientalist, and self-orientalizing tendencies, and is therefore necessarily jumbled, shuffled, and agitated by these political and cultural thrusts. More of a "war of positions" made up of contrasting and shifting voices than a monolinguistic and unified narrative, and less linear or unidirectional than circular, this story realistically resists stable and totalizing definitions. The story is incomplete at this historical moment. The challenge of discussing the media representations of the epidemic in Asia and women's ways of communicating about and resisting it is to highlight the provisional and jumbled nature of competing voices in the First World/Third World divide, as well as the racial and gender divides. I propose treating the representational voices as moving vectors that travel inside and alongside the forces of power, despair, confusion, and community empowerment that the global AIDS pandemic has forged. The conceptualization of the mobile, traveling voices enables us to think of them as temporary, mimetic, and adaptive.

In the first section of this chapter, I will discuss the rhetorics in the First World media about "Asian AIDS" in general and "AIDS in Thailand" in particular (what may be construed as "media orientalism"). I will focus on the episodic nature of the rhetoric, characteristic of what Homi Bhabha (1992) calls the "ambivalent colonial impulse," void of any simple, unified sense of racial, sexual, or economic superiority. Here, I will attempt to enact an imaginary dialogue that takes place in the (equally imaginative) sphere of "postcolonial theory" and "subaltern studies." I weave together a kind of tapestry of narratives, vignettes that are drawn from the abyss of media orientalism. These narratives have a tendency to cross over to each other, so that no voice (including my own) tells a definitive story, so that every voice poaches. I want to use the tapestry to suggest that the historic and specific elements of the HIV/AIDS epidemic in Asia hinge on how the global vectors of the transnational trafficking of capital, bodies, desires, pleasures, and ideologies are constantly translating and retranslating this very historical moment of crisis in the Asian region, particularly Asian women's lives. Next, I describe the critical response to the pandemic by Asian women and their feminist allies in other developing countries and in the First World, focusing on how women organize to combat the epidemic and the structural conditions that are connected to it. I conclude with some theoretical remarks about the question of the political meaning of "Third World women" in Western feminist scholarship and intervention in the moment of a devastating pandemic. It is my hope that this discussion will help to clearly depict for readers the questions of Asian AIDS and Asian women's organizing, particularly for those of us in the West.

TAPESTRIES

The language of critique . . . opens up a space of translation: a place of hybridity, figuratively speaking, where the construction of a political object that is new, *neither the one nor the other,* properly alienates our political expectations, and changes, as it must, the very forms of our recognition of the moment of politics.

—Homi Bhabha
(emphasis his)

"Asian AIDS" emerged in the mid- to late 1980s. In the very same period, global development has deeply transformed the East and South Asian regions into new economic centers modeled after Euro-American economies. The historical parallel makes the celebration of "Asian capitalism" a highly ambiguous and deeply anxious event. In his best-selling book, Julian Weiss writes:

The Asian Century *has* arrived. It is an unexpected shooting star in the night sky of world events from which great possibilities emerge. The "Asian Century" concept embodies far more than economics. It is the kernel of new geopolitics, a basic realignment in an information age and postindustrial era. The shape of the next century is being cast in the Pacific. (1989: p. vi)

Terms in global capitalism such as "divergent investment," "free trade," and "bilateral cooperation" now carry ironic connotations in the narrative of economic development on the one hand and AIDS on the other. These terms are ironic because by considering the phenomenon of international trafficking of women alone (e.g., as mail-order brides, domestic servants, and sex workers), terms such as "free trade" take on a double meaning, involving the transaction of two kinds of commodity—namely the woman's body and money, and therefore invariably intensifying the global trafficking of another kind: the HIV/AIDS epidemic. The triumphant tone in the global stories such as that provided by Julian Weiss, in effect, masks that dangerous interconnection among the sexualized body, capital, and an epidemic.

In the global AIDS narrative, the Third World is seen simultaneously as the culprit or the origin of the modern plague as well as its victim. To the First World—and the First World always seems to be the vantage point from which we speak—"they" gave us AIDS, "their" AIDS is now killing their own people, and "they" try to deny both. In the international AIDS story, this triangular indictment—this triple assault—shapes the meaning of the name "AIDS in the Third World."

In 1992, *The New York Times* published its first in-depth report on AIDS in Asia (Shenon, 1992). The headline, "AFTER YEARS OF DENIAL, ASIA FACES SCOURGE OF AIDS," immediately cues the reader to a familiar narrative elsewhere: the narrative of AIDS in Africa and government denial. In fact, the article opens its report about Asian AIDS with a comparison with African AIDS. The journalistic coverage of Third World AIDS therefore rests heavily on past narratives, to the extent that the existence of AIDS in Asia is constructed by way of stories from another time, another place, and another discursive space. This coupling of Asia and Africa, however, has historical structural basis within the classic global narrative of post–World War II development that has cast the Asian and African countries as the vast testing ground for Western economic and social development. From the neocolonial point of view, the tragic duo of economic depravity in the past becomes the misfortunate pair of sexually and medically underdeveloped worlds in the 1980s and 1990s. In this context, one may say that the figure of "the Asian" is imagined as that of "the African."

The *New York Times* article features a photograph of an Asian male AIDS patient in an AIDS ward in Bangkok. The patient is lying in a hospital bed, his body wasted and completely covered with tattoos. He looks at the camera, caught in the ambivalent gaze of the foreign journalist. Once again, the AIDS patient is unmistakably marked by signs of macabre: extreme weight loss, bedridden, swollen face, helpless, and near death. But this image has more: a body of an Asian AIDS victim covered with tattoos. The tattoos provide the signifier of an infectious environ; mystic orientalism is recoded as contamination. In this double exoticism, we are reminded once again of the discursive folding of the Asian onto the African through the horrified but ambivalent gaze.

This gaze directed at the other is exactly what Franz Fanon remembers, in his much-quoted rendition of the highly charged racist scene:

> My body was given back to me sprawled out, distorted, recoloured, clad in mourning in that white winter day. The Negro is an animal, the Negro is bad, the Negro is mean, the Negro is ugly; look, a nigger, it's cold, the nigger is shivering, the nigger is shivering because he is cold, the little boy is trembling because he is afraid of the nigger, the nigger is shivering with cold, that cold that goes through your bones, the handsome little boy is trembling because he thinks that the nigger is quivering with rage, the little white boy throws himself into his mother's arms: Mama, the nigger's going to eat me up. (Fanon, 1991, p. 80)

In this traumatic scene from Fanon, the black subject caught in the white gaze appears to be an ambivalent text of projection and introjection, what Homi Bhabha calls "the masking and splitting of 'official' and phantasmatic knowledges" (1992, p. 327). Might we see the same psychic process at work in the delivery of the image of the Asian man with tattoos? In the folding together of the black and Asian objects in colonial discourse, the Fanonian transfer may look something like this, *deceptio visus*:

> Look, an Oriental AIDS victim; he is contaminated; he is shivering; the Oriental AIDS victim is shivering because he is contaminated; the colonial subject trembles because he is afraid of the Oriental AIDS victim; he is shivering with contamination, that contamination that goes through your bones; the handsome little colonial subject is trembling because he

thinks that the Oriental AIDS victim is quivering with a deadly raging virus; he throws himself into his nation's arms: "Mama, the Oriental AIDS victim quivering with the deadly raging virus is going to eat me up."

The AIDS epidemic has reached crisis proportions in Thailand. Since the first cases of HIV infection in Thailand were reported around 1984, the figures of newly reported cases have been steadily soaring. In 1994, National Public Radio claimed that one in every 50 Thais is now infected with HIV, and the ratio could climb to one in fifteen infected by the end of the decade (National Public Radio, 1994). The Economist *reported that in 1989, with only limited diagnostic technologies, Thailand had already accounted for half of all the cases of HIV infection in all of Asia (*The Economist, *February 4, 1989). Both the World Health Organization and the Public Health Ministry of Thailand have projected that if public awareness and education can change drug use and sexual behavior rapidly and positively, the rate of HIV infection will peak in the mid- to late 1990s and the cumulative number of HIV cases by the turn the century will be four million (Rhodes, 1991). The World Health Organization estimates that at least ten million Asians will be infected by the year 2000 and that AIDS will kill more people in the Asian region than in any other (Shenon, 1992).*

In Thailand, the growing awareness of the serious consequences of the HIV pandemic has built an impressive system producing large quantities of statistical information and other nonquantitative forms of knowledge about the epidemic in the country. This is evident in the sentinel surveillance system initiated in 1989 that reports seroprevalence in a number of target groups in all provinces every two years. Information about the impact of the epidemic on specific subpopulations has been supplemented with cohort and follow-up studies that have been carried out among military recruits, commercial sex workers, pregnant women, and newborns. Dutch researcher Han ten Brummelhuis (1993) suggests that contrary to popular belief, Thailand could claim to be one of the first countries where the HIV/AIDS epidemic is systematically documented with the greatest detail and reliability. He observes that "[n]o [W]estern country will be able to compete due, among other things, to ethical and juridical constraints in blood testing" (p. 3).

Brummelhuis (1993) also suggests the first AIDS cases since 1984 could be traced to foreign contacts, although not in all instances with complete certainty. He writes, "There is no evidence to establish the first route in this intercountry transmission. Probably, it happened almost simultaneously: Thais who had sexual contacts abroad bought the virus back home, Westerners having sex with Thais took it to Thailand, and HIV entered Thailand also through sharing of drug use equipment between foreigners and Thais" (p. 3). He argues that since 1988, a pattern has developed that makes it difficult to apply Western epidemiological categories in terms of exclusively heterosexual, homosexual, and bisexual behavior. He mentions, for instance, the case of a male AIDS patient who had sex with his male foreign employer with the consent of his wife (p. 3). As reported in the International AIDS Conference in Berlin, any attempt in the Thai situation to isolate specific risk groups is rapidly becoming obsolete. The obsession to focus only on female prostitutes and single males has occluded the steady rise of incidence among married men and their wives.

The Thai profile is also complicated by the internal mobility of its people, largely migrants from the rural north to the urban centers in the south and southeast. The concentration of HIV infection in the northern region of Thailand may be changing due to the internal migration patterns. Nearly 50 percent of all AIDS/ARC cases reported in 1993 are from five provinces in the upper north representing only 4.7 percent of the Thai population (Brummelhuis, 1993, p. 4).

A poster in a bar in the Philippines near a United States military base has this poem, greeting the customers:

> A tiny little shade of light
> A little bed with sheets so white
> A little loving in the gloom
> A little pair of lips, so warm and wet
> A little whisper, "Please not yet"
> A little pillow from the head
> Slipped beneath the hips instead

A little effort to begin
A little help to get it in
A little arm that grips me tight
Then I ask, "Does it feel all right?"
She smiles and says, "It feels so good"
And I reply, "I knew it would"
Two little legs around me wind
Two slanted eyes look into mine
A little movement to and fro
A little whisper, "give me more"
Two little hearts beat as one
Two little lovers having fun
A little hunch, a little sigh
A little phrase, "You come, GI?"
A little effort to repeat
A little spot upon the sheets
A little bath when you are through
A little drink or two
A little sleep and finally then
A little breakfast at half past ten
And as you dress and put on your hat
You look back and say . . .
"Did I fuck 'that'????!!!!"

Similar, but more concise, messages about the *delicatesse* can be found on baseball hats, T-shirts, and bumper stickers.

The Thai national planning authorities officially designated 1987 as Visit Thailand Year. Many events were planned to attract a record number of foreign tourists. It was the same year that the Thai government began to take actions to address the impact of the AIDS crisis to Thailand. The conflict between dealing with AIDS and promoting tourism became apparent. The Thai government was determined to play down the scope of AIDS. The rationale: to avoid public panic and hysteria.

Today, it has become customary for service girls and bar boys in the entertainment districts to wear on their necks an ID card—known as the "green card"—issued by the local health officials stating their HIV test results, proving to their local and foreign clients that they were safe, without being offered a reciprocal proof from the clients.

The United States Pacific Command, a massive military complex, spans over five major Asian countries and the vast area of Micronesia. With 300 bases and facilities stationing about 330,000 servicemen and women, this military complex has had a profound economic impact on the host countries. A whole host of small businesses is stimulated and sustained by the presence of the military personnel; these businesses would not have survived had it not been for the whole economy of sexual labor (Sturdevant and Stoltzfus, 1992). In Thailand, next to the production of rice, prostitution is the largest industry.

In addition, the modern tourist industry in Southeast Asia is modeled after the rest and recreation (R & R) centers that were established during the Vietnam War. The understanding of the specific shape in which the AIDS crisis is taking in the 1990s cannot be separated from the understanding of what transpired in the war of the 1960s and 1970s as well as the global economic tales of the 1970s and 1980s.

In the realm of the military, sexual relations always take on particular meanings. The military depends on certain presumptions about masculinity in order to sustain soldiers' morale and discipline. It goes without saying that the construction of militarized masculinity goes hand in hand with the construction of feminized poverty and sexual submission.

In the previously mentioned *New York Times* article, a long report spanning more than a full page, no mention is made of the historical conditions in which Southeast Asia finds itself, nor any mention of the militarization of the region. In one very short passage, the encounter between foreign military personnel and local Cambodians is briefly mentioned in this way:

> A United Nations peace settlement, reached late last year, ended Cambodia's isolation and brought a torrent of foreigners and thousands of United Nations peacekeeping troops. They were met on the streets of Phnom Penh by hundreds of prostitutes who had left their impoverished native villages in search of work in the capital. (Shenon, 1992, p. A1)

The key linguistic turn in the passage lies in the three simple words "They were met," skillfully suggesting that the encounter between the soldiers and native Cambodians is initiated by the prostitutes, by which the soldiers are seduced. A nine-part series on AIDS in Asia broadcast on National Public Radio in 1994 explored a wide range of related subjects, including the economic impact of AIDS on Thailand and India, the "problematic" local sexual customs, the educational efforts to curb the spread of HIV, and the tragic plight of young women sold to prostitution. Yet no mention was made of the prevailing presence of foreign military forces in the countries.

If you were to write a storybook about contemporary Southeast Asia, you may consider telling the story of a brothel:

Outside the brothel, there would be a big red sign with only an "A" written on it. The bar down the street with the "Off limits" sign issued by the local Social Hygiene Clinic backed by the military authority would look deserted. But here, there would be navy officers interacting with tourists from their home countries, reminiscing about old times. The owner of the business would be busy greeting the customers, some of whom are here for their favorite waitresses, others are looking for their loyal male servers. The women might be dressed in bright saris and gaudy jewelry, or simply miniskirts topped with T-shirts with the Coca-Cola or Florida palm tree prints. The male servers might wear nothing except a G-string, always smiling.

The story might be illustrated with narratives of the women and men who describe how they end up in this brothel. They might express their anger at how their bosses cheat on their wages, all the while worrying about the children, parents, siblings, and lovers whom they try to support with their meager earnings. Several of them would tell stories about the sexual practices of these foreign men, what turns them on, what makes them come back for more. In these stories, you would hear their subtle analyses of how the American, British, French, Australian, and United Nations troops, and tourists from Japan, Hong Kong, and the United States came to occupy their city and country.

You might also tell the stories, the longing stories, of the soldiers and tourists who patronize the brothel. They would describe how homesick they are when they are thinking about their friends and wives in their own countries, and how they know, but are no longer bothered by, the fake loyalty and submissiveness displayed by their temporary Asian partners. You might have a character or two who are especially brazen about their sexual prowess. Some of the tourists, however, might be more serious in their quest for the unique beliefs, cultural codes, and even ethics of the Asian body in bed.

In this brothel, the male patrons, especially the soldiers, would learn how to be men in front of each other as far as their class, race, and sexual performance are concerned.[1]

In the popular representations of Asians, we appear in the timidity of our bodies, unable to express our pleasures, and reveled in the obscure religious complexity of our pains. Such representations cast us as the handmaids of bourgeois history, the servants of some larger economic machine, as servants, cheap labor, and whores.

The orientialist imagination sees South and Southeast Asia as societies worthy of embarrassment, if not ridicule: there is the image of the cheap sexual labor on the one hand, and the idea of a sexually "craved" race on the other. Therein lies the double humiliation rooted in a diasporic economy, and in the political, religious, and psychical repression associated with the Asian character.

In general, the U.S. media assures us that in Asia, AIDS is spread by Asian-to-Asian heterosexual contact, not by contact with foreigners. Stories of female prostitutes are told to suggest their ignorance and helplessness when it comes to protecting themselves and their foreign customers. Scattered throughout the First World media's sporadic coverage of Asian AIDS are images of and obligatory references to the Asian society and the cultural traits of the Asian people: they are poor, underdeveloped, reserved, custombound, complacent, superstitious, and war-stricken. Moreover, there are tales of Thai and Indian men who drink profusely, visit brothels regularly, and bring home AIDS and other sexually transmitted diseases to their wives. Visiting brothels, we are told, is a cultural sign of Asian masculinity, a local custom, even an ethic. Here, media orientalism delivers an ethnicization of the virus. In this ethnic turn, AIDS in Asia is constructed as a crisis internal to the Asian world, cultures, peoples, indigenous character—in short, its "Third Worldness."

The impotence of the Asian character, it seems, may have been the reason for the West to call into question the ability of the Asian region to deal with AIDS, a crisis associated with drug use and sexual labor. A sexual and narcotic crisis, in a tautological turn, confirms the cultural marker of "Asian" as the tragic by-product of civilization, unable to control our fate and reduced to narcotic and sexual indulgences.

The metaphors of depravity, filth, darkness, repression, and illness have once again delivered the Orient to the West.

"Excuse me, how much is an Asian body worth?"

"THE CARE OF THE SELF"

The intervention of the Third Space of enunciation, which makes the structure of meaning and reference an ambivalent process, destroys [the] mirror of representation in which cultural knowledge is customarily revealed as an integrated, open, expanding code.

—Homi Bhabha (1994, p. 37)

In this section, I want to provide a modest, provisional map of women's organizing efforts to cope with HIV/AIDS in Thailand and more broadly in Third World countries.[2] Here, as in many other contexts, women's organizing need not be equated with any visible activist movements, even when overlapping occurs. Especially in the context of Third World women's organizing, many of their important efforts point to a broad range of community, relational, and personal interventions, not all of which are necessarily articulated in "political" or even "feminist" terms, not the least in terms conceived in the Western world. The map I am drawing here is provisional for two important reasons. First, women's organizing is a continuously changing and growing reality due to the shifting patterns of resource coordination between and within regions and nations. Second, the contour and momentum of women's organizing changes according to new cultural and political considerations of "gender" and "sexuality" in the interwoven contexts of multinational capitalism, nationalism, neocolonialism, and self-orientalism.

I take it as self-evident that at this particular moment in our attempt to understand "global AIDS," the discussion about non–First World conceptualizations of gender and sexuality in conjunction with women's resistance against the structural conditions associated with HIV/AIDS is a newly emergent discourse.[3] We are only beginning to learn how the cultural systems of gender and sexuality work separately and with each other in specific historically, culturally, and religiously shaped nations in the developing world affected by the HIV/AIDS pandemic. I also take it as self-evident that "women's organizing" as a practice as a whole involves multiple women's constituents across the First/Third World divide. Women's organizing must always be treated as an ongoing negotiation—and sometimes contestation—between and among Third World and non–Third World women and their allies.

By and large, international and local organizing for Third World women to cope with the HIV/AIDS pandemic remains marginal. This is not because there have not been new and sometimes innovative programs focusing on Third World women's needs in HIV/AIDS. In fact, numerous transnational programs and local grassroots organizing for women formed around the triadic focus of the AIDS campaign—biomedical research, sex and drug use education, counseling and support—have emerged in many African, Asian, Latin, and Caribbean countries, especially in the past five years. Such organizing remains marginal often because there is a lack of coordination across various institutions and groups to sustain long-term interventions. Anyone who has been involved in community organizing around HIV/AIDS understands how resources are strained when efforts are unnecessarily duplicated and inefficiently spread among those in need. But more debilitating is the continued ideological separation of women's behavior, women's identity, and the cultural context of women's lives displayed by Western scientists and policymakers who often dominate the organizing effort. Such an ideological separation can render the knowledge gained from quantitative data (i.e., obtained through knowledge, attitudes, beliefs, and practices assessments [KABPs]) and qualitative cultural research incompatible. Women's organizing efforts may be marginalized because this incompatibility can create a perception that the knowledge surrounding Third World women with AIDS is "incoherent," "insufficient," and in extreme cases, "irrelevant." When difficulty arises in trying to legitimize knowledge about women with HIV/AIDS, direct and negative impacts can be immediately felt in the attempt to gain funding for organizing efforts. As Cindy Patton reminds us, many women's groups are organized organically and therefore do not perceive themselves as eligible for funding (1994, p. 135). The inability of mainstream researchers to hear the complexity of women's stories may therefore contribute to a cycle of delegitimation at the level of knowledge as well as the level of funding and resource coordination.

Despite these many obstacles, women's organizing continues to flourish. At the level of global initiatives, both Third World and non–Third World women have vigilantly lobbied for the destigmatization of commercial sex work in many developing countries. In the work of the World Health Organization's Global Program on AIDS (GPA), which remains one of the major global initiatives dealing with women, women participants have successfully pointed out that the useful educational efforts developed for and by sex workers cannot be effectively transferred to nonprostitute women's communities if women's needs continue to be viewed from the separated categories of sex-workers and "normal women." The effort to destigmatize sex work, which can be historically traced back to the work of European and North American activist movements organized by sex workers,[4] makes visible the discourse about the complexity and risks of street life as something well-connected to larger socioeconomic realities for women. Such a discourse is now present within the WHO-GPA and has promoted a better understanding of prostitution as a structural condition linked to poverty and patriarchal economics. This understanding is critically central for a country such as Thailand and the Thai women affected by HIV/AIDS.[5]

Other international efforts in which women have played a part include the work of nongovernmental organizations (NGOs). Third World women experience multiple challenges in their involvement in NGOs. In large international NGOs such as the International Council of AIDS Service Organizations (ICASO), the Global Network of Positive People (GNP+), or even the Red Cross, Third World women are often marginalized because participation in such groups often assumes certain language skills and access. Western-style meeting and deliberation procedures that are often conducted in English form a barrier to participation by women from developing countries.

Reflecting on the skepticism of many Third World participants in such large organizations, political scientist Dennis Altman (1994) laments, "However sincere the commitment of grassroots organization and empowerment, the creation of global community/PWA networks creates its own elites, who necessarily are representative only in the most indirect and paternalistic ways" (p. 151). Yet women continue to establish and manage smaller-scale NGOs that are often local projects at the grassroots level. Once a program experiences effectiveness in the local community, however, it is difficult to transfer to or even be recognized by other communities. In fact, women involved in small local projects sometimes do not perceive their work as having the status of "program" or their organization as an NGO and thus making them eligible for grant support (Patton, 1994, p. 125).

One significant type of NGO that does not receive sufficient attention by scholars and critics despite many women's deep involvement is the church-related grassroots group. We often underestimate the role of local women in these organizations in providing emotional support, empowerment strategies, life skills, and shelters for many women in developing countries. To be sure, local women's participation in missionary-oriented groups, for instance, carry with them mixed enthusiasm due to certain imposing postures of the Christian or Catholic church. Yet, women have been able to use their skepticism to generate provisional adaptation strategies so as to gain access to well-funded church-based NGOs which can provide them with financial and community support.

One of the most outspoken church-based NGOs involved in HIV issues for young women is the international body called The Campaign to End Child Prostitution in Asian Tourism (ECPAT).[6] Formed in 1991 through a number of Christian bodies in Asia, ECPAT has concentrated its work in Thailand and has been a resourceful connection for many local Thai women. Through an opposition to tourist-related sexual exploitation of Asian children, ECPAT has evolved into a moderate kind of international activist group making visible the connection of sex tourism to international racism and misogyny

against underage women. Besides mounting awareness and educational campaigns at the local and international arenas for local families and young girls, ECPAT also seeks legal measures to stop Western men from descending into Thailand to engage in sex trade with
children. The ECPAT's lobbying effort has reached Washington and
successfully helped to launch the Child Sexual Abuse Prevention Act
as part of the crime bill signed by President Clinton in 1994. The Act
specifies new measures to identify and indict individuals and travel
agencies in the United States involved in sex tourism to Asia. More
important, it has also evoked bilateral cooperation from the Thai
government. ECPAT reports in December 1995 that the Office of the
Attorney General in Thailand has begun to seriously investigate the
phenomenon of sex tourism. The mixture of ideological motivations
that undergird ECPAT's vigilance may well be a form of external
imposition that privileges law enforcement in the expense of more
complex cultural understandings. Yet, ECPAT has promulgated a
highly visible international discourse about global racism and sexism
and connected it to the HIV pandemic. Third World women can
benefit if NGOs such as ECPAT can serve as a springboard for an
oppositional voice to international racial and gendered exploitation
practices and a leader for a genuine discussion of alternative developments in the Third World.

   Today, the single most important form of organizing does not lie
in well-organized, institutionalized bodies but in women's informal
groups. Research on informal communities of women sharing
street-smartness, self-care information, medically related planning
skills, and relationally based support remains scarce. Yet the social
power that women experience in such communities can combat the
erosion of women's status in the social structure. It is particularly
important that this kind of informal connection be linked to effective institutions in order to generate spaces for both information
acquisition and the sharing of life skills and self-esteem.

   One such institution in Thailand that has successfully served as a
bridge for women sex workers' need for education about AIDS,
social and political awareness about exploitation, and social support
is the activist group named EMPOWER (Education Means Protection of Women Engaged in Recreation).[7] EMPOWER is organized
by local feminists, foreign women, and former prostitutes. It is

situated at the heart of the Patpong district in Bangkok, the commercial center for sex work provided to local Thai men and a large number of foreign tourists. EMPOWER provides structured support for bar girls such as teaching them English in order to protect themselves from foreign men and publishes AIDS education brochures. EMPOWER has also become a guerilla activist movement that ties together many Thai women's multiple identities as wives, sex workers, sisters, experts of street life, appropriators of resources, mutual educators, strategists when dealing with men, and informal leaders in the fight against AIDS and the structural problems connected to the epidemic.[8] Women's organizing at the international and local institutional levels must be matched by the EMPOWER-style movement in order to bring about political and social change through the capturing of economic capital as well as women's unique cultural capital.[9]

Above, I have only sketched a tentative picture about the multiple facets of women's organizing against AIDS. With no claim of comprehensiveness, I nonetheless hope to highlight the quality of active negotiation as the principle ethos of women's organizing. I want to conclude with a brief discussion of two additional areas of intervention for women organizing against AIDS in the global sphere.

To organize a movement that would radically transform public health for women in the Third World means confronting the "developmentalist crisis" brought about by the global economic structure. At this broad level, middle-class women from both the First and Third Worlds can form coalitions and NGOs that can exert pressure on international economic and policy bodies (such as the World Bank and WHO). The recent Fourth World Conference on Women held in Beijing (October 1995) saw the attempt to renetwork women from the affluent north area of China and the developing south. Discussion about public health concerns during the conference linked women's health with several hegemonic phenomena: uneven distribution of wealth in the global economy, the demise of the state, the weakening of social movements that address the needs of the disenfranchised, the decentralization of transnational programming on world health (such as the weakening of the coordinated approach within WHO-GPA), the environmental crisis, and the resurgence of patriarchal forces globally and locally (e.g., in the guise of religious fundamentalism and cultural nationalism). A sustained critique of such global phenomena would require more coordination among women economists, feminist cultural scholars, feminist social movement activists, women health professionals, and women leaders in global and local efforts to control AIDS. The work of important coalitions such as Development Alternatives with Women for a New era (DAWN) must be continued.

DAWN represents a network of women from the economic South who organized themselves during the Third United Nations Conference on Women (held in Nairobi in 1985) in order to begin research and analysis of key development issues affecting women. Their analysis over the past ten years has resulted in a number of important platform documents demanding structural change in global development (e.g., Sen and Grown, 1987; Wiltshire, 1992; Correa, 1994). Their most recent platform document presented during the Beijing conference, *Markers on the Way: The DAWN Debate on Alternative Development* (1995), contains a strong feminist critique of the crisis of global development and a comprehensive set of recommendations for change. Unfortunately, DAWN made no mention of the global HIV pandemic affecting women from the developing countries. It must link the debate on alternative development to the crisis of AIDS. It must draw the connection of the crisis of global development to the devastation of AIDS in all three areas of its analysis toward a feminist-oriented alternative developmentalism: government reform, gendering human development, and strengthening civil society.

One of the additional sites of intervention for women's organizing that would articulate their effort to the critique of globalization is the mass media. Strategic co-optation of the news media by First World AIDS activists such as ACT UP's ongoing media campaigns (Crimp and Rolston, 1990) can be adopted by AIDS activists in the developing countries. Needless to say, the adaptation of such a strategy raises the question of access to local and global media. One may recall that in 1989, there was a different grassroots social movement that managed to stage its political campaign for the entire world to see: the student uprising in Tiananmen Square. Media analyst McKenzie Wark (1994) described this charged moment in which the disenfranchised gained access to the representational arsenal of the global media:

> The people who came to Tiananmen Square were not likely to be seeking a system in which an elected government represents them. They were more likely there to express the fact that since the present autocracy doesn't represent them, they will represent themselves. . . . Since representation turned out to be a key issue between the democracy movement and the government, this idea of self-representation is of no small importance. The intersection of an absence of a vector along which to represent themselves, and the spontaneous creation of self-representation in posters and T-shirts and poses for foreign cameras is one story that one can tell about this event, and an interesting one, given the creativity in extreme situations that the democracy movement displayed for their government, Beijing residents, and international media audiences to see. (p. 98)

Witness, also, the most recent organizing by women's groups in Okinawa, Japan to protest the presence of the U.S. military bases there. The atrocity of the raping of a young Japanese schoolgirl by three U.S. servicemen plunges world media into a shocking revelation of an existing sexual economy everybody knew but only a few First World journalists were willing to cover. Outraged, women's groups from Okinawa launched a world media campaign to expose the story of the military's economic as well as sexual domination. On January 26, 1996, the Japanese Women's Appeal published a full-page statement in *The New York Times* urging the U.S. military to pull out of Okinawa and other Asian regions and countries.[10] The event of the rape and the international self-representation by Japanese women activists makes painfully clear that military masculinity is one of many forms of global sexual exchange coinciding with (if not contributing to) a raging global pandemic.

Like the Chinese students in Tiananmen Square and the Japanese women of Okinawa, the Thai women in military bases and sex tourist sites can create a kind of media vector through the existing media power to open up a discourse about self-representation at the local level and plug themselves into the global media outlets for the international viewers (such as CNN).

The HIV/AIDS crisis in Thailand and many other developing countries has once again thrusted women's reality to the foreground. The survival of the gendered body across the transnational flow of desire in various commodity forms supported by global capitalism and the decentralization of world health would critically depend on how the multiple forms of social activism explored above. The work of grassroots organizations such as EMPOWER, the international women's consortiums such as DAWN, the critical analysis of the media representation of the global AIDS crisis by academic scholars, and the theoretical work on gender, sexuality, race, and class by First and Third World feminist cultural scholars must mutually inform and challenge each other if we want a dramatic arrest of the global pandemic. Meanwhile, these efforts must be carefully employed from within an ongoing political discourse in which First and Third World feminists and their allies endeavor to talk to and across their differences, engaging in the political moment of critical translations.

BETWEEN THE LINES

International AIDS-control efforts, which have by and large focused on epidemiological surveillance, have only recently acknowledged the devastation of South and Southeast Asia by the AIDS pandemic, especially in Thailand, India, and the Philippines. Meanwhile, the press of the developed world has been anxiously silent about it. The handful of media reports from the United States, as we have seen, have created a classic orientalist heterosexual "Asian AIDS." This reinaugurates the postcolonial discourse of global economic development and precolonial fantasies about militarized and leisurized masculinity, both firmly etched in the spatial and temporal movement and class-based consumption of interracial desire and pleasure in the form of *sanuk*. (The term *sanuk* in Thai language connotes "fun"—coyly coded as casual sexual exchange.) Such discourses and fantasies are a paradoxical mode of knowledge in which South and Southeast Asia appears as an ambivalent territory: it is something that is always already known and wholly predictable, and something that must be eagerly reinvented and repeated.[11] In this kind of neocolonial moment, "South and Southeast Asia" and "Asian AIDS" follow the same paths of imaginings that gave rise to "Africa" and "African AIDS" in the 1980s, but with a difference.[12] Besides positing (and eagerly repeating) the conceptual superiority of the developed world over the economically disadvantaged countries by way of correlating heterosexuality with the danger of exotic microbes, the very label of "Asian AIDS" reinscribes Euro-American bodies and desires—the traveling *farang* (the figure of the ornate but vulgar male foreigner, in Thai language)—as part of the resonating narrative of disaster now experienced by the peoples of South and Southeast Asia.

The grand narratives of Pacific militarism and Asian economic development in the 1990s, coinciding with the historical narrative of Thailand as "concubine" to the West that was first articulated in the European literature of the early twentieth century, continue to invent a certain global conception of Thai sexuality as the primary site of exotic maladies evolving into the AIDS disaster. Yet in continuing this orientalist impulse, these narratives bring into focus the world's attention on the scandal of promiscuous pleasure that was once hailed by the military/industrial/tourist complex as its justifiably naughty rights. Seen in this way, South and Southeast Asia in the ruins of AIDS functions as a giant confessional, a space in which open secrets, half-truths, dodges, and sometimes outright lies and denial are most productive, and therefore, a space most capable of mystification. In the neocolonial construction of "Asian AIDS," what is historically and geopolitically marginal and in need of control turns out to be symbolically and psychosexually central. As with Africa, "Asian AIDS" is about the global distribution and trafficking of resources, desire, and power. But unlike it, the First World's construction of "Asian AIDS" reverberates with a charged, suggestive, nagging silence.

Telling the story of "Asian AIDS" is no easy task. The effort to recast the political meaning of "Third World women" by First World feminists, impressively punctuated by Chandra Mohanty's groundbreaking article, "Under Western eyes: Feminist scholarship and colonial discourses" (1994) has met new challenges as HIV/AIDS violently reshapes the lives of Third World women in colo-

nial and postcolonial settings. Mohanty's description of the hege-
mony of Western scholarship, which criticizes such scholarship's
tendency to universalize the category of "Third World women" as
ahistorical, singular objects of Western political theory, magnifies
today in the international discourse about Third World AIDS. The
professional stability of this discourse in conferences and publications continues to depend on the deployment of archaic archetypal
images of women in the developing countries, sometimes by feminist researchers themselves. Yet, the global pandemic has continued
to effect a kind of revolt against undialectical thinking. Taking heed
of Mohanty's suggestion that "the definition of 'the Third World
woman' as a monolith might well tie into the larger economic and
ideological praxis of 'disinterested' scientific inquiry and plural-
ism" (1994, pp. 215-216) means that, in the context of global AIDS,
we need to demand dialectical constructions of Third World
women's realities as always a negotiated reality across the First/
Third World divide. The effort to recast the meaning of "Third
World women" is thus part of the overall project of feminist resistance against a pandemic that is being inscribed deeper and deeper
into the global/local matrix.

Feminist resistance, when spoken here (in North America) and
now (in advanced capitalism), signals disjunction, slippage, and
high self-consciousness resulting from the complex struggles
between Third World and non–Third World interventions over the
plight of the gendered body in AIDS. Feminist resistance, when
organized "there," is therefore always already an overdetermined
discourse—a committed but reluctant partner to the West—because
it is positioned as both the locus and the receiver of such disjunction, slippage, and self-consciousness in the First World. As a
result, Third World women's organizing against HIV/AIDS has to
craft the gendered body as a site of dialectical contestation waged
with the affectivity of street-smartness, skepticism, rage, anxiety,
and local understanding of women's self-esteem on the one hand,
and with the efficiency of institutional organizing along the lines of
transnational capital and research flow on the other hand. The body
therefore navigates within the global/local nexus with shrewd determination.

A feminist response to the HIV/AIDS pandemic in the international arena entails a critical negotiation between the two spaces of resistance described above. Any attempt to mount an educational campaign about HIV/AIDS for Third World women in the name of international feminism, for instance, would have to understand the nature of both First World colonizing tendency (e.g., "Use our model of safe sex.") and Third World cultural and ideological adaptive tendency (e.g., "We will use your model of safe sex provisionally."). Moreover, such ideological thrusts must not be viewed as static and deterministic but as transitory since they are in the constant process of continuing self-revision. AIDS in the Third World and the transitory nature of organizing in response to the crisis teach us that pure resistance in the form of anticolonialism, antidevelopment, or antiglobal capitalism cannot exist for either First or Third World feminisms without committing the mistake of delinking feminisms from the material specificities of women's lives. Writing about the global HIV/AIDS pandemic in feminist terms would therefore require us to situate our own voices in a juncture of a permanently awkward kind.

NOTES

1. This passage is inspired by Enloe's (1992) excellent essay on the military construction of masculinity.

2. Much of the material on women's organizing in Thailand was obtained through personal correspondences with various individuals and organizations in Thailand and their allies in the United States. Special thanks to Nicola Bullard of the ECPAT-Bangkok, Ellis Shenk of ECPAT-USA (New York), Chularat Phongtudsirikul of the YMCA (Chiangmai, Thailand), Kathryn Inoferio of the Center for Global Education at Augsburg College (Minneapolis), the staff of the Women's Information Center at the Foundation for Women (Bangkok). Kent Klindera has also offered precious help and advice.

3. Rosalind C. Morris's important article, "Three sexes and four sexualities: Redressing the discourses on gender and sexuality in contemporary Thailand" (1994), remains one of the most illuminating works on Thai gender and sexuality. The volume *Nationalisms and Sexualities* (Parker et al., 1992) is also a significant book that explores diasporic and subaltern configurations of gender and sexuality in many developing countries. See also Bishop and Robinson (forthcoming), Jackson (forthcoming), and Tannenbaum (1995).

4. See Delacoste and Alexander (1987) and McClintock (1993).

5. For an excellent discussion of the general patriarchal conditions responsible for Asian women's poverty, see Enloe (1990) and Truong (1990).

6. For more information, contact Ellis Shenk, ECPAT-USA, 475 Riverside Drive, Room 612, New York, NY 10115. (212)-870-2427; and Nicola Bullard, ECPAT-Bangkok, 328 Phyathai Road, Bangkok 10400. (662)-2153388.

7. For more information, write to EMPOWER, 57/60 Tiwanon Road (Ban Tuek Center), Muang Nonthaburi, Thailand 11000. (662)-526-8311.

8. For a more descriptive account of the activities of EMPOWER and the kinds of informal relational dynamics among women based on the organization, see Odzer (1994).

9. Besides EMPOWER, women's activist groups similarly organized around commercial sex work, HIV/AIDS, and anticolonialism in Asia include "Talikala" and "Gabriele" in the Philippines. See Altman (1994, p. 48) and Enloe (1990, pp. 39, 88).

10. For more information, contact the Japanese Women's Appeal, Reimei Building, 1-36 Kanda Jimbo-cho, Chiyoda-ku, Tokyo 101, Japan. Fax: 81-3-3293-0574.

11. Homi Bhabha (1992) has argued that the notion of ambivalence constitutes the force of colonial stereotype, because the vacillation between the "already known" and the "endlessly repeated" produces the combined effect of predictability and probability, thereby ensuring the sign of the colonial other as one of excess. I suggest that the desire for the colonial other in the developing world assumes just such excess, especially in economic and cultural terms.

12. Some of the best discussion of the popular constructions of "African AIDS" to date are Patton (1990, pp. 77-97), Treichler (1989), and Watney (1994).

REFERENCES

Altman, D. (1994). *Power and Community: Organizational and Cultural Responses to AIDS*. London: Taylor & Francis.

Bhabha, H. (1992). The other question: The stereotype and colonial discourse. In Screen (Ed.), *The Sexual Subject: A Screen Reader in Sexuality*, 312-331. London and New York: Routledge.

Bhabha, H. (1994). The commitment to theory. In Homi Bhabha (Ed.), *The Location of Culture*, 19-39. New York: Routledge.

Bishop, R. and Robinson, L. (forthcoming). *Night market: Thailand in Post-Colonial Sexual Cartographies*. New York: Routledge.

Brummelhuis, H. T. (1993). *Between Action and Understanding*. Paper presented in the Fifth International conference on Thai Studies, London, July.

Correa, S. (1994). *Population and Reproductive Rights: Feminist Perspectives from the South*. London: Zed Press.

Crimp, D. and Rolston. A. (1990). *AIDS Demo Graphics*. Seattle: Bay Press.

DAWN. (1995). *Markers on the Way: The DAWN Debate on Alternative Development*. A monograph distributed during the Fourth World Conference on Women, Beijing, China.

Delacoste, F. and Alexander, P. (Eds.). (1987). *Sex Work: Writings by Women in the Sex Industry*. Pittsburgh: Cleis Press.

Economist. (1989). Thailand: AIDS homes in, *310*, (February 4) (7558), 37.

Enloe, C. (1990). *Bananas, Beaches, & Bases: Making Feminist Sense of International Politics.* Berkeley: University of California Press.

Enloe, C. (1992). It takes two. In S. Sturdevant and B. Stoltzfus (Eds.), *Let the Good Times Roll: Prostitution and the U.S. Military in Asia*, 22-27. New York: The New Press.

Fanon, F. (1991). The fact of blackness. In F. Fanon (Ed.), *Black Skin, White Masks, 109-140.* London: Pluto Press.

Jackson, P. (forthcoming). Kathoeys<>Gay<>Man: The historical emergence of gay male identity in Thailand. In L. Manderson and M. Jolly (Eds.), *Sites of Desire/Economies of Pleasure: Sexualities in Asia and the Pacific.* Chicago: University of Chicago Press.

McClintock, A. (1993). Sex Workers and Sex Work (special issue). *Social Text*, 37.

Mohanty, C.T. (1994). Under western eyes: Feminist scholarship and colonial discourses. In P. Williams and L. Chrisman (Eds.), *Colonial Discourse and Post-Colonial Theory: A Reader, 196-220.* New York: Columbia University Press.

Morris, R. (1994). Three sexes and four sexualities: Redressing the discourses on gender and sexuality in contemporary Thailand. *Positions: East Asia Cultures Critique*, 2, (1), 15-43.

National Public Radio. (1994). AIDS in Asia. (Nine-part series). Washington, DC February 17-March 6, 1994. Executive Producer: Ellen Weiss. Transcript inquiry: (202)-414-3232.

Odzer, C. (1994). *Patpong Sisters: An American Woman's View of the Bangkok Sex World.* New York: Blue Moon Books.

Parker, A., Russo, M., Sommer, D., and Yaeger, P. (Eds.). (1992). *Nationalisms and Sexualities.* New York: Routledge.

Patton, C. (1990). *Inventing AIDS.* New York: Routledge.

Patton, C. (1994). *Last Served?: Gendering the HIV Pandemic.* London: Taylor & Francis.

Rhodes, R. (1991). Death in the candy store. *Rolling Stone*, November 28, 62-70,105,113-114.

Sen, G. and Grown, C. (1987). *Development, Crises, and Alternative Visions: Third World Women's Perspectives.* New York: Monthly Review Press.

Shenon, P. (1992). After years of denial, Asia faces scourge of AIDS. *The New York Times*, November 8, A1,A8.

Sturdevant, S. and Stoltzfus, B. (1992). Disparate threads of the whole: An interpretive essay. In S. Sturdevant and B. Stoltzfus (Eds.), *Let the Good Times Roll: Prostitution and The U.S. Military in Asia, 300-334.* New York: The New Press.

Tannenbaum, N. (1995). *Buddhism, Prostitution, and Sex: Limits on the Academic Discourse on Gender in Thailand.* Paper presented at the Conference on Gender and Sexuality in Modern Thailand, Canberra, Australia.

Treichler, P.A. (1989). AIDS and HIV infection in the Third World: A First World chronicle. In B. Kruger and P. Mariani (Eds.), *Remaking History.* Dia Art

Foundation Discussions in Contemporary Culture, Number 4, 31-86. Seattle: Bay Press.

Truong, T. (1990). *Sex, Money, and Morality: Prostitution and Tourism in Southeast Asia*. London: Zed.

Wark, M. (1994). *Virtual Geography: Living with Global Media Events*. Indianapolis: Indiana University Press.

Watney, S. (1994). Missionary positions: AIDS, "Africa," and race. In S. Watney (Ed.), *Practices of Freedom: Selected Writings on HIV/AIDS, 103-120*. Durham, NC: Duke University Press.

Weiss, J. (1989). *The Asian Century*. New York: Facts on File.

Wiltshire, R. (1992). *Environment and Development: Grassroots Women's Perspectives*. A DAWN monograph.

Chapter 11

To Desire to Direct Differently: Women Producer/Directors of AIDS Films

Linda K. Fuller

In feminist cinema, there is already a way of desiring—in difference—that is "spoken" in feminist films. It is not simply a matter of "learning" to speak a new language, nor of deploying new cinematic strategies, but of a desiring process itself that emerges from a locus of difference. "Desiring differently" posits another logic (logic of an Other?) whose terms and positions are precisely—feminine.

—Sandy Flitterman-Lewis
To Desire Differently (1990, p. 2)

Having performed an exhaustive study of AIDS films (Fuller, 1993,1994b,1996a), it struck me that I have been looking at the wrong side of the camera; instead of simply focusing on the content

The author would like to acknowledge the following individuals and organizations for their help in this project: Gary Crowdus, Cinema Guild; Jonathan Lee, Fear of Disclosure Project; Scott Meckling, Program Manager, Out on the Screen; Elizabeth Meister, Dyke TV; Ilana Navara, Membership and Outreach Coordinator, Media Network; Ann Poritzky, Senior Communications Specialist, and Willie Church, Research Specialist, CDC National AIDS Clearinghouse; Leslie R. Wolfe, President, Center for Women Policy Studies; and the many distributors and agencies who have helped coordinate producer/directors and their various videos. Most of all, she certainly wants to thank the interviewees for their input and enthusiasm.

of motion pictures dealing with the disease, it is time to consider the creative process behind those images. Women producer/directors, it is argued here, have particularly keen perspectives—of PWAs (people with AIDS), of their caretakers, their families, and their public(s). This chapter reviews the literature on film producers and directors, offers some comments on feminist filmmaking and HIV/ AIDS filmmaking, and gives reportage on interviews with 18 women AIDS filmmaker/videographers.

REVIEW OF THE LITERATURE

Most research on producers and/or directors focuses, not surprisingly, on men. Consider the title of a 1971 book by Muriel Cantor, a highly respected sociologist from American University: *The Hollywood TV Producer: His Work and His Audience*, which discusses how producers are influenced by their professional values, viewing audiences, the network, colleagues, and film buyers.

Typically, producer/director studies have focused on television (Anderson, 1975; Fuller, 1990, 1994a; Tunstall, 1994), portraying them either as powerful creative sources of programming or as the confounding tools of network policy. Gaye Tuchman (1974), for example, discusses the pattern of economic determination of commercial programming, stating the basic rule: "Plan programs that will attract a large audience (as indexed by rating services) so that the audience may be sold profitably to commercials advertisers" (pp. 119-120). Newcomb and Alley (1982), on the other hand, discovered producers able to personalize their work, labeling them as "self-conscious artistic producers" (p. 70).

Alternative media producer/directors have received scant attention: Faulkner (1971) on studio musicians, Caughie (1981) on authorship, Downing (1984) on outlets, Juhasz (1994) on AIDS videos, or Fuller (1996b) on relationships. Regarding independent feminist film in particular, Kaplan (1983, p.196) outlines some of the contradictions dominating alternate cinematic strategies and practices:

1. Filmmakers have had to rely for funding on the very system they oppose.

2. In the case of anti-illusionist films, directors have been using cinematic strategies that are difficult for the majority of people, who are raised on narrative and commercial films.
3. Having made the films, directors have not had any mechanism for the distribution and exhibition of their films on a large scale.
4. The culminating contradiction is that filmmakers whose whole purpose was to change people's ways of seeing, believing, and behaving have only been able to reach an audience already committed to their values.

Diverse viewpoints are increasingly appearing in the literature, especially regarding Black filmmakers. Recognizing the difficulty of defining Black film, Madubuko Diakite (1980) offers this attempt: "The finished film that was inspired and directed by a Black filmmaker, regardless of the amount of non-Black assistance, money, or censorship involved" (p. v). Mark A. Reid (1993) discusses "Black womanist film," which he sees as a critical form of resistance. Ed Guerrero (1993), who celebrates the emergence of a number of filmmakers who are taking responsibility for "framing blackness" in their own terms, makes this telling point: "What all this means, specifically for African Americans (and extrapolated to a wide range of *other* minorities) is that in almost every instance, the representation of black people on the commercial screen has amounted to one grand, multifaceted illusion" (p. 2).

More recently, with a growing interest in women and film—particularly their cultural construction therein, an alternative tradition has been evolving that includes both studies of women filmmakers and their feminist evaluative perspectives (Kay and Peary, 1977; Erens, 1979, 1990; Kuhn, 1982; Kaplan, 1983; McCreadie, 1983; Mayne, 1984; Gentile, 1985; Foster, 1995; Krasilovsky, 1997). As first expressed by both Claire Johnston (1973) and Laura Mulvey's legendary 1975 essay, "Visual Pleasure and Narrative Cinema," the joyous declaration of difference continues to develop. "Feminist films are part of a unique aesthetic/political movement rooted politically in contemporary feminism (especially the younger, liberationist branch of the women's movement) and aesthetically in independent film traditions as they developed in America," declares Jan

Rosenberg (1983, p. 7). "Understanding how the feminist film movement grew out of the women's movement provides a necessary preface to understanding the feminist film movement itself."

Apropos to the title of this book, a number of scholars are celebrating women's ways of communicating (Bovenschen, 1977; Erens, 1979; Rosenberg, 1983; DeLauretis, 1984; Doane, Mellencamp, and Williams, 1984; Rose, 1986; Doane, 1987; Penley, 1988; Fischer, 1989; Flitterman-Lewis, 1990; Basinger, 1993; Penley and Willis, 1993). Envisioning "women's art as engaged in an oppositional struggle with the patriarchal tradition," Fischer (1989, p. 9) provides a clear outline to the many divergent approaches that various women filmmakers and film critics have taken, such as a feminine aesthetic, counter-heritage, re-visions, counter-cinema, and/or feminist deconstructions.

At the same time, an entire book genre is emerging that features profiles of various women filmmakers (e.g., Betancourt, 1974; Smith, 1975; Slide, 1977; Heck-Rabi, 1984; Corliss, 1986; Quart, 1988; Acker, 1991; Cole and Dale, 1993; Sklar, 1994). These developments suggest that women in general, feminist filmmakers in particular, are capable of offering unique perspectives on HIV/AIDS.

FEMINIST FILMMAKING

Writing in 1974, Jeanne Betancourt reported finding that, "A new group of filmmakers with a feminist consciousness are making movies. Their films, most of them short documentaries, are united only by the shared consciousness of the women who made them. They take as their themes the qualities of life that concern women, the oppressions that women share with all oppressed groups, or the problems women have particularly as women" (pp.vi–vii). More than two decades later, her words still hold true.

In a foreword to Ally Acker's *Reel Women* (1991, p. xv), film reviewer Judith Crist reports how difficult it is to get statistics on the number of women and minorities in the motion picture industry. Of the Directors Guild of America, which she considers a leader in helping improve this situation, she says they have a continuing growth,

But the figure is still only at 18 percent, some 1,620 of its 9,000 members. Women constitute 13 percent of the production managers, 23 percent of the first assistant directors, 33 percent of the second assistant directors, 38 percent of the associate directors in tape, and 23 percent of the stage managers. The Producers Guild of America reports that 50 of its 416 active and inactive members are women and that there's been a steady growth in their numbers in recent years. The Writers Guild of America reports that 38 percent, some 3,914 of its 10,300 members are women, but this includes those who write for both television and film or television exclusively, as well as newswriters. There's no breakdown of screenwriters.

Pointing out that with the sole exception of Dorothy Arzner, who worked in the motion picture industry from the beginnings of sound in the 1920s and on into the 1940s (Johnston, 1975), Barbara Koenig Quart (1988) echoes that woman directors have only recently emerged as feature filmmakers: "It is no longer unusual for five or six films by women directors to be playing simultaneously in Manhattan theatres, films as often from Europe or elsewhere as from America, since the phenomenon is international" (p. 1). "With this veritable explosion of films, we are witnessing nothing less than a new world for women, all the more dramatic given the sad early history of women directors."

HIV/AIDS FILMMAKING

The importance of the feminist filmmaking vision is underscored by Juhasz (1993), who has described how television documentaries have tended to juxtapose images of innocent female "victims" with "scientific facts" about AIDS, typically including women in their stories only as corollaries, such as the wife or girlfriend of a gay man. In mainstream media, she writes, "Somehow AIDS has become just one more systematic oppression in our society, exaggerating and multiplying the compromised positions under which many women already live their lives" (p. 150).

It is important to note that a disturbingly high number of Blacks consider AIDS as part of a white-inspired conspiracy to eliminate them.[1] AIDS as ideology also appears in works by Lester (1989), Pearlburg (1991), MacKinnon (1992),[2] Treichler (1993),[3] Squire (1993), Patton (1994), and Fuller (1996c), to name a few. Alisa Lebow (1993) celebrates an emerging crop of lesbian videomakers, "Whose work grew out of the AIDS activist movement, and who have developed an elaborate defense of down and dirty video activism. Seeking to blur the line between video art and documentary, (they) have developed distinctive voices and styles and are firmly rooted in the documentary tradition" (p. 19). Tangentially, Richard Dyer (1988) provides a fascinating discussion on related filmic concerns for vampirism, and Martin Norden (1990) calls for cinematic sensitivity regarding the physically "different."

This chapter seeks a more complete understanding of women filmmakers who have decided to focus on the HIV/AIDS pandemic. Eighteen female filmmakers/directors whose work addresses the HIV/AIDS pandemic were interviewed. Their insights about both filmmaking and HIV/AIDS enhance our understanding of women creating new discourses.

SURVEYING WOMEN PRODUCER/DIRECTORS OF AIDS FILMS

Methodology

The first step involved trying to determine where to find women who had produced and/or directed films concerning AIDS. A visit to New York City in the spring of 1995 with Ilana Navara of Media Network was particularly helpful, as were the many independent film resources cited in my study of community television (Fuller 1994a). As can be seen in Appendix I: "Contacts," nearly 100 agencies were identified, approached, and sent the letter reproduced in Appendix II: "AIDS-Related Agencies." While approximately a dozen were returned for new addresses or no addresses known, a number were helpful for further networking.

Thirty letters were sent on October 18, 1995 to potential interviewees, along with a sample list of questions that might be asked (see Appendix III: "Potential Producer/Director Interviewees" and

Appendix IV: "Survey Instrument"). Within a matter of days, the process had begun, with women producer/directors calling either to set up dates and times for interviews or actually participating in the interview process. As can be seen in Appendix V: "Filmography/ Videography," and detailed below, their contributions to the field have been prolific. The legend listed on the filmography/videography (C—Cinematographer; D—Director; E—Editor; P—Producer; V—Videographer; W—Writer), placed after each artist's name to indicate the role she played in a film, also attests to their wide areas of expertise. Appendix VI: "Distributors" is included in case readers would like to order any of the films and videos cited here.

Semistructured telephone interviews[4] reported here took place between October 20 and December 21, 1995. Averaging about five to ten minutes, although some ran longer, they can be classified as very open-ended. Even though a number of possible questions were included in the survey instrument, interviewees were assured that the key issue was whether they were interested first in AIDS and then got involved in filmmaking, or vice versa. Regarding the demographic information, they were simply encouraged to contribute whatever data they wanted to supply. Many of the interviewees were particularly pleased to know that nothing would be printed here without their approval.

The Filmmakers/Videographers

Mimi Plevin-Foust

Three years after her friend Raul Llorens was diagnosed with AIDS, Mimi was so impressed with both his attitude and his vigorous health that she decided to collaborate with him on a documentary about long-term AIDS survivors. The result is *Wide Time: Surviving AIDS* (1996). Based on the Mexican saying, "Life may not always be long, but it can be wide," the film profiles six dynamic women and men who have beaten the odds and survived full-blown AIDS from six to fifteen years. Their stories are intercut with interviews of doctors and researchers, revealing the psychological and medical strategies both long-term AIDS and cancer survivors share. Shot in both New York City and Berlin, the film, according to Mimi,[5] offers courageous examples along with solid information, providing models of spiritual and psychological health from people who have clearly learned to appreciate life.

Anne Lewis

Everyone in the southern Appalachian area knew Belinda, a young mother with a great sense of humor, a deep commitment to the community, and an abiding love of music. It was independent filmmaker Anne Lewis, though, who decided that her story—contracting AIDS from a medical mishap during the birth of her second child—needed to be captured. Shooting for *Belinda* began a year before Belinda died, before she relinquished her seat on the National Commission on AIDS to Magic Johnson. But when Anne began researching archival material on the disease beginning with the year 1984 and even up to 1992, she found little news coverage on the topic of people with AIDS. So she formed her own vision of Belinda the activist, who helped choose much of the music for the film and helped transfer her case from the personal to the political. With a grant of $39,000 to produce the film from the Robert Wood Johnson Foundation, as well as another grant from the Public Welfare Foundation, the 30-minute tape has meant a great deal to many different people in this rural area of Kentucky. Anne is especially pleased that it has been well received by a number of kids. She tells a poignantly tragic story about the time she took it to Louisville, though: an HIV-positive woman called her ahead of time, asking for permission to attend the showing.[6]

Juanita Mohammed

She's a "people person." Juanita had been a housing inspector in Brooklyn and had worked at a health clinic. Everywhere, she was becoming aware of the AIDS crisis, and decided to volunteer at Gay Men's Health Crisis (GMHC). Only then did she get involved with video work—first, working with WAVE (The Women's AIDS Video Enterprise, an innovative educational project aimed at empowering women in communities disproportionately affected by the disease). There, she worked with Alexandra Juhasz on *We Care* (1989), which was aimed at care providers for PWAs, and eventually built up her skills to form her own mother-daughter production company. In 1992, Juanita was hired by GMHC to work in their audiovisual department, where she remains to this day. She is the proud co-producer of *Two Men and a Baby* (1992), about two gay black men adopting the HIV-positive son of one's sister, and *Part of Me* (1992), about a Latina lesbian with AIDS, a former IV drug user who has become an impassioned AIDS educator. She also was responsible for *Words to Live by* (1993), an educational tape funded by the Board of Education that was put together by teens for other teens. "Due to bureaucratic slipups, the commitment level of their teenage participants, and the interference of school employees, Mohammed shot the tape over only seven days, partly during school time, partly on weekends" (Juhasz, 1990, p. 38), resulting in an ideal mix of divergent teenage dialogues and depictions. Still a "buddy" to many PWAs, including about 30 in her neighborhood who don't want to join a formal organization, Juanita is particularly sensitive to women's roles here. "They think about the time, and the money, and then put themselves last," she bemoans.[7] Hopefully, her many positive, educational tapes will encourage and educate not only fellow women of color, but all women.

Vivian Kleiman

"What film does best is create an emotional connection with the viewer," states this filmmaker/media activist.[8] A graduate of the University of California/Berkeley, Vivian traveled widely and then returned to the West Coast in 1976 to found Cultural Research & Communication, Inc., a nonprofit organization whose goal is to use media forms to help promote critical thinking. After working with Marlon Riggs on several documentaries, Vivian's contribution to the topic of AIDS evolved when she read about men offering extra money to sex workers for unsafe sex. "I got that shiver," she shares—and decided she had to work with that population of sex workers. *My Body's My Business* (1992), which works to keep women on the streets safe, is the result of outreach and rap sessions with a number of people. Not wanting to exploit or sensationalize the topic, Vivian's video offers straightforward dialogue dealing with issues like how to slip condoms onto customers and how to deal with the empowerment that comes from hearing fellow sex workers declare, "No amount of money is worth my life." It has been extremely successful—not only on the festival circuit, but even more important, as a story of women empowered to gain a voice.

Jennifer Lytton

Setting off to make her mark with a degree in Religious Studies, Jennifer has worked in distant countries such as India and Vietnam, and has been involved in professions ranging from rape crisis counseling to bereavement training to health care. Today, this 20-something AIDS educator combines her loves of social services and art in media literacy for healthcare workers. For Media Network's "Seeing Through AIDS" program, she works to incorporate already produced AIDS media into their clinical practice and outreach, teaching media literacy in the context of psychosocial issues relative to AIDS, such as socialization, negotiating safer sex, addiction, death and dying, family communication, staff burnout, and living with HIV and pediatric AIDS.

For New York Hospital's Center for Special Studies, Jennifer is currently working on a video tentatively called *Disclosure Project* that is aimed at an audience of parents who are HIV positive but have not yet told their children. There are a lot of issues to explore, especially for families who have difficulty in communication. "It's easier to talk to a room of strangers than one person in my family, and I have to tell someone, even if it is a video camera" she's been told by one participant, who speaks for so many of the others.[9]

Patricia Livingstone

Legally deaf and blind from Ushers Syndrome, filmmaker Patricia Livingstone felt compelled to make a video about her younger cousin and his relationship with his mother when he found out he had AIDS at age 26. He died just 18 months ago. Working with a crew who did the camerawork, she endeavored to show the healing power of love between a mother struggling with her own battle with cancer and the illness of her son. Patricia has had to persevere despite her own physical limitations, the disinterest of social service agencies, and her own grief. As we spoke on the telephone, Patricia, using special amplifiers on her end, shared how each step in the process of making the film mirrored her own experiences in dealing with her cousin's illness—from initial fears about AIDS to finally saying goodbye.[10] At this point, the tape still needs some off-line editing, and Patricia is seeking funding to finish it.

Jeanne Blake

As a medical reporter covering the early days of the AIDS epidemic in the 1980s for WBZ-TV in Boston (back when it was being called "GRID"), Jeanne clearly recalls that first story and the impact that the young man with AIDS had both on her and on the viewing audience; this was supposed to be something people were getting in the bigger cities such as New York or San Francisco, but here it was in Boston; it was scary. Since then, she has covered some 500 such stories. In 1986, she helped produce a documentary about a man the television station had followed with their cameras for 16 months. It was called *The Paul Cronan Story: Living with AIDS*. The viewer response was tremendous, with some 1,000 people calling and writing extremely empathic letters. "It was a defining moment," Jeanne recalls[11]. At the same time, she was invited to speak to schoolchildren across Massachusetts; from those powerful conversations came her book, *Risky Times: How To Be AIDS-Smart and Stay Healthy* (Workman, 1990, 1995)—which has sold some 200,000 copies to date, and is now also available in Spanish. In 1993, she coproduced a documentary that aired on PBS stations, *Sex Education in America: AIDS and Adolescents*—for which she raised the funds, did preproduction and production, scriptwriting, and served as the correspondent. Having been told that she has a gift for reaching young people, Jeanne's most recent project is the award-winning *In Our Own Words: Teens & AIDS* (1994), which she produced, directed, and wrote for Media Works. A journalist who openly claims she feels fortunate every day, Jeanne and her work sets an example for anyone interested in public health issues.

Deborah Wasser

A graduate of Harvard and then film school, Deborah's focus these days is on finishing up *Legacy*, a documentary devoted to the life of AIDS activist and songwriter Michael Callen. Not only did Callen start the first PWA health group, he also exemplified the revolutionary concept of surviving joyously; as such, he was an inspiration in the way he fought the disease in his own personal way—mainly through song. Appropriately, the documentary is something of an "AIDS operetta," including much of Callen's own music. The audience for it has changed, Deborah told me,[12] making the 26-minute film more of a live musical than simply a life's recounting. A full-time filmmaker/producer, Wasser also played a powerful role in the 1993 4-hour documentary, *A Time of AIDS*, which ran on the Discovery Channel. She reviewed an amusing event: doing research on the film for the British in their archives, she was unable to find any footage on gay bathhouses, so substituted some old porno films from the 1970s. A high-powered and obviously talented artist, Deborah will undoubtedly contribute much more to the field of feminist filmmaking.

Barbara Hammer

A decade ago, Barbara was teaching film at Columbia College in Chicago, but found it too stifling. Barbara's work is abstract and personal, and as a 40-something at that point, she knew something was lacking in her life. Through a class she instructed in feminist film, she got involved in a discussion on AIDS, and around the same time met the photographer Jan Zita Grover who introduced her to Simon Watney and his work on the hysteria surrounding the disease. That information was particularly pivotal. Soon thereafter, Barbara took control, deciding to dedicate her energies as a media artist to helping other women use computers and cyberspace for their unique expressions. "When I work as an artist, I have to work to challenge myself," she said,[13] typically dedicating herself to working with and for the "marginalized," and to making the "invisible" visible. Some 52 films and 26 videos later, she was imminently leaving to voluntarily teach High-8 video to women in the South African townships of Capetown and Johannesburg, funded by the National Lesbian Association ASTRAEA. Having just returned from judging The Yamagata International Documentary

Film Festival in Japan, Barbara Hammer's global vision is without parallel.

Meg Saegebarth

Meg's MBA had helped land her a spot on Wall Street. Her career was booming when she decided to volunteer for the Children's Hope Foundation. That led to being a counselor at the Birch Summer Project camp in Upstate New York for HIV-positive families, an experience that opened up a whole new world for her. Meg was so impressed with the kids' spirits that she decided to do a video about them—even though she had no background in filmmaking. Many people could not understand why she loved these kids so much, and so many had misconceptions that Meg was determined to educate them. The issue of access was solved through friendship with a woman on the Pediatric AIDS Committee at ACT UP, who introduced her to families who agreed to have their children be part of the video. In the end, Meg personally recruited all the children; all were over age eight and knew their status. Aimed at sixth-graders, the film is so real and so alive and so unique that Meg hopes many people will see it. What she also hopes is that this project will direct her to another career, where she'll be able to continue to make a difference.[14]

Gini Reditker

With a longtime interest in women's health, Gini was disturbed when she read an article in *The New York Times*, some six or seven years ago, about the frighteningly high number of babies who were HIV positive. "Why hadn't the women's movement taken up this issue?" she mused[15]—and then answered her own question, knowing it was the stigma involved. A self-taught filmmaker, she collaborated with Amber Hollibaugh to produce *Heart of the Matter*, which premiered with great success at the 1994 Sundance Film Festival, winning the festival's Freedom of Expression award. Aimed at women in particular—feminists, HIV-positive women, women of color, church women, and others, the film's main point is to draw attention to the problems surrounding AIDS and its attendant sexism; the film bills itself, in fact, as "the first film to consider AIDS as a women's issue." By appealing universally to women, Gini's work truly does address the universality of women's roles.

Jean Carlomusto

Reflecting upon her media activism with AIDS in the 1980s and 1990s, Jean was considering her prolific contributions to the cause, stating, "Making media was part of the movement . . . we were making history." As many of her fellow artists are feeling depressed by the dwindling interest, she believes it is the ultimate challenge to continue to do AIDS-related work. Having grown up in a family that always loved film and movies, it makes sense that Jean became a filmmaker/videomaker at age 18. She is mainly interested in documenting history and using progressive political process methods. Beginning as a volunteer at GMHC, she became increasingly concerned about representations of PWAs as pariahs, and decided to do something about it. First, she worked as a collective member for *Testing the Limits* (1987); next came a reaction to the Women's Committee of the AIDS Coalition To Unleash Power (ACT UP)'s protest to a *Cosmopolitan* article offering dangerously misleading information to women about unsafe sex, *Doctors, Liars and Women* (1989), which she coproduced and directed with Maria Maggenti for GMHC. *Voices from the Front* (1991), which Jean also coproduced, continued a profile on New York City AIDS activists, including both local and national stories underlining both the personal and political community effects of the disease. Her most recent piece is *What About My Kids?* (1994), which deals with HIV-positive women's worries about legal issues regarding custody of their children. Meant to work hand in hand with support services, Jean considers the film a "balancing ramp into the system."[16] The idea is that after seeing it, women will have a clearer idea of what they're getting into. And with all else, this vital filmmaker also finds time to teach video production to young people—a process she considers her most important intervention, as it aims to encourage burgeoning filmmakers with a sense of self-reliance.

Beverly Peterson

"Video letters" for women dying of AIDS to leave as legacies for their families are Beverly's incredible contribution to the cause. Armed for a second career after getting a BFA from Cooper Union Art School, then studying filmmaking at NYU, her first foray was *Totally Vulnerable*, a 1988 piece striking in its day because it dealt with healthy, hopeful AIDS patients discussing one's rights to die. That was followed by *Defining Life* (1990), featuring the story of John, a man living with AIDS, and his concerns about dying with dignity. Dealing with the right to die, the film was recorded just days before John committed suicide. Soon thereafter, volunteering for Project Hospitality in their homeless program, Beverly became captivated both by the organization and its clients and decided to help a woman make a film portrait to pass on to her daughter, and another for a second women whose daughter she would never know; thus, *Sandra's Web* (1996) was born. It since has been shown at the first annual Northampton Film Festival, and is scheduled to be shown on HBO. But don't just think about AIDS, Beverly cautions: "If you focus on the virus, you've lost—the virus will eat everything you have."[17] And she doesn't only aim to keep perspective in her filmmaking: she and her husband have adopted the 11-year-old son of one of her video letter senders!

Paula Mozen

After Paula's distributor sent me a review copy of *No Rewind* (1993), Paula's snappy, award-winning video featuring teens talking out about HIV/AIDS awareness, I could better understand why Paula wanted me to see it before having her interview. Multicultural, myth breaking, and candid, the film deals with the topic—including an hilarious scenario of teens trying to put a condom on a cucumber. The film's title came from the kids themselves ("So they're the experts," Paula explains).[18] The film particularly focuses on Robert, a gay, black, HIV-positive male, and Antigone, a straight, white, young woman whose lack of self-esteem and subsequent unprotected sex now find her also HIV-positive. The film depicts their lives revolving around regular teen activities and concerns. Using stories, peer educators, instruction, and rap songs, *No*

Rewind evolved as Paula's Cinema Studies master's thesis from San Francisco State. And what a video it is, having appeared at more than 30 film festivals, and winning the following awards: Blue Ribbon, American Film and Video Association; CINE Eagle, Council on International and Nontheatrical Events; Silver Apple, National Educational Film and Video Festival; Dore Schary Award for Human Relations, First Place for Documentary; Regional Emmy, Academy of Television Arts & Sciences, College Television Awards Competition; First Place for Documentary, Utah Short Film and Video Festival, and many more. But most of all, it has reached the 12- to 18-year-old audience Paula targeted, offering both social and sexual advice.

Cynthia Roberts

Cynthia and her husband, Greg Klymkiw, saw the theater adaptation of Hillar Liitoja's *Last Supper* in which their AIDS-infected friend Ken McDougall portrayed an AIDS patient who committed doctor-assisted suicide. Cynthia and Greg had a mutual revelation: "This is a movie."[19] Longtime fans of the DNA Theatre in Toronto, Cynthia and Greg had only known Ken as a person who had used his body so effectively to choreograph theatrical statements. At the end, Ken was restricted to a sickbed and the "real time" shooting of the film took place in a hospice. Ken died four days after the video was completed,[20] yet he was seen almost dancing from his deathbed. Special because it celebrates sex, *Last Supper* went on to win a Teddy Award for best feature at the Berlin Film Festival, and has appeared at more than 30 festivals on every continent. The two Canadian filmmakers feel especially good that their film has been well received by both straight and gay audiences, as it is essentially a story of a lovely relationship.

Ann L. Poritzky

As the senior communications specialist at the CDC National AIDS Clearinghouse, my appeal for women producer/directors of AIDS films landed on Ann's desk. When she called me, we talked about the video she has been coordinating: *HIV/AIDS Clinical*

Trials: Knowing Your Options. A marketing person with zero experience in filmmaking, Ann, as part of a team effort, has played multiple roles such as scriptwriter, conceptual planner, interviewee recruiter, and audience targeter extraordinaire. As she phrases it, "I'm the one there to see that the information in the film is accurate, the correct messages are conveyed, and that the people from the primary target audiences appear in the video."[21] The video was sponsored by the AIDS Clinical Trials Information Service (ASTIS). The video has been developed to help people learn what HIV/AIDS clinical trials are and how to make decisions about participating in clinical trials. This video has been developed for all people living with HIV/AIDS. The people who appear in the film are primarily women and people from racial and ethnic minority groups because they have been underrepresented in HIV/AIDS clinical trials. Ann hopes that a film follow-up will be made in Spanish.

Rita DeSouza

As the Executive Director of the statewide agency, Alaskans Living with HIV, Rita learned about this project from a friend in Oakland, California, and contacted me about the videos she has produced. She told me, "Some are about prevention education, some about Alaskan Native people who have died from AIDS and other various themes."[22] When we spoke, she elaborated further: coming from San Francisco, where she was feeling burned out by the AIDS scourge—having lost lots of friends, including a brother, Rita moved to Juneau and decided to use her filmmaking talents toward helping others. The "goose-bumpy" *Sitka Trilogy* is just one result, and she has some 200 tapes of raw footage waiting to be made into more films. Coming from a Buddhist viewpoint, Rita has been easily assimilated and accepted into the native community; for example, when Ryan White's mother Jeannie came to Alaska, Rita escorted her around for a media blitz into areas where other outsiders would hardly have ever gone. Her explanation for this success: "I'm heartfelt."

Charline Boudreau

Originally getting involved in the AIDS issue by forming the women's coalition of ACT UP in Montreal, Charline has been prolific in producing relevant videos: *Liaisons Perillueuses* in 1991, *Le Ravissement* and *Step out Smartly*, both in 1993. The last tapes were produced at the Banff Center for the Arts, where Charline was invited to participate in a three-month program focusing on the production of AIDS-related public service announcements. She managed to skirt the broadcasting censorship issue by overshooting and editing two versions of these pieces: one for media broadcast, the other for the "festival" circuit.

The media, according to Boudreau, have always focused on the gay aspect of the AIDS issue. The fact is that women are, and have been, the fastest rising group since the 1980s. Even as we speak, women are dying of "unknown causes" because there is so little research done on how women manifest AIDS symptoms. In other words, Boudreau suggests, when gay men were the most affected, they drew enormous amounts of attention to themselves and to the issue, i.e., "the crisis." But now that gay men are within acceptable statistical parameters, the *need* to fight for attention has apparently ceased. Gay men did not bother to extend their knowledge and structure to others (e.g., women, non-white, non-western peoples, etc.). The task at hand then is to shift the focus from AIDS as a *gay issue* to AIDS as a serious issue for women—not only a health concern, but one that affects our political, socioeconomic, and cultural lives."[23]

Findings/Comments

First, some statistics on demographics. All but one of the 18 interviewees disclosed their ages without prompting; they ranged from a low of 27 to a high of 55; their average age was 39.5 years old. While eight stated that they were white, only one said she was black. Only one said she was Hispanic, while three added that they were Jewish. Of the two Canadians, one declared herself Acadian. Five of the women were married (three of them referred to children), one mentioned having a male partner/father of their two-year-old, six said they were lesbians (two of whom had been previously married), and one was single—if that number doesn't add up to 18, it's because the others didn't mention marital status.

While the standard wisdom has been that lesbians are the "safest" population in the pandemic, Marguerite Moritz (1994) pointed out that, "Because the media had consistently used the word *gay* to refer to both men and women, lesbians were implicated in the AIDS crisis even though they are among the lowest risk subgroup for the disease, a fact that rarely was reported" (p. 66). Yet according to Cole and Cooper,

> Lesbians need HIV education. They are in waiting rooms across America—waiting. More and more HIV infection among lesbians is showing up in clinics across America, yet lesbians remain an enigma to most health professionals and continue to be excluded from HIV/AIDS education. A lesbian can become HIV-infected the way any woman can: some lesbians engage in oral, vaginal, and anal intercourse with men by choice, force or necessity; some use drugs and share needles, some have blood transfusions, some are artificially inseminated, and some exchange blood and vaginal secretions during sexual contact with women. (1990/1991, p. 18)

For our purposes, Alisa Lebow's (1993) comments are particularly pertinent:

> There is an entire crop of lesbian videomakers, including Ellen Spiro and Jean Carlomusto, whose work grew out of the AIDS activist movement, and who have developed an elaborate defense of down and dirty video activism. Seeking to blur the line between video art and documentary, both have developed distinctive voices and styles and are firmly rooted in the documentary tradition, even as they seek to expand its limit. (p. 19)

In education and training, the 18 interviewees again represented a wide range, from film school or MFAs, or journalism degrees to being self-taught or in the process of learning about video. Their occupations included the following: writer, teacher, multimedia coordinator, self-described filmmaker/videographer, market researcher, media activist, AIDS educator, medical reporter, media artists (2), and freelancer, with a number of over-lapping self-descriptions. Most labeled themselves "feminist filmakers."

While a number of the 18 women producer/directors were AIDS volunteers, such as being AIDS buddies or serving on AIDS task forces or in various agencies in addition to their video work, they also reported doing volunteer work in other areas, such as Big Sister, school systems, collaborative video projects, serving on non-profit boards, tutoring English as a second language, and other social service areas. Snyder and Omoto (1992a, 1992b), surveying motivations of AIDS volunteers in Minneapolis, identified five main reasons: to express their basic values (e.g., "Because of my humanitarian obligation to help others"), to express their commu-nity concerns and solidarity (e.g., "To help members of the gay community"), to help gain knowledge (e.g., "To learn about how people cope with AIDS"), to foster personal growth (e.g., "To chal-lenge myself and test my skills"), and to enhance their self-esteem (e.g., "To feel better about myself").

CONCLUSIONS

This chapter presents a profile of producer/directors of AIDS films who are as rich and diverse as their backgrounds and perspec-tives. After interviewing them, it seemed to me that they emerge as women first, filmmakers second. In response to the key question of whether they got involved in the first place because of AIDS or because they were filmmakers looking for themes, the interviewees chose the latter—but only by a slight margin. Seven of the women interviewed for this survey became producer/directors out of a con-cern for the AIDS issue, while the eleven others were filmmaker/ videographers who happened on issues and stories crying out for visual representation.

AIDS films produced and/or directed by women provide insight not only into women's ways of acknowledging AIDS, but also into feminist film and gender issues in filmmaking. Interviews with women producer/directors give access to their thoughts about HIV and their motivations for producing and directing AIDS films. This genre could be the harboring of a new era of feminist filmmaking.

Appendix I

Contacts

ACLU AIDS Project
ACT UP
AIDS Action Council
AIDS Clinical Trials Information Service
AIDS Education and Prevention
AIDS Film Initiative
AIDSFILMS
AIDS Information Office, Centers of Disease Control
AIDS National Interfaith Network
AIDS Treatment Data Network
Aims Media
Alliance for Community Media
American Film Institute
American Foundation for AIDS Research
Alternative Views/Austin Community TV
Angles: Women Working in Film and Video
Arts Over AIDS
Asian Cinevision
Association of Independent Video and Filmmakers
Audio-Visual Resources for Social Change
Bay Area Video Coalition
Black Entertainment TV
Body Positive
Broadway Cares
California Newsreel
Chicago Access Corp.
Cine Festival
The Cinema Guild
Creative Coalition
Design Industries Foundation for AIDS/DIFFA
DIVA-TV/ACT-UP

Downtown Community TV
Dyke TV
Equity Fights AIDS
Fanlight Productions
Fear of Disclosure Project
Film in the Cities
Filmmakers Library
Flying Focus Video Collective
Frameline
Gay and Lesbian Alliance Against Defamation (GLAAD)
Gay Men's Health Crisis (GMHC)
Gran Fury
International Radio and TV Society
The Kitchen
Latino Collaborative
Media Alliance
Media Coalition
Media Network
The Names Project AIDS Memorial Quilt
National Academy of Cable Programming
National AIDS Clearinghouse (NAC)
National AIDS Hotline
National Alliance of Artists' Organizations
National Alliance for Media Arts and Culture
National American Public Broadcasting Consortium
National Association of Artists Organizations
National Association of People With AIDS
National Bi-Programming Consortium
National Black Programming Consortium
National Cable TV Asso.
National Coalition of Independent Public Broadcasting Producers
National Commission on Acquired Immune Deficiency Syndrome
National Endowment for the Arts' AIDS Working Group
National Gay and Lesbian Task Force
National Lawyers Guild AIDS Network
National Leadership Coalition on AIDS
National Minority AIDS Council
National Resource Center on Women and AIDS

National Videotape Exchange
The 90's
Not Channel Zero
Office of the National AIDS
Paper Tiger TV/Deep Dish
Photographers & Friends United Against AIDS
Public Broadcasting System
Public Interest Video Network
The PWA Health Group
San Francisco Community TV Corporation
Select Media/Educational Film and Video
Testing the Limits Collective
Third World Newsreel
Union for Democratic Communications
United States Conference of Mayors AIDS Program
Video Data Bank
Video Project
Videoteca del Sur
Visual AIDS
Water Bearer Films
Woman Vision
Women Organized to Respond to Life Threatening Diseases
    (WORLD)
Women's Access Coalition
Women Express, Inc.
Women in Film and Video New England
Women Make Movies

Appendix II:

Letter to AIDS-Related Agencies

October 18, 1995

Dear AIDS-involved organization:

Since you are on the forefront of AIDS concerns, it struck me that perhaps you might be interested in participating in a project I'm doing with Nancy Roth of Rutgers University, to be published by The Haworth Press:

Women and AIDS: Negotiating Safer Practices,
Care, and Representation

For my contribution, I plan to speak directly with people who have chosen to work with film and/or video about the topic—especially, producer/directors of AIDS films. I have constructed a survey that takes approximately 5 to 10 minutes, and would like to have names, addresses, and telephone numbers of persons I might interview— preferably by telephone. I can send a copy of an outline of the kinds of questions we might cover, ranging from personal information to the actual work (s), when, where, and why.

As I would like to include as many producer/directors of AIDS films and videos as possible, may I ask you to let me know of anyone you think I should contact for this project? Of course I will be happy to share my results with you, and nothing will be used without participants' permission. I am including some examples of my most recent publications.

Needless to say, I thank you in advance for any leads you might have on this critical topic, and I wish you all the best.

Sincerely,

Linda K. Fuller

Appendix III

Letter to Potential Producer/Director Interviewees

October 18, 1995

Dear

Because, like you, we feel so committed to doing something about the growing phenomenon of women and AIDS, Nancy Roth of Rutgers University and I are co-editing a book to be published by The Haworth Press:

> *Women and AIDS: Negotiating Safer Practices,*
> *Care, and Representation*

For my contribution, I would like to speak directly with women who have chosen to work with film and/or video about the topic— which is why I would like to talk to you. Tentatively called "To Desire to Direct Differently: Women Producer/Directors of AIDS Films," my chapter aims to report on various projects from a range of approaches to the same topic.

Toward that end, I would very much like to interview you—prefer- ably by telephone. I am enclosing an outline of the kinds of ques- tions we might cover, ranging from personal information about you to what you have worked on, when, where, and why. Estimating our conversation might last 5 to 10 minutes, please let me know when it would be most convenient to talk. Listed below are various ways you can contact me so we can set up the best time for the interview.

As I would like to include as many women producer/directors of AIDS films and videos as possible, may I also ask you to let me know of anyone else I should contact for this project? Of course I will be happy to share my results with you, and nothing will be used without your permission. I am also including samples of my most recent publications.

Let me finish by saying how much I look forward to working with you on this long overdue, exciting project.

Yours in sisterhood,

Linda K. Fuller

Appendix IV

Survey Instrument

Name:

Address:

Phone/FAX:

Women Producer/Directors of AIDS Films: A Survey

A. *Demographics*—some personal information

1. Age:
2. Race/ethnicity:
3. Marital status/sexual orientation:
4. Education/training
5. Occupation/employment:
6. Volunteer involvement:
7. Self-label (e.g., feminist, activist):
8. Future career goals:

B. *Content*—some information about your AIDS films/videos

1. What AIDS films/videos have you been involved with? (List them all, including title, year, producer, distributor, time, and your role)
2. Why did you want to deal with the subject of AIDS cinematically?
3. Who has been pivotal to you in this process?
4. Have you quit any AIDS-related projects you had started? If so, why?
5. How would you describe your approach to filmmaking?
6. Did any of your films/videos have to be negotiated? If so, why?

C. *Your background*—some information about your AIDS involvement

1. How did you happen to get involved with the topic of AIDS?

2. Are you a member of any AIDS-related advocacy group(s)?
3. What has been your personal involvement with HIV/AIDS?

D. *Audience*—some information about your intended audience

1. Did you have a particular audience in mind for your AIDS film(s)?
2. Did you want to speak to a wide or specialized audience?
3. What age group(s) did you want to appeal to? Gender? Race? Interests?
4. What kind of feedback have you received about your film(s)?

E. *Personal responses*—some information about what this has meant for you

1. Generally, what has been your overall reaction to your IDS film(s)?
2. What kind of things have you learned from it/them?
   a. Technical and/or nontechnical training?
   b. Anything about yourself?
   c. Anything about HIV/AIDS? About PWAs?
3. How might you critique your film(s), both positively and negatively?
4. How do you think you get along with your production crew?
5. Do you think your production(s) have affected your status in any way?
6. Did your film(s) help fulfill any of your wider goals?
7. What do you envision to be your future involvement with AIDS films?

Please feel free to add any further comments about either this subject and/or this survey. Thank you!

Appendix V

Filmography/Videography

Date	Program	Artist/Role	Distributor
1986	*Paul Cronan Story: Living with AIDS*	Jeanne Blake (Reporter)	Media Works
1986	*Snow Job: Media Hysteria of AIDS*	Barbara Hammer (P/D/V/E)	Frameline
1987	*Testing the Limits: NYC*	Jean Carlomusto (Collective member)	Testing the Limits
1988	*Doctors, Liars, and Women*	Jean Carlomusto (Co-P)	GMHC
1989	*Marlon Riggs— Tongues Untied*	Vivian Kleiman (C)	PBS
1989	*Totally Vulnerable*	Beverly Peterson (P/D/E)	No longer in distribution
1989	*We Care*	Juanita Mohammed (Co-P)	WAVE
1990	*Defining Life*	Beverly Peterson (P/D/E)	Filmmakers Library
1991	*Voices from the Front*	Jean Carlomusto (Co-P/D)	Media Network
1992	*Belinda*	Anne Lewis (P)	Appalshop
1992	*My Body's My Business*	Vivian Kleiman (P/D)	Cult Res & Comm
1992	*Part of Me*	Juanita Mohammed (Co-P)	Distributor unknown
1992	*Two Men and a Baby*	Juanita Mohammed (Co-P/D)	GMHC
1993	*Liaisons Perillueuses*	Charline Boudreau (P/D)	C. Boudreau
1993	*No Rewind*	Paula Mozen (P/D/E)	Film Library
1993	*Le Ravissement*	Charline Boudreau (D/E)	Frameline

Date	Program	Artist/Role	Distributor
1993	*Sex Ed in America: AIDS & Adolescents*	Jeanne Blake (Co-P/W)	Media Works
1993	*Step out Smartly*	Charline Boudreau (P/D)	C. Boudreau
1993	*A Time of AIDS*	Deborah Wasser (AP)	Discovery Channel
1993	*Words to Live By*	Juanita Mohammed (P)	Distributor unknown
1994	*Heart of the Matter*	Gini Reditker (Co-P/D)	C. Boudreau
1994	*Last Supper*	Cynthia Roberts (D/Co-P)	Hryhory Yulyan
1994	*Out in South Africa*	Barbara Hammer (P/D/V/E)	Women Make Movies
1994	*Sitka Trilogy*	Rita DeSouza (P/D)	Muddy Pond
1994	*What About My Kids?*	Jean Carlomusto (P/D)	GMHC, Brooklyn Legal Service
1995	*In Our Own Words: Teens & AIDS*	Jeanne Blake (P/D/W)	Media Works
1996	*HIV/AIDS Clinical Trials*	Anne L. Poritzky (Coord.)	CDC Natl. AIDS Clearinghouse
1996	*Sandra's Web*	Beverly Peterson (P/D/E)	HBO
1996	*Wide Time: Surviving AIDS*	Mimi Plevin-Foust (Co-P/D)	Not yet selected
In progress	*Disclosure Project*	Jennie Lytton (P/D)	NY Hospital
In progress	*Everybody's Children*	Meg Saegebarth (EP)	Not yet selected
In progress	*Legacy*	Deborah Wasser (P/D/W)	Distributor unknown
In progress	*Mother and Son*	Patricia Livingstone (P)	Newton TV Foundation

Legend: C – Cinematographer;   D – Director;   E – Editor;   P – Producer;
V – Videographer;   W – Writer;   Co-P – Co-producer;   Coord. – Coordinator;
EP – Executive Producer;   AP – Associate Producer

Appendix VI

Distributors

Appalshop, 306 Madison St., Whitesbury, KY 41858

Charline Boudreau, 935 Marie-Anne East, Montreal, Quebec, Canada H2J 2B2

CDC National AIDS Clearinghouse, P.O. Box 6003, Rockville, MD 20849-6003

Changing World Productions, 71 West Broadway, New York, NY 10007

Cultural Research & Communication, 2600 Tenth St., Berkeley, CA 94710

Film Library/No Rewind, 22-D Hollywood Avenue, Hohokus, NJ 07423

Filmakers Library, 124 East 40th St., Suite 901, New York, NY 10016

First Run/Icarus Films, 153 Waverly Place, 6th floor, New York, NY 10014

Frameline, 346 Ninth St., San Francisco, CA 94103

Gay Men's Health Crisis (GMHC), 129 West 20th St., New York, NY 10011

Home Box Office (HBO), 1100 Avenue of the Americas, New York, NY 10036

Hryhory Yulyan Motion Pictures, 164 Bellwoods Ave., Toronto, Ontario, Canada M6J2PH

Media Network, 39 West 14th St., Suite 403, New York, NY 10011

Media Works, P.O. Box 15597, Kenmore Station, Boston, MA 02215

Muddy Pond, c/o Alaskans Living with HIV, 174 S. Franklin #208, Juneau, Alaska 99801

The Newton TV Foundation, 1608 Beacon St., Waban, MA 02168

Out on the Screen, 8455 Beverly Blvd., #309, Los Angeles, CA 90048

Testing the Limits Collective, 31 West 26th St., 4th floor, New York, NY 10010

Video Data Bank, School of the Art Institute, Columbus Drive and Jackson Blvd., Chicago, IL 60603

Women Make Movies, 462 Broadway, Suite 500, New York, NY 10013

NOTES

1. See a number of polls and surveys cited in Ed Guerro (1993, p. 160), many of which can also be found in Andrew Hacker's book, *Two Nations: Black and White, Separate, Hostile, Unequal* (1992, p. 49).

2. MacKinnon (1992) states, "Whatever the perception of AIDS, it is new, or at least its name and perception are new . . . AIDS suffering and AIDS deaths are a fact . . . It is a construction whose medical meaning has been determined by 'experts' interpreting data in a particular, exclusive way" (p. 13).

3. Regarding NBC's 1985 AIDS drama, *An Early Frost*, Treichler (1993) discusses not only how gayness was watered down, but also adds, "Boilerplace biomedical AIDS information constitutes a second take-home message" (p. 174).

4. For more on the methodology of self-structured interviews, see Smith (1995).

5. Telephone conversation with Mimi Plevin-Foust, October 20, 1995.

6. Telephone conversation with Anne Lewis, October 23, 1995.

7. Telephone conversation with Juanita Mohammed, October 24, 1995.

8. Telephone conversation with Vivian Kleiman, October 31, 1995.

9. Telephone conversation with Jennie Lytton, October 31, 1995.

10. Telephone conversation with Patricia Livingstone, October 31, 1995.

11. Telephone conversation with Jeanne Blake, November 3, 1995.

12. Telephone conversation with Deborah Wasser, November 3, 1995.

13. Telephone conversation with Barbara Hammer, November 3, 1995.

14. Telephone conversation with Meg Saegebarth, November 7, 1995.

15. Telephone conversation with Gini Reditker, November 10, 1995.

16. Telephone conversation with Jean Carlomusto, November 10, 1995.

17. Telephone conversation with Beverly Peterson, November 10, 1995.

18. Telephone conversation with Paula Mozen, November 10 and 21, 1995.

19. Telephone conversation with Cynthia Roberts, November 20, 1995.

20. Roberts' production notes include this description: "By the time of the shooting, Ken was absolutely bedridden and weighed about 68 pounds. He was skin and bones. Every movement he made was painful because he did not have flesh to cushion him . . . There was hardly anything left of his eyelids. He could not completely close his eyes which naturally rolled back into his head. His body was wasted, but his mind was sharp and his will was like iron" (p. 5).

21. Telephone conversation with Ann Poritzky, November 27, 1995.

22. FAX from Rita DeSouza, December 3, 1995. We spoke on December 5, 1995.

23. Telephone conversation with Charline Boudreau, December 21, 1995.

REFERENCES

Acker, A. (1991). *Reel Women: Pioneers of the Cinema 1896 to Present.* New York: Continuum.

Anderson, C. (1975). *Video Power: Grass Roots Television.* New York: Praeger.

Basinger, J. (1993). *A Woman's View: How Hollywood Spoke to Women, 1930-1960.* New York: Alfred A. Knopf.

Betancourt, J. (1974). *Women in Focus.* Dayton, OH: Pflaum.

Blake, J. (1990/1995). *Risky Times: How to Be AIDS-Smart and Stay Healthy.* New York: Workman.

Bovenschen, S. (1977). Is there a feminine aesthetic? *New German Critique,* 10 (Winter), 111-137.

Cantor, M. G. (1971). *The Hollywood TV Producer: His Work and His Audience.* New York: Basic Books.

Caughie, J. (Ed.). (1981). *Theories of Authorship.* London: Routledge and Kegan Paul.

Cole, J. and Dale, H. (1993). *Calling the Shots: Profiles of Women Filmmakers.* Kingston, Ontario: Quarry Press.

Cole, R. and Cooper, S. (1990/1991). Lesbian exclusion from HIV/AIDS education: Ten years of low-risk identity and high-risk behavior. *Siecus Report,* December/January, 18-23.

Corliss, R. (1986). Calling their own shots: Women directors are starting to make it in Hollywood. *Time* (March 24), 82-83.

DeLauretis, T. (1984). *Alice Doesn't: Feminism, Semiotics, Cinema.* Bloomington, IN: Indiana University Press.

Diakite, M. (1980). *Film, Culture, and the Black Filmmaker: A Study of Functional Relationships and Parallel Developments.* New York: Arno.

Doane, M. (1987). *The Desire to Desire: The Woman's Film of the 1940s.* Bloomington, IN: Indiana University Press.

Doane, M., Mellencamp, P., and Williams, L. (Eds.). (1984). *Re-vision: Essays in Feminist Film Criticism.* Frederick, MD: University Publications of America and the American Film Institute.

Downing, J. (1984). *Radical Media: The Political Experience of Alternative Communication.* Boston: South End Press.

Dyer, R. (1988). Children of the night: Vampirism as homosexuality, homosexuality as vampirism. In S. Radstone (Ed.), *Sweet Dreams: Sexuality, Gender, and Popular Fiction, 47-72.* London: Lawrence and Wishart.

Erens, P. (Ed.). (1979). *Sexual Stratagems: The World of Women in Film.* New York: Horizon Press.

Erens, P. (Ed.). (1990). *Issues in Feminist Film Criticism.*

Faulkner, R. R. (1971). *Hollywood Studio Musicians: Their Work and Careers in the Recording Industry.* Chicago: Aldine-Atherton.

Fischer, L. (1989). *Shot/Countershot: Film Tradition and Women's Cinema.* Princeton, NJ: Princeton University Press.

Flitterman-Lewis, S. (1990). *To Desire Differently: Feminism and the French Cinema.* Urbana, IL: University of Illinois Press.

Foster, G. A. (1995). *Women Film Directors: An International Bio-Critical Dictionary.* Westport, CT: Greenwood.

Fuller, L. K. (1990). Producers of Programming for Noncommercial Television. *Medienpsychologie, 4,* 302-314.

Fuller, L. K. (1993). *AIDS as (Filmic) Entertainment*. Paper presented to the Eastern Communication Association. New Haven, CT.

Fuller, L.K. (1994a). *Community Television in the United States: A Sourcebook on Public, Educational, and Governmental Access*. Westport, CT: Greenwood.

Fuller, L. K. (1994b). *Doubly Excluded from the Dialogue: Depictions of Women in AIDS Films*. Paper presented to the Gender and Communication Division, International Association for Mass Communication Research, Nineteenth General Assembly, Seoul, Korea.

Fuller, L.K. (1995). Introduction. In L.K. Fuller and L. McPherson Shilling (Eds.), *Communicating About Communicable Diseases*, vii-xii. Amherst, MA: Human Resource Development Press.

Fuller, L.K. (1996a). Filmic fictions: Depictions of AIDS in motion pictures. In L.K. Fuller (Ed.), *Media-Mediated AIDS*, 89-104. Amherst, MA: Human Resource Development Press.

Fuller, L.K. (1996b). *Media-Mediated Relationships: Straight and Gay, Mainstream and Alternative Perspectives*. Binghamton, NY: The Haworth Press.

Fuller, L.K. (1996c). *WWAs: Women with AIDS*. Paper presented to the Speech Communication Association, San Antonio, TX.

Gentile, M.C. (1985). *Film Feminists: Theory and Practice*. Westport, CT: Greenwood.

Guerrero, E. (1993). *Framing Blackness: The African-American Image in Film*. Philadelphia: Temple University Press.

Hacker, A. (1992). *Two Nations: Black and White, Separate, Hostile, Unequal*. New York: Scribners.

Heck-Rabi, L. (1984). *Women Filmmakers: A Critical Reception*. Metuchen, NJ: Scarecrow Press.

Johnston, C. (Ed.). (1973). *Notes on Women's Cinema*. London: British Film Institute.

Johnston, C. (Ed.). (1975). *Dorothy Arzner: Towards a Feminist Cinema*. London: British Film Institute.

Juhasz, A. (1990). The contained threat: Women in mainstream AIDS documentary. *The Journal of Sex Research, 27* (1), 25-46.

Juhasz, A. (1993). Knowing AIDS through the documentary. In C. Squire (Ed.), *Women and AIDS: Psychological Perspectives*, 150-164. Newbury Park, CA: Sage.

Juhasz, A. (1994). So many alternatives: The alternative AIDS video movement. *Cineaste, XXI*, (1-2), 37-39.

Kaplan, E.A. (1983). *Women & Film: Both Sides of the Camera*. London: Metheun.

Kay, K. and Peary, G. (Eds.). (1977). *Women and the Cinema: A Critical Anthology*. New York: E.P. Dutton.

Krasilovsky, A. (1997). *Women Behind the Camera: Conversations with Camerawomen*. Westport, CT: Praeger.

Kuhn, A. (1982). *Women's Pictures: Feminism and Cinema*. London: Routledge and Kegan Paul.

Lebow, A. (1993). Lesbians make movies. *Cineaste, XX*, (2), 18-23.

Lester, B. (1989). *Women and AIDS: A Practical Guide for Those Who Help Others.* New York: Continuum.

MacKinnon, K. (1992). *The Politics of Popular Representation: Reagan, Thatcher, AIDS, and the Movies.* Rutherford, NJ: Fairleigh Dickinson Press.

Mayne, J. (1984). The woman at the keyhole: Women's cinema and feminist criticism. In M. Doane, P. Mellencamp, and L. Williams (Eds.), *Re-vision: Essays in Feminist Film Criticism*, 49-66. Frederick, MD: University Publications of America and the American Film Institute.

McCreadie, M. (1983). *Women on Film: The Critical Eye.* Westport, CT: Praeger.

Moritz, M.J. (1994). The gay agenda: Marketing hate speech to mainstream media. In R. K. Whillock and D. Slayden (Eds.), *Hate Speech*, 55-79. Thousand Oaks, CA: Sage.

Mulvey, L. (1975). Visual pleasure and narrative cinema. *Screen, 16* (3), 6-18.

Newcomb, H.M. and Alley, R.S. (1982). The producer as artist: Commercial television. In J.S. Ettema and D.C. Whitney (Eds.), *Individuals in Mass Media Organizations: Creativity and Constraint*, 69-89. Beverly Hills: Sage.

Norden, M.E. (1990). Victims, villains, saints, and heroes: Movie portrayals of people with physical disabilities. In P. Loukides and L.K. Fuller (Eds.), *Beyond the Stars: Stock Characters in American Popular Film*, 222-233. Bowling Green, KY: Popular Press.

Patton, C. (1994). *Last Served? Gendering the HIV Pandemic.* London: Taylor & Francis.

Pearlburg, G. (1991). *Women, AIDS, & Communities: A Guide for Action.* Metuchen, NJ: Women's Action Alliance and The Scarecrow Press.

Penley, C. (Ed.). (1988). *Feminism and Film Theory.* New York: Routledge, Chapman, and Hall, Inc.

Penley, C. and Willis, S. (Eds.). (1993). *Male Trouble.* Minneapolis, MN: University of Minnesota Press.

Quart, B.K. (1988). *Women Directors: The Emergence of a New Cinema.* Westport, CT: Praeger.

Reid, M.A. (1993). *Redefining Black Film.* Berkeley: University of California Press.

Rose, J. (1986). *Sexuality in the Field of Vision.* London: Verso.

Rosenberg, J. (1983). *Women's Reflections: The Feminist Film Movement.* Ann Arbor, MI: UMI Research Press.

Sklar, R. (1994). *Movie-Made America: A Cultural History of American Movies, Revised and Updated.* New York: Vintage.

Slide, A. (1977). *Early Women Directors.* New York: A.S. Barnes.

Smith, J.A. (1995). Semi-structured interviewing and qualitative analysis. In J.A. Smith, R. Harre, and L. Van Langenhove (Eds.), *Rethinking Methods in Psychology*, 9-26. Thousand Oaks, CA: Sage.

Smith, S. (1975). *Women Who Make Movies.* New York: Hopkinson and Blake.

Snyder, M. and Omoto, A.O. (1992a). Volunteerism and society's response to the HIV epidemic. *Current Directions in Psychological Science*, (1), 113-115.

Snyder, M. and Omoto, A.M. (1992b). Who helps and why? The psychology of AIDS volunteerism. In S. Spacapan and S. Oskamp (Eds.), *Helping and Being Helped: Naturalistic Studies.* Newbury Park, CA: Sage.

Squire, C. (Ed.). 1993. *Women and AIDS: Psychological Perspectives.* Newbury Park, CA: Sage.

Treichler, P.A. (1993). AIDS narratives on television: Whose story? In T.F. Murphy and S. Poirier (Eds.), *Writing AIDS: Gay Literature, Language, and Analysis,* 161-199. New York: Columbia University Press.

Tuchman, G. (Ed.). (1974). *The TV Establishment: Programming for Power and Profit.* Englewood Cliffs, NJ: Prentice-Hall.

Tunstall, J. (1994). *Television Producers.* London: Routledge.

Sentimentality, Race, and *Boys on the Side*

Katie Hogan

Blanche was unimpressed by the tears, and Grace's Mammy-save-me eyes. Mammy-savers regularly peeped out at her from the faces of some white women for whom she worked . . . . She never ceased to be amazed at how many white people longed for Aunt Jemima. They'd ease into the kitchen and hem and haw their way through some sordid personal tale. She'd listen and make sympathetic noises.[1]

The fictional character in the above quotation is Blanche White, a middle-aged, black domestic worker whose opinions of her employer, Grace, are expressed in Barbara Neely's award-winning mystery novel, *Blanche on the Lam* (1992). Well aware of the construction of the black woman as "mammy" and "Aunt Jemima," Blanche humorously exposes what film historian Donald Bogle (1994) calls the enduring fantasy of "black women as nurturing, caretaking marvels. . . . helping poor white women untangle the knots in their lives" (pp. 358-389).

Blanche pretends to "listen and make sympathetic noises," but readers know her true feelings of contempt and dislike, feelings which only increase as the story progresses and it is revealed that Grace is a psychotic killer (Neely, 1992). Neely's fictional Blanche "performs" the role of mammy out of economic necessity, but this never stops her from having her own opinions and leading an independent life. Blanche's insightful critical commentary suggests how sentimentality, or the production of tears, functions as a smoke screen behind which lies the struggle and rage of poor women and women of color. In short, Blanche makes clear the link between women's sentimentality and the invisibility of black women in representation.

The lives of working-class women of color have rarely been the focus of popular fiction or of screenplays and productions of commercial Hollywood films. Until the late 1960s, most black actors in Hollywood films were still unabashedly cast as happy, childlike dancers, singers, or musicians, or as affable maids and servants who functioned as human props and foils to the white stars (Bogle, 1994). In Shirley Temple movies, for example, the adorable curly-haired girl forged a relationship with her black dance teachers and servants. In Mae West movies, the outrageously sexy star, beloved by both gay men and feminists, was shown surrounded by adoring black maids who answered to her every "beck and call" (Bogle, 1994). Even Hattie McDaniel's dignified performance of Mammy in *Gone with the Wind* (1939) reinforced the notion that, as Bogle puts it, "black shoulders were made to cry on" (p. 153). McDaniel's performance threatened to steal the show as she plays a powerful surrogate mother-mammy whose outspoken, bossy, domineering manner is respected (Bogle, 1994). But as with most black female roles, Mammy is not allowed to possess a complex life of her own. Her only means of expression are through her influence and care of the suffering yet "difficult" Scarlett O'Hara. Unfortunately, this all-too-familiar cultural fantasy of the black woman as "the mighty nurturer" continues to structure the kinds of roles black female actors play in contemporary American films (Bogle, 1994).

For example, aside from the controversial film *The Color Purple* (1985), Whoopi Goldberg has been repeatedly cast in films in which she is the sole black character surrounded by an all-white cast (Bogle, 1994). In addition to this lonely, outcast status, Bogle argues that Goldberg is often presented in an updated version of the mammy/servant role. In *Ghost* (1990), for example, Goldberg plays a whacky psychic medium who is compelled to reunite a grief-stricken white woman with her dead, yuppie boyfriend (Bogle, 1994). In *The Long Walk Home,* Goldberg plays a domestic servant who "humanizes" her white, Southern employer, and in *Clara's Heart* she assumes the role of a beautifully dressed, wise, live-in,

Jamaican maid who nurtures a neglected, rich, white boy (Bogle, 1994). While Goldberg is always portrayed as the moral center in these films, and as in *Clara's Heart,* her own personal struggles are somewhat developed and realized, she is consistently without a separate, developed romantic/personal life of her own. Unfortunately, her role as Jane DeLuca in Herbert Ross's 1995 film, *Boys on the Side,* follows this dominant pattern of the "updated mammy" (Bogle, 1994, p. 298).

Hailed by *The New York Times* film critic Janet Maslin (1995) as "one of the strongest Hollywood movies to deal with AIDS thus far" (p. C3), *Boys on the Side* (1995) breaks ground as the first commercial film with well-known actors—Whoopi Goldberg, Mary-Louise Parker, and Drew Barrymore—to both address the neglected issue of women and AIDS and to present an out, black lesbian character. The film attracted a mixed audience, but it was marketed as a women's/gay film. The target audience included lesbians and bisexual women anxious to see a major star play "gay," and heterosexual women and gay men attracted to the "women's" bonding theme as well as the topic of AIDS. The story begins with Jane, played by Goldberg, as an angry, isolated, unsuccessful lead singer for an all-white, all-male rock band. In the opening scene, Jane is singing a rendition of Janis Joplin's "Piece of My Heart" before an indifferent audience in a seedy New York nightclub. One of the club's intoxicated patrons, a young white woman, is laughing and flirting with her male date, and disturbing Jane's concentration. Insulted by this woman's rude behavior, Jane boldly approaches her after the set. The woman immediately assumes that Jane is a "waitress" who has come to clear away the bottles and glasses. Jane explains that she is the singer in the band and humorously confronts the woman's annoying behavior.

Jane's character here, as in the first thirty minutes of the film, is smart, confrontational, and sarcastic. She swears unflinchingly at a New York city cab driver, she wears a black leather jacket, and she's forceful and opinionated. When Jane's co-worker informs her that the band has lost their gig at the club, this seventeen-year veteran in the music club scene swiftly decides to quit the band and move to Los Angeles in search of new work and a new life. She answers an ad for a ride share placed in the newspaper by Robin, played by Mary-Louise Parker, and she and Robin meet for lunch.

Robin and Jane are the archetypal odd couple. Whereas Jane is abrasive, tough, and direct, Robin, a successful real estate agent, is controlled, ultra feminine (she's often dressed in soft cashmere and angora) and fastidious. With great reluctance (and with no real options), Jane agrees to the ride share with Robin, whom she calls "the whitest woman on the face of the earth."

The movie charts the growth and transformation in Jane's and Robin's unlikely friendship as they travel across the country accompanied by Jane's cute, but goofy friend Holly, played by Drew Barrymore. Together, the three women bond as they confront Holly's experiences with domestic violence, Robin's struggle as a woman with AIDS, and Jane's encounters with racism and homophobia. The film ends with Robin's death from AIDS, the birth of Holly's interracial baby, and with Jane in pretty much the same position as when the story started: without a job, a girlfriend, or a viable cultural community.

SENTIMENTAL FEMINISM

The standard feminist interpretation of women's sentimental texts—films as well as fiction—is that they are politically inspired attacks on patriarchal domination. The interrelated genres of sentimentality, melodrama, romance fiction, and women's "weepies" were of great interest to feminist literary and film critics in the late 1970s and early 1980s. This was a time when feminists were reclaiming and rediscovering women's texts and lives. For instance, The Feminist Press reissued Susan Warner's *The Wide, Wide World* (1987). Other writers, such as Fanny Hall and Louisa May Alcott, were the focus of much feminist scholarly activity. In 1982, Tania Modleski's application of feminist theory to the interpretation of romance fiction, Gothic novels, and soap operas opened up an avalanche of cultural criticism on popular culture from an explicitly feminist perspective.

Prior to this time, texts associated with women or with "femininity" were either ignored or dismissed as commercialized, mass audience "trash" by both male and female critics. In the field of literary criticism, most literary historians pigeonholed Harriet Beecher Stowe, Louisa May Alcott, and other popular women writers as "minor" and unimportant, a response that Jane Tompkins challenges in her well-known 1985 study, *Sensational Designs*. Tompkins' book not only uses feminist literary criticism to challenge the gender politics of canon formation, but she also argues that Harriet Beecher Stowe's *Uncle Tom's Cabin* was a great piece of American literature. Dismissed by literary critics for years as "popular," "maudlin," and lacking in literary skill, Tompkins (1985) reads Stowe's influential novel as possessing a uniquely feminine "sentimental power" (pp. 122-146). Tompkins argues that nineteenth-century sentimentality was more than a genre, it was a national project, one that "reorganized[d] culture from the woman's point of view" and thus served as the basis of the future women's liberation movement (1985, p. 124). In fact, Tompkins claimed that the novel's sentimental power put an end to slavery.

In the early 1990s, the feminist critic Shirley Samuels broadened the discussion of feminism and sentimentality even further by editing a collection that reads sentimentality from a number of new perspectives. The overall theme of *The Culture of Sentiment* (1992) is that sentimentality is neither good nor bad; rather, it is a complex aesthetic, cultural, language-oriented practice that requires careful, theoretically informed analysis (Samuels, 1992). Armed with critical perspectives such as poststructuralism, Marxism, new historicism, and African-American criticism and theory, Samuels' anthology exploded the ingrained prejudice that sentimentality was a one-dimensional, simple-minded middle-class woman's practice. One of Samuels' contributors, Lynn Wardley, argues that the sentimental genre is a cross-cultural genre with roots in West Africa (Wardley, 1992).

Feminist literary critics continue to see women's sentimental and popular writing as intertwined with women's films, television programs, and other examples of popular culture. The gender politics involved in both the production and critique of texts labeled "sentimental" (e.g., soap operas, love stories, and domestic narratives) are even more under scrutiny today in the field of cultural studies. And although contemporary feminist scholarship on sentimental aesthetic practice has become more critically engaged and less celebratory than scholarship of the early 1980s, it maintains its original position that revisionary understandings of women's writing and experiences under patriarchy are central to feminist criticism. Despite innovations, complexities, commitments, and advanced theoretical understandings of sentimentality, including Wardley's argument that the culture of sentiment derives not from white, Christian, America, but from West African spiritual practices, the sentimental aesthetic practice of American texts—whether visual or written—still tends to explicitly favor the experiences of white, middle- and upper-class women. The result is that these texts aggressively construct and produce "woman" and femininity as decidedly white and middle class.

The feminist critic Hazel Carby argues that the typical nineteenth-century sentimental plot involves a white, privileged female character who gets to die a sentimental death, while the black female character, who survives her numerous violations and mistreatment, is deemed less womanly for doing so. As Carby states, the black woman's ability to endure slavery, rape, and the humiliation of servitude renders her ineligible for the ranks of true womanhood—"the true heroine would rather die than be sexually abused" (Carby, 1987, p. 34). This racialized sentimental legacy, also known as the "cult of true womanhood," structures some popular twentieth-century cultural and artistic work as well.

As Helen Taylor (1986) points out in "*Gone With the Wind:* The mammy of them all," some white feminists have consistently celebrated the novel and film in terms of Scarlett O'Hara's determination, leadership, and instances of gender nonconformity while black feminists "are left to point to the political problems" (p. 114). Taylor explains that such white feminist celebration would require "both turning a blind eye to [the novel's and film's] white supremacist, Southern propaganda, and entering into an unholy alliance with the crudest Southern chauvinism and the activities of the Ku Klux Klan" (Taylor, 1986, p. 115). Simply put, what some feminist critics and readers interpret as women's resistance to domination, other feminist critics and readers interpret as reactionary racial stereotypes and ideology. This tension within a white feminist sensibility that challenges patriarchal dominance, yet capitulates to stereotypical constructions of racial, economic, and sexual inequalities and identities has been vigorously challenged by numerous critics, including bell hooks, Hazel Carby, Patricia Hill Collins, Barbara Smith, to name just a few. However, the tendency among feminist critics to isolate gender from the material influences and details associated with race, class, and sexual identities still remains a stumbling block in feminist criticism and theory. As Margaret L. Anderson and Patricia Hill Collins (1995) put it, the "mantra" of race, class, and gender become hackneyed when they are perceived as metaphoric "voices," "voices" which are too often "disembodied from particular historical and social conditions—a framework that has been exacerbated by postmodernist trends in feminist theory" (p. xiii). In fact, I would argue that the paucity of work on women and AIDS in feminist theory and criticism is connected to the overall influence of postmodern feminist theory's inclination to subordinate the body to the mind (Hogan, 1997).

The demand for a multicultural feminist approach to the discourses on AIDS is particularly important because while race, class, gender, and sexual identities and AIDS are inextricably linked in the politics and experiences of people with the disease, many examples of AIDS discourse separate the two. Sentimentalized constructions of AIDS are especially prone to this "separation" abuse. In order words, the conjunction of feminist interpretations of the culture of sentiment on the one hand and the issue of women and AIDS are either miles apart or complicitous with the silences on women and AIDS. Feminist criticism on sentimentality needs to address the legacy of coding sentimentality as white and middle class as well as the consequences of using a discourse which literally renders many women invisible.

The question of sentimentality as a form of invisibility in the construction of AIDS is explored by Perri Klass in her intricate novel, *Other Women's Children* (1990). Part meditation on the political effects of using sentimental literature to represent childhood death, and part story of an overworked, overwhelmed pediatrician and mother who is caring for a three-year-old African-American boy who is dying of AIDS, the narrator of *Other Women's Children*, Amelia Stern, unravels the racialization of sentimentality. For instance, in a powerful chapter "Has There Even Been a Child Like Eva," Stern wonders why Topsy, the undernourished, mistreated slave girl in Stowe's *Uncle Tom's Cabin* is not granted the fanfare of a sentimental death, while Little Eva, the well-fed, well-cared for white girl gets to be "more angel than earthly" (Klass, 1990, p. 98). Klass's narrator concludes that only the child who is judged as inherently more valuable and noble, Little Eva, is granted a sentimental death, and in this way the novel exposes the racial politics of the sentimental aesthetic; Little Eva is exalted, but only by foregoing an accurate picture of the bodily realities of Topsy's life.

The details and conditions of class difference are similarly marginalized by sentimental discourse when Mary-Louise Parker plays a working-class injection drug user with AIDS in the made for television drama, *A Place for Annie* (1994). Like Whoopi Goldberg's Jane in *Boys on the Side*, Parker's character in *A Place for Annie* is unrealized, yet in this television drama, Parker's character is neither used as a mythical moral/nurturing center of the film nor is she a symbol of lost motherhood and heterosexual union. In this story, Parker gives up her HIV-positive infant daughter for adoption, but then tries to regain custody once the daughter is in recovery. In her first appearance on the television screen, she's angry, agitated, and depicted as irresponsible, as she parades through the social worker's office wearing a miniskirt, a low-cut, tight-fitting blouse, and high heels. A chain smoker, she constantly holds a lit cigarette. This woman's inevitable death from AIDS will not be presented, step-by-step, with visitations from an angelic dead child or with a devoted girlfriend by her side, as in *Boys on the Side*.

In *A Place for Annie*, the emphasis is on getting Mary-Louise Parker's HIV-positive baby, Annie, away from her—once Annie sheds her mother's infected immune system, she becomes HIV negative—and into the hands of a "better" mother, the pediatric nurse played by Sissy Spacek. The focus is clearly not on the woman suffering from AIDS, as it is in *Boys on the Side*. In fact, Parker's dying woman is shunted off to an AIDS hospice near the end of the program, so that the focus can remain on the baby as victim of a pathological, drug-infested, working-class mother, whose miniskirts and smoking offend the middle-class viewer. It is instructive to compare and contrast Little Eva and Topsy, Jane and Robin, and the two constructions of a woman with AIDS played by Parker in order to consider how one character's death is represented with sentimental flourish while the other's death is unworthy of any representation.[2]

In terms of woman and Aids, white and middle-class sentimentality interferes with women's understandings of their own risk for HIV infection. I want to emphasize again that the fundamental question I am posing is not whether *Boys on the Side* presents an "acceptable" feminist message; the questions are how are "woman" and "feminism" constructed in this film, what is sentimentality's role in these constructions, and what are the consequences in terms of representation, political life, and women's lives? In *Boys on the Side*, the three female characters bond in terms of a feminism that is based primarily on gendered inequalities. The inextricable enmeshment of gendered, sexualized, racialized, and economic inequalities and identities of women are constantly denied.

THE DESEXUALIZATION OF WHOOPI

The formidable *New York Times* film critic, Janet Maslin, and the *Gay Community News* film reviewer, Elizabeth Pincus both refer to the use of sentimentality and the production of tears in *Boys on the Side*, but neither critic explores the political consequences of the sentimental genre on the presentation of Goldberg's Jane. Unlike Neely's character, Blanche White, who clearly understands the association between sentimentality and the construction of black women as mammies and servants, Maslin, more in line with academic feminists such as Tompkins, sees the film's sentimentality as presenting a charming and poignant tale of women's solidarity and power. In fact, from Maslin's (1995) perspective, *Boys on the Side* is a successful film: "sharp, funny," and one that "creates an unexpected groundswell of real emotion" (p. C3). Comparing it to *Thelma and Louise* (1991) and *Terms of Endearment* (1983), Maslin celebrates *Boys on the Side* for its ability to "blur lines of race and gender with surprising ease" (p. C3).

Blurring lines of race and gender, however, is not the same as acknowledging and honoring difference, and this is a distinction that Maslin (1995) and the movie seem to miss. "Blurring" race and gender also fails to decenter whiteness—Goldberg's character, despite the "blurring," is still marginalized (Hartman, 1996). Maslin

(1995) does note, however, that Goldberg's Jane is "the quintessential outsider as the film begins" and that Goldberg herself is "Hollywood's most uncategorizable star" (p. C3). This inexplicable loneliness and outsider status seem irrelevant to Maslin, who declares that *Boys on the Side* has finally provided Goldberg with "a role that suits her talents" (p. C3). Since Goldberg has been consistently cast in all-white films in which her main activity is to nourish troubled white people—similar to her role in *Boys on the Side*—one wonders what Maslin has in mind here.

In a sort of quick afterthought, Maslin (1995) does comment on the "small irony" that *Boys on the Side* "depicts [AIDS] in terms of a straight white woman" and on the unfortunate decision to present Jane's sexuality "in terms of metaphor and wisecracking rather than actual physicality" (p. C3). But for viewers with even the slightest awareness of the politics of AIDS in America, this choice will not be surprising—a white, straight, middle-class woman, even one who contracts HIV through a one night stand with a bartender, is more likely, given racial, class, and sexual politics, to garner sympathy than a black or working-class woman who contracts HIV in the exact same way.

Robin's inevitable death from AIDS takes on broad, heroic meanings: she symbolizes lost youth, unrealized young motherhood, and the impossibility of heterosexual love and marriage. For example, after a tearful watching of *The Way We Were* (1973)—Robin can't get HBO in her room so she asks Jane if she can watch it in her, and Jane joins her—Robin confesses that she's not "very liberated . . . I want a husband with a decent job. I want two kids, a boy and a girl, in that order. And a salt-box Colonial with three bedrooms, a sunporch, a stairway with a white bannister, and a convertible den" (Maslin, 1995, p. C3). Through her association with Jane, Robin develops a feminist consciousness, but it's one that foregrounds motherhood, marriage, and monogamy above all else. Robin can symbolize what counts as the American Dream in a way that Jane cannot.

One could argue that the film focuses on Robin as the woman with AIDS instead of Jane for precisely this reason: a black woman with AIDS is yet another, defeated, pathetic, cringing victim of "social tragedy." According to American mythology, Jane could never mourn the impossibility of a husband with a decent job, a salt-box Colonial, and the sorrow in not having children. She could only represent *the black woman with AIDS.* The screenwriter's refusal to give Jane an interior life of her own, one composed of desires, rage, dreams, memories, pleasure, fears, flaws, as well as a visible community, makes this clear. Neither the tragic role of the heterosexual woman with AIDS nor the devoted lesbian friend/ mammy can liberate Jane from subtle second-class citizenship in this film. This is because, in the case of Jane, the outcast status of AIDS is competing with already preexisting outcast social identities of blackness and lesbianism, whereas Mary-Louise Parker's Robin can domesticate AIDS; she can make having AIDS seem heroic and consequently more palatable for a mass audience.

Had Maslin been more in touch with the politics of AIDS and representation, and better informed about women and AIDS—had she known, among other things, that black women comprise 57 percent of the cases of all U.S. women with AIDS, and that in 1993, a study conducted in San Francisco indicated that HIV seropreva-lence was more than three times higher among lesbian and bisexual women than for all women—perhaps her discussion of the "small irony" of Robin and the elision of Jane's "actual physicality" would have been more complex (WORLD, 1995).

To Elizabeth Pincus, *Boys on the Side* may be "brash" and "ballsy," with Whoopi Goldberg "bursting onto the screen as a full-blown, not-shy-of-the-'L'-word lesbo," but the film's desexual-ization of Goldberg's lesbian character is a real disappointment to Pincus (1995). Pincus angrily argues that Goldberg "is granted a platonic crush on the movie's tragic heterosexual, turning a hereto-fore bawdy romp into a picture that's maudlin and sterile" (1995, p. 26). Sharing Pincus's frustration are several lesbian viewers who voiced their discontent on America On-Line: "The lesbian was cynically rendered unlucky-in-love as to make her more palpable for a general audience. Wouldn't the movie have done just as well if Whoopi Goldberg's love life was healthy?" "In film, lesbians are usually a sexual void"; "My friend said she was sick of seeing Hollywood portray lesbians as 'women who always fall in love with straight women'"; "I am also tired of unrequited lesbian love stories."

While these viewers' frustrations with the film's inability to "cough up a viable love interest for Goldberg" seems accurate, it is revealing that none address the desexualization of Goldberg in terms of racial politics: the fact that Jane is a black woman surrounded, for the most part, by white people (Pincus, 1995, p. 26). Pincus, unlike Maslin and the viewers quoted above, questions the film's overly idealized multiracial, intergenerational sisterly solidarity, which she dismisses as "hokey" and "def[ying] belief" (Pincus, 1995, p. 26). But Pincus's discussion of lesbian representation overlooks the process of what Wahneema Lubiano refers to as racialized gender (1992). Pincus, like Maslin, fails to consider that the black lesbian character, Jane, is stripped of a romantic life, not only because of her sexual identity, but also because she is black. Jane is certainly neither celibate nor indifferent, as her wistful, sexual-emotional longing for the heterosexual Holly and Robin makes evident. But the fact that she is a black woman may also explain her nonexistent love life.

Jane's lack of "actual physicality" exists within the larger historical framework of the black woman as innately immoral, or, as Evelynn Hammonds puts it, the historical framework of the black woman as "the embodiment of sex" (Hammonds, 1994, p. 132). As a black lesbian, Jane experiences her sexuality as a "deviant sexuality [which] exists within an already preexisting deviant sexuality" (Hammonds, 1994, p. 137). She is unconsciously associated with historical narratives of black women's sexuality as illicit and taboo. As Hammonds argues, from "the production of the image of a pathologized black female 'other' in the eighteenth century" to the myth of the "loose," hypersexual black female that was produced during and after slavery and Reconstruction, representations of black women's sexuality have been fraught with silence, unease, and racist mythologies (Hammonds, 1994, pp. 132-133).

One strategy developed by late nineteenth-century and early twentieth-century black women social reformers was to counter the myth of the black woman as the "embodiment of sex" with the image of black women as "super-moral"—an image that still has far-reaching impact on contemporary representations of black women, as Donald Bogle's history of black actors in film suggests (Hammonds, 1994; Bogle, 1994). The fact that neither Maslin nor Pincus come close to the kind of critical insight on racial narratives that Hammonds and Neely's fictional Blanche White provide is striking. From Blanche White's perspective, the "pure soapsuds" aspect of *Boys on the Side*, while potentially moving and empowering to white audiences, may not be experienced as such by women of color (Pincus, 1995, p. 26). In short, homophobia clearly contributes to the desexed, nurturing Jane, but homophobia and racism are inseparable, as Hammonds's theoretical work on black women's sexuality makes clear. Pointing again to the history of blacks in American cinema, Donald Bogle (1994) explains that in almost all of her movies, Goldberg is consistently denied an on-screen romance: "The very idea of Whoopi Goldberg as a romantic film personality was unacceptable to certain audiences. Filmmakers seemed to view her as an asexual creature from another universe" (p. 298).

WHOOPI AS MAMMY FIGURE

While audiences and filmmakers may feel uncomfortable with Whoopi as a heterosexual or homosexual romantic personality, they are, predictably, very at ease with her in films with a "covert nurturing theme" (Bogle, 1994, p. 331). Jane is repeatedly depicted as comforting and emotionally attentive to both Robin and Holly, yet rarely the recipient of their tenderness and care. And while it is true that Whoopi plays Jane as an opinionated, forceful woman, Jane is so busy responding to these two women that her own needs are pushed aside. With each scene, Jane's initial preoccupation with finding work in Los Angeles as a musician and with healing her own broken heart evaporates as she's "naturally" pulled into the dilemmas of Robin's and Jane's circumstances.

For example, during their road trip, Robin is reminded of her sad childhood. She, her parents, and her baby brother—who was diagnosed with cancer when he was six years old—traveled across the United States just before Robin's father left his family. Robin remembers the three of them standing by the roadside, the mother taking photos of her two young kids. Jane unknowingly adds salt to Robin's wounds when she makes a sarcastic comment about Robin's using their current roadtrip to "walk down memory lane." When Jane learns that Robin's brother died of cancer, she quickly feels guilty and ashamed of her flip remark. Shortly after Robin's disclosure, Robin becomes severely nauseous and Jane finds her vomiting in the women's room in a diner where they've just eaten. Up to this point, Jane has been extremely skeptical of accompanying Robin on her "walk down memory lane." But it is at this juncture in the story that Jane begins to undergo a slow transition from the hard, tough, antisentimentalist, antiromanticist to a woman of exquisite feeling and caretaking.

Next, shortly after their dramatic and narrow escape from Holly's brutish and violent boyfriend, Holly begins to have second thoughts and considers returning to this drug-addicted, physically abusive man. Even though Jane is appalled by Holly's decision to return to Nick, she stays by her side and watches Holly cry. Frustrated, Jane walks into the bathroom to enlist Robin's help, only to find Robin collapsing onto the cold floor. Jane's attention shifts from Holly to Robin, who is immediately rushed to the hospital in an ambulance. The next scene depicts the exhausted and worried Jane sitting in a hospital waiting room, the sweet little Holly sleeping in her lap, as the doctor informs Jane that Robin has AIDS. In the following scene, Jane is shown comforting Robin as she cries and pulls at the tubes in her nose and arms.

Three months later, the three women are living together in a beautiful house in Tucson, Arizona, and Jane has hooked into a lesbian bar/community. However, in addition to the constant stress and anxiety associated with Robin's AIDS diagnosis, Robin's and Jane's idealized friendship deteriorates due to misunderstandings and Jane's "crush" on the heterosexual Robin. Meanwhile, the pregnant Holly becomes involved with an idealistic, naive, Republican cop, who turns Holly over to the authorities once he learns that Holly may have been involved in the murder of her battering boyfriend, Nick. Maslin refers to this part of the plot and the courtroom sequence that follows as clumsy and "contrived." But the courtroom drama allows Jane to come out as "gay" in response to an arrogant, feminist-bashing, homophobic prosecutor, and it provides Robin with the opportunity to present her ideas on feminism and sisterly solidarity before she dies. Significantly, when Robin shows up in Philadelphia to testify on Holly's behalf, she tells her estranged friend, Jane, "You are my family and I love you." Jane responds by bending over and picking up Robin's luggage.

While white female caretaking is often constructed in AIDS discourse as involving HIV-negative women whose love and tenderness rescue the stigmatized male from the realm of total abjection, no one performs this symbolic function for HIV-infected women of color on a representational—or political—level. The white middle-class female character may even possess a nonconventional trait, such as the imaginative, eccentric, drug-addicted Harper Pitt of Tony Kushner's *Angels in America*, or the funky lesbian Helpmates in Paul Monette's novel, *Halfway Home*, and Nisa Donnelly's *The Love Songs of Phoenix Bay*, but these female characters are nevertheless constructed in terms of the traditional idea of the good woman as the woman who cares.[3] In other words, they act as "white" mammies, but because of their class and race privileges, they are more often constructed as slim, ethereal "ministering angels" rather than as the sentimentalized figure of the hefty, black mammy. In *Boys on the Side*, it is a slender white middle-class woman with AIDS and a black, unattractively dressed, desexualized lesbian who serve as moral compass and role models to an AIDS-phobic audience and society. Yet, in both configurations of women and caretaking, the black woman's experience of being HIV infected or living with AIDS is erased. Every experience except that of "Mammy" is elided.

As critic Ann Cvetkovich argues in her work on women's sensation novels, the lavish emotional display of suffering in these texts is not amiss because it expresses manipulative, "feminine" culture (a patriarchal view); or because it provides women readers with the opportunity for fantasy, identification, and potential consequences of the construction of the figure of the suffering woman" (Cvetkovich, 1992, p. 98). Sentimental novels potentially empower female readers by urging them to recognize how patriarchal culture represses women's pain, but they also suggest that the expression of feeling is in itself the way to alleviate the conditions of oppression—"relief would be if she could only articulate her feelings" argues Cvetkovich (1992, p. 98). By contrast, Blanche White's relief does not occur when her boss, Grace, articulates her feelings—in fact, Grace's articulation of her feelings is experienced by Blanche as one more instance of exploitation. Blanche's unraveling of the politics of the suffering white woman supports Cvetkovich's

(1994) argument that the privileging of emotional articulation alone "cast[s] social problems as emotional ones in order to construct emotional solutions" when, in fact, the solutions most desperately needed are economic, social, and political reform (p. 131).

BLACK WOMEN AND AIDS

Blanche's analysis of "Mammy savers" uncovers a key mechanism in the production of silence about black women and AIDS in this film (and in American culture at large): through the spectacle of white, middle-class women's tears. The sentimentalized Mammy or Aunt Jemima figure provides this powerful angle of vision. In other words, Blanche's perspective brings to the fore how the black woman as mammy distracts attention away from the material realities of black women's sexuality and health. Because the sentimentalized mammy figure is, by definition, selfless, asexual, and concerned only with the lives of others, she serves as the perfect cover-up in a movie that both wants to be "progressive"; yet, at the same time, cannot or will not deal with AIDS in black women.

As Evelynn Hammonds (1994) observes, in terms of representation in the AIDS epidemic "black women are victims that are once again the 'other,' the deviants of the deviants, regardless of their sexual identities and practices" (p. 141). In like manner, Imani Harrington (1992) places her personal experiences as a black woman with AIDS alongside the history of racism in America: "Here in America I am the 'alien,' the 'foreigner' with the AIDS virus. My people have been set apart, divided and dam near conquered in this society . . . Our culture, tradition and languages have never been accepted" (p. 180).

While *Boys on the Side* avoids the all-too-familiar "negative" images of black women with AIDS as bad mothers, pathetic drug users, and murderous prostitutes, it is crucial to recognize how the weight of these historically entrenched "negative" stereotypes are the flipside of the super-moral, sentimental, black mammy. Again, as Hammonds (1994) argues, "visibility in and of itself neither erases a history of silence, nor does it challenge the structure of power and domination, symbolic and material, that determines what can and cannot be seen" (p. 141). A black lesbian can be "seen" in

Boys on the Side, but only in terms of a subtle, contemporary reworking of the sentimental, desexualized mammy figure who is isolated from communities of color and denied a sexual/romantic relationship. She is represented in such a way that the underlying structure of domination that exacerbates black women's invisibility in the U.S. AIDS epidemic is *not* challenged.

Similarly, women and AIDS can now be "seen" in a commercial Hollywood film, but only through the limited perspective of white, middle-class, heterosexual sentimentality. What is missing in the film is the working-class and black female body infected with HIV, as well as a dramatization of the issue of power between white and black women. Instead, these issues are silenced by the spectacle of a supposedly neutral and "natural" feminist emotionality, complete with an updated beloved black servant figure and a feisty, dying, white heroine. Emotional femininity may be an "imperative task of gender," as Susan Brownmiller (1986) attests, but it is class and race inflected task that some women are expected to perform at other women's expense.

Similar to much of the well-meaning (and effective) white abolitionist fiction and nonfiction of the nineteenth century, which challenged slavery, while at the same time reproducing racial, class, and gender stereotypes, representations of black women in *Boys on the Side* reproduce, rather than challenge, the very racial and gender stereotypes the film anxiously tries to avoid (Carby, 1987). Equally important, it sets forth a popular definition of feminism that places the experiences of white, middle- and upper-class women at the center of analysis while relegating the experiences and identities of everyone else to that of incidental player (hooks, 1984).[4]

CONTACT WITH DEPARTED SPIRITS

Although I have been interpreting sentimentality as oppressive to Jane, and indicative of an outdated view of feminism, the emotionality of sentimentality, coupled with its standard view of death as a "crossing over" or "homecoming" may require more careful consideration. For these, qualities of emotionality and death as a crossing over convey a more complex representation of the actual individual emotional suffering caused by HIV/AIDS than do biomedical constructions, right-wing moralizing, and even political/activist renderings of the disease. For example, Harriet Beecher Stowe's famous Little Eva was known as "more angel than ordinary," and when she "crossed over," it was felt that her spirit had never really belonged to the earth. So, too, we find themes of a child's innate otherworldliness in *Boys on the Side*. During Robin's last hospital stay shortly before she dies, her deceased baby brother, Tommy, visits her. He is on the other side or her hospital room window, staring and waving. Mary-Louise Parker plays this scene with expert skill, with just the right mixture of fear, intrigue, disbelief, and desire. The effect is moving, and will especially comfort viewers whose lives have been torn apart by AIDS. The scene provides a consoling vision, one that diffuses the extreme fear and anxiety of death.

Likewise, the choreographer David Rousseve uses images of death as "crossing over" in his AIDS dance theater piece, *The Whispers of Angels* (1995). Similar to Stowe's lavish deathbed scenes in *Uncle Tom's Cabin* (1951), and to the supernatural communion between the dying Robin and her already dead little brother in *Boys on the Side*, Rousseve presents visitations with departing spirits as an imaginative way to offer solace and comfort his beleaguered audience.[5] Rousseve centers his piece on human beings making the transition from life to death because he is deeply attracted to this process. In addition to a chorus, the choreographer includes several dancing angels, many of whom are people who have died of AIDS: "Angels help with the idea of losing people, of people crossing over, The concept soothes me: death is a continuum with life. Angels are a source of comfort, an unabashedly spiritual thing" (Zimmer, 1995, p. 63). For Rousseve's part in the dance, he plays a black gay man dying of AIDS who, just as he dies, is miraculously reunited with his estranged, dead father. The idea of the continuum between life and death which makes death a "crossing over"; the highly emotional reconciliations between the dying gay man and his estranged, dead father; the belief that when we die we become angels, are all stock images and ideas found in sentimental aesthetic practice. Rousseve deepens his use of these traditions when he explains that the notion of death as a "crossing over," and as a productive homecoming, are fundamental ideas of the black church. Similar to the ideas of critic Lynn Wardley, who argues that notions of transcendence and spirituality found in nineteenth-century American sentimental writing unwittingly posses a complex "infusion" and "cross-cultural influence" of West African spirituality, Rousseve merges the hopefulness of the black church's death as crossover theme into his contemporary dance theater on AIDS. Both Wardley and Rousseve offer a hopeful view of sentimental transcendence while also challenging a Eurocentric view. Death as a glorious, long-awaited homecoming, as well as the belief that objects and places posses a spiritual animation are not naturally or inevitably Christian, white, middle-class, Euro-American inventions.

As the same time, Rousseve, unlike Wardley, points out that "crossing over" and becoming an angel must not act as a "tranquilizer" for the audience. Existence may, in fact, be better once we have "crossed over," but that promise must not interfere with the business of helping people who struggle in their bodily lives. Rousseve refers to a critic who recently confronted his work's vision by saying that "it doesn't help us in the here and now to say you're going to be an angel" (Zimmer, 1995, p. 63). Rousseve agrees.

It is highly unusual to find such a balanced view of sentimentality, a view that does not use emotional intensity as spectacle to drown out the material, political, social, and economic context of AIDS. Rousseve explains that the use of angels in his piece is a "paradox," and that he himself holds a conflicted view of sentimental spirituality. Death does, from this imaginative perspective, have some meaning, as it ushers us into a better place where we can still communicate with those who have left us and with those whom we have left. Yet, as the same time, Rousseve maintains a skepticism about the very view that he cherishes and lavishly displays in his dance. "The black church," he explains, "has been criticized, rightfully, for being tranquilizing. . . . That's the paradox of the piece: people cross over, they're still with us, but things are still screwed up. They're dying all around us" (Zimmer, 1995, p. 63).

With this last statement, Rousseve offers a contradictory view of his own sentimental practice, a complexity that *Boys on the Side* and many other pieces on AIDS lack. He openly considers how concepts such as crossing over and reunion with departed spirits can, and do, distract us from the problems of the living. However, the advantages of Rousseve's and Herbert Ross's constructions of AIDS as transformative are obvious to anyone who has been made to feel invisible by either intellectualization and medicalized discourse.

Ann Cvetkovich specifically argues for a balance between free, emotional expression/mourning, and political action in response to AIDS, not an eradication of emotional expression. She would not condemn the moving vision of Rousseve's dance piece or its skillful ability to evoke an emotional response; nor would she scoff at the desire for contact with the dead or for the sisterly solidarity expressed in *Boys on the Side.* It is not the representation of suffering per se that is at issue; it is the way in which emotional suffering is used to obscure other complexities and experiences. In fact, Cvetkovich (1992) warns against an approach to AIDS that would deny the full expression of emotion:

> The most effective activism might require both mourning *and* militancy, the recognition both of what can be changed because AIDS is not simply a biological problem but a social one, and of what cannot be changed in the face of death. The repression of mourning because of the need to confront without sentimentality how sexism, racism, and homophobia structure the incidence and treatment of AIDS might constitute a dangerous avoidance of the reality of suffering, an avoidance that creates not just individual psychic distress but political difficulties. The expression of feeling and activism need not be at odds, although they often are when affect is represented or experienced as natural or inevitable (p. 127).

For Cvetkovich, the problem lies not in human emotion itself, but in the trivialization of human emotion and in passing off suffering and emotional expression as an ahistorical, decontextualized, "natural" activity.

CONCLUSION: SENTIMENTALITY AND AIDS

The limitations of a sentimental construction of AIDS stem from sentimentality's ambivalence toward difference and its preoccupation with a homogenous and universal transcendence—a view that can potentially render the experiences of many people with AIDS as irrelevant and invisible, especially poor women and women of color. However, the point in giving a closer inspection of sentimentality is not to dismiss it as trivial or lacking in artistic skill or to denigrate the enormously complex and subtle process of emotional articulation. Few people with personal experience with AIDS would easily reject one of the few available discourses that allow people with AIDS and those who love them some release—no matter how flawed.

My purpose is to adopt as a feminist-inspired AIDS criticism what the writer Dorothy Allison (1994) calls the ability to "read books cynically" (p. 16). Cynical reading does not, as is so often argued, rule our inspired, passionate claims for the power of imagination, themes of hopefulness, and visions of social/political change (Rorty, 1996). The complex inspiration and solace that aspects of the sentimental—in particular, the spiritual notion of death as crossover—provides must be acknowledged. Rousseve's use of the "crossing over" theme, and Robin's visitations from her baby brother point to some of these moments.

In addition, *Boys on the Side* does succeed in breaking the resounding silence on women and AIDS in mainstream film. The first Hollywood film to address AIDS, *Philadelphia* (1993), includes a woman character in a minor, incidental way—the most prevalent construction of women in AIDS discourse, even when women themselves are HIV infected. *Boys on the Side* eschews this positioning of women in the AIDS pandemic by giving the film's central role to a woman character, who falls outside the ideological "risk group" fabrication. We watch her swallow her AZT, struggle with nausea, and prepare for death. Again, for audience viewers who have personal/political experience with HIV/AIDS in women, the story is powerful. Robin's deep human fear of mortality and physical pain; her intense feelings of social isolation; her desperate need for her mother; her longing for romantic and sexual love; the painful and vivid memories of the loss of her six-year-old brother to cancer; and Jane's overall reaction to Robin, which suggests that Robin is not the first friend Jane has lost to AIDS, are all representational issues with which feminist criticism must reckon.

On the whole, in critiquing AIDS narratives from a "cynical," debunking perspective, I want to move criticism away from the dangerous notion that since AIDS is so unambiguously devastating and rooted in the boy, the multifaceted AIDS communities of the world should just be grateful for whatever Hollywood—or any other venue—has to give. For while the culture of sentiment does manage to make feelings the center of its project, and the expression of pain and the longing for a better afterlife its most consoling vision, sentimentality too often achieves this vision by shifting our attention away from the bodily conditions of people's lives. In this way, sentimental aesthetic practice has always been in cahoots with a conservative agenda, even in its more liberal guises. *Boys on the Side* relies heavily on a watered-down, nostalgic notion of universal feminist solidarity to address the enormously painful issue of women and AIDS and to present a hopeful, humane vision of care-taking. But in doing so, it sometimes reinforces the stereotypes of women as inevitable, "natural" carers, and insidiously constructs black women as comic maids and sentimentalized mammies.

In an effort to "denaturalize" sentimentality and its inseparable twin, sympathy, I have argues that one person's sentimentality is another person's oppression. The all-too-real emotional and physical pain experienced by people with AIDS demands that critics of this literature begin asking questions about the political effects of framing this illness/event in terms of sentimental expression and transcendence. Sympathy for people with AIDS is too often presented as an end in itself, even in the most well-meaning narratives, and so the help needed to change the political, social, and economic conditions that exacerbate AIDS are ignored or trivialized. Furthermore, the sentimentalization of AIDS—the discourse that presents people as victims who "deserve" sympathy—has not received sufficient critical scrutiny. As Carol Schilling (1994) remarks, "the moral dilemmas implicit in acts of representation, especially problems regarding the moral efficacy of sympathy" are fundamental issues in AIDS criticism (p. 110).

In James Baldwin's (1995) essay, "Everybody's Protest Noval," he blasts sentimentality for its snuffing out of "true" emotion. Rather than a language of genuine feelings, Baldwin sees sentimentality as a process of dehumanization. He characterizes sentimentality as "the mark of dishonesty, the inability to feel" (p. 14). He says that "the wet eyes of the sentimentalist betray his aversion

to experience, his fear of life, his arid heart; and it is always, therefore, the signal of secret and violent inhumanity, the mask of
cruelty" (p. 14). As Hazel Carby shows, scores of black female
characters have been dehumanized, made invisible, and belittled in
white women's sentimental literature. Blanche White's critique of
sentimentality, similar to Baldwin's also focuses on violence—each
time her self-absorbed employer breaks into tears, Blanche's invisibility and oppression are intensified.

On the whole, Whoopi Goldeberg's Jane, unlike Barbara Neely's
Blanche, loses her critical ability to resist the transformative effects
of sentimental power. Goldberg's Jane has been extremely skeptical
of Robin: her physical appearance, her taste in music—Carole King
and the Carpenters—and her penchant for women's romances and
"weepies," such as *The Way We Were* (1973) and *An Officer and a
Gentleman* (1982). But before too long, Jane is humming, and even
singing and playing, Carpenters songs, symbolizing that these two
otherwise incompatible women/cultures have forged a bond despite
insurmountable odds. In fact, the more Jane becomes immersed in
the world of Robin, the less she seems like the independent, East
Village musician we meet when the movie opens.

At one point, however, it is Jane who emerges as a strong influence on Robin. In this scene, she persuades the prudish, uptight Robin
to utter the word "cunt," liberating Robin from her sexually repressed
training—"You free, Miz' Scarlett, you free!" Jane is "humorously"
constructed as the hypersexual black woman while comically paro-
dying the figure of the sentimentalized mammy. But by the movie's
end, Jane changes from a wisecracking skeptic to a loving, desexualized "sister," while Robin lets go of her homophobia and admits in
front of an entire courtroom that she's not gay, but "at times, I understand the inclination." The initial racial-cultural tension with which the
film opens and the continual focus on the "working out" of that tension—although at Jane's expense—is the film's underlying project.

NOTES

1. Barbara Neely, (1992). *Blanche on the Lam.* New York: Penguin, p. 39.

2. Dorothy Allison's *Bastard Out of Caroling* (1992), described by one
reviewer as "One of those unusual books that show childhood abuse without sentimentality or simplicity," subtly and brilliantly explores the class politics of senti-

mentality. For instance, Bone, the "white trash" lead character and narrative voice, has just left the emergency room, where she was treated for multiple fractures and broken bones. The attending physician suspects child abuse and confronts Bone's mother. The mother is offended and whisks her child away, but on the ride home, Bone begins to have fantasies of passionate rescue, confrontation, forgiveness, and dramatic death: "I would pull up from my sickbed. I would look right into [her abuser's] eyes, into the lamp of his soul. Yes, I would say. Yes. I forgive you. Then probably I would die" (p. 116). Allison draws from all the stock conventions of sentimentality here, complete with Christian forgiveness and heroine's sudden death after she pardons her abusive stepfather. Allison's lampooning of the sentimental aesthetic construction of violence is effective and very moving.

3. In general, women of all races, classes, ages, and religions are often constructed in AIDS discourse as didactic role models to a heartless AIDS-phobic society instead of as complex women located in diverse communities who are struggling with homophobia, racism, and sexism, as well as with AIDS. Even when a woman herself is HIV positive, the extent of women's actual experiences in the epidemic is often treated as peripheral and incidental.

4. For white, straight women, the messages of *Boys on the Side* are all too familiar: sex is dangerous for women; penis-vagina intercourse is the only sexual activity that "counts"; most men are liars and beasts who will do anything to get laid; women are more nurturing, responsible, and emotionally sensitive than men; women are, unfortunately, uninteresting sexual partners; lesbians are, paradoxically, both completely devoid of sexuality and scary, sexual predators—as one America On-Line respondent said, "I enjoyed *Boys on the Side*, but I am tired of lesbians being portrayed as dangerous shark-types that will attack and devour any woman in sight."

However, one of the more puzzling contradictions arises when considering how the film's detailed presentation of Robin's demise from AIDS is juxtaposed with the antics of Drew Barrymore's Holly, a sexually active childlike woman who's never heard of safer sex or contraceptives—she's eight weeks pregnant when the film opens and won't consider abortion because "it's murder." Janet Maslin describes Holly as possessing the luscious flirtiness of a 1940s pin-up girl, but her position in this film is a bit more sinister. The film ends with Holly married to a Republican cop who, miraculously, accepts her interracial baby. What is contradictory about the representation of Robin and Holly is that one character suggests that yes, even white, heterosexual, educated women contract HIV and develop AIDS, while this same message is then repeatedly undermined by Holly, who has more unsafe sex than any other character in the entire film, and never once considers HIV through a one-night stand. On one level, Holly can be read as comic relief from the "heavy" issues so that the movie itself can have a sexy and fun side (Hartman, 1996). But the underlying effect is that pleasure and danger are not addressed simultaneously in this film; instead, they are split off, as are race, class, and gender, as if they existed in separate universes, a binary that Carol S. Vance, editor of the groundbreaking anthology on women's sexuality, *Pleasure and Danger* (1984), says stems from antifeminist societal expectations. "It is all too easy to cast sexual experience as either wholly pleasurable or dangerous; our culture encourages us to do so" (p. 5).

    5. Also see Tony Kushner's *Angels in America—Part One: Millennium Approaches* and A*ngels in American—Part Two: Perestroika.*

BIBLIOGRAPHY

Alcott, L.M. (1983). *Little Women*. New York: Signet.

Allison, D. (1992). *Bastard Out of Carolina*. New York: Dutton.

Allison, D. (1994). A Questions of Class. *Skin: Talking about Sex, Class & Literature,* 13-36. New York: Firebrand Press.

Andersen, M.L. and Collins, P.H. (1995). *Race, Class, and Gender: An Anthology*. Belmont, CA: Wadsworth.

Baldwin, J. (1995). Everybody's protest novel. In *Notes of a Native Son*. Boston: Beacon Press.

Betterton, R. (Ed.). (1987). *Looking On: Images of Femininity in the Visual Arts and Media*. London: Pandora.

Bhavnani, K. (1993). Talking racism and the editing of women's studies. In D. Richardson and V. Robinson (Eds.), *Thinking Feminist: Key Concepts in Women's Studies*. New York: The Guilford Press.

Bogle, D. (1994). *Toms, Coons, Mulattoes, Mammies, and Bucks: An Interpretive History of Blacks in American Films,* (Third Edition). New York: Viking.

Boys on the Side. (1995). Screenplay by Don Roos. Directed by Herbert Ross. With performances by Whoopi Goldberg, Mary-Louise Parker, Drew Barrymore, Matthew McConaughery, Anita Gilette, James Remar, Amy Aquino, Dennis Boutsikaris, and Estelle Parsons. Warner Brothers.

Brownmiller, S. (1986). *Femininity*. London: Paladin Books.

Cvetkovich, A. (1991). *Mixed Feelings: Feminism, Mass Culture, and Victorian Sensationalism*. New Brunswick, NJ: Rutgers University Press.

Hammonds, E. (1994). Black (w)holes and the geometry of black female sexuality. *More Gender Trouble: Feminism Meets Queer Theory differences, 6* (2, 3).

Harrington, I. (1992). American quarantine: Isolation, alienation, deprivation. In A. Rudd and D. Taylor (Eds.), *Positive Women: Voices of Women Living with AIDS*. Toronto: Second Story.

Hogan, K. (1997). Where experience and representation collide: Lesbians, feminists, and AIDS. In D. Heller (Ed.), *Cross Purposes: Lesbian Studies, Feminist Studies and the Limits of Alliance*. Indiana: University of Indiana Press.

hooks, bell. (1984). Feminism: A movement to end sexist oppression. In _____ (Ed.), *Feminist Theory: From Margin to Center*, 17-31. Boston: South End Press.

Klass, P. (1990). *Other Women's Children*. New York: Random House.

Lubiano, W. (1992). Black ladies, welfare queens, and state minstrels: Ideological war by narrative means. In T. Morrison (Ed.), *Race-ing Justice, En-gendering Power,* 323-361. New York: Pantheon.

Marshment, M. (1993). The picture is political: Representation of women in contemporary popular culture. In D. Richardson and V. Robinson (Eds.), *Thinking Feminist: Key Concepts in Women's Studies.* New York: The Guilford Press.

Maslin, J. (1995). Another buddy story, with a twist or two. Review of *Boys on the Side. The New York Times*, February 3, C3.

Modleski, T. (1982). *Long with a Vengeance: Mass-Produced Fantasies for Women.* London: Methuen.

Neely, B. (1992). *Blanche on the Lam.* New York: Penguin.

Pincus, E. (1995). Side dish. Review of *Boys on the Side. Gay Community News* (Winter), 25-26.

"A Place for Annie," (1994). *Hallmark Hall of Fame.* ABC. WABC, New York. May 5.

Rorty, R. (1996). The necessity of inspired reading. *The Chronicle of Higher Education*, February 9, A48.

Samuels, S. (Ed.). (1992). *The Culture of Sentiment: Race, Gender, and Sentimentality in 19th Century America.* New York: Oxford University Press.

Savran, D. (1995). Ambivalence, utopia, and a queer sort of materialism: How *Angels in America* reconstructs the nation. *Theatre Journal, (47)*, 207-227.

Schilling, C. (1994). Book Review of *Confronting AIDS through Literature: The Responsibilities of Representation. Modern Language Studies, 24*(3), 110-112.

Stowe, H.B. (1981). *Uncle Tom's Cabin or, Life Among the Lowly.* New York: Penguin Books.

Taylor, H. (1986). *Gone with the Wind:* The mammy of them all. In J. Radford (Ed.), *The Progress of Romance: The Politics of Popular Fiction.* London: Routledge & Kegan.

Tompkins, J. (1985). *Sensational Designs: The Cultural Work of American Fiction, 1790-1860.* New York: Oxford University Press.

Vance, C.S. (Ed.). (1984). *Pleasure and Danger: Exploring Female Sexuality.* Boston: Routledge.

Wardley, L. (1992). Relic, fetish, femmage: The aesthetics of sentiment in the work of Stowe. In S. Samuels (Ed.), *The Culture of Sentiment: Race, Gender, and Sentimentality in 19th Century America.* New York: Oxford University Press.

Warner, S. (1987). *The Wide, Wide, World.* New York: The Feminist Press.

WORLD. (1995). Women and AIDS: Get the facts! *WORLD: Women Organized to Respond to Life-Threatening Diseases: A Newsletter by, for, and about Women Facing HIV Disease*, 56, December 4-5.

Zimmer, E. (1995). Angel in Brooklyn. Review of *The Whispers of Angels. Village Voice*, December 5.

Index

Order Your Own Copy of
This Important Book for Your Personal Library!

WOMEN AND AIDS
Negotiating Safer Practices, Care, and Representation

_____ in hardbound at $39.95 (ISBN: 0-7890-6014-0)

_____ in softbound at $19.95 (ISBN: 1-56023-882-8)

COST OF BOOKS_____

OUTSIDE USA/CANADA/
MEXICO: ADD 20%_____

POSTAGE & HANDLING_____
(US: $3.00 for first book & $1.25
for each additional book)
Outside US: $4.75 for first book
& $1.75 for each additional book)

SUBTOTAL_____

IN CANADA: ADD 7% GST_____

STATE TAX_____
(NY, OH & MN residents, please
add appropriate local sales tax)

FINAL TOTAL_____
(If paying in Canadian funds,
convert using the current
exchange rate. UNESCO
coupons welcome.)

☐ **BILL ME LATER:** ($5 service charge will be added)
(Bill-me option is good on US/Canada/Mexico orders only;
not good to jobbers, wholesalers, or subscription agencies.)

☐ Check here if billing address is different from
shipping address and attach purchase order and
billing address information.

Signature_____

☐ **PAYMENT ENCLOSED: $**_____

☐ **PLEASE CHARGE TO MY CREDIT CARD.**

☐ Visa   ☐ MasterCard   ☐ AmEx   ☐ Discover
☐ Diner's Club

Account #_____

Exp. Date_____

Signature_____

Prices in US dollars and subject to change without notice.

NAME _____

INSTITUTION _____

ADDRESS _____

CITY _____

STATE/ZIP _____

COUNTRY _____ COUNTY (NY residents only) _____

TEL _____ FAX _____

E-MAIL_____
May we use your e-mail address for confirmations and other types of information? ☐ Yes   ☐ No

Order From Your Local Bookstore or Directly From
The Haworth Press, Inc.
10 Alice Street, Binghamton, New York 13904-1580 • USA
TELEPHONE: 1-800-HAWORTH (1-800-429-6784) / Outside US/Canada: (607) 722-5857
FAX: 1-800-895-0582 / Outside US/Canada: (607) 772-6362
E-mail: getinfo@haworth.com
PLEASE PHOTOCOPY THIS FORM FOR YOUR PERSONAL USE.

BOF96